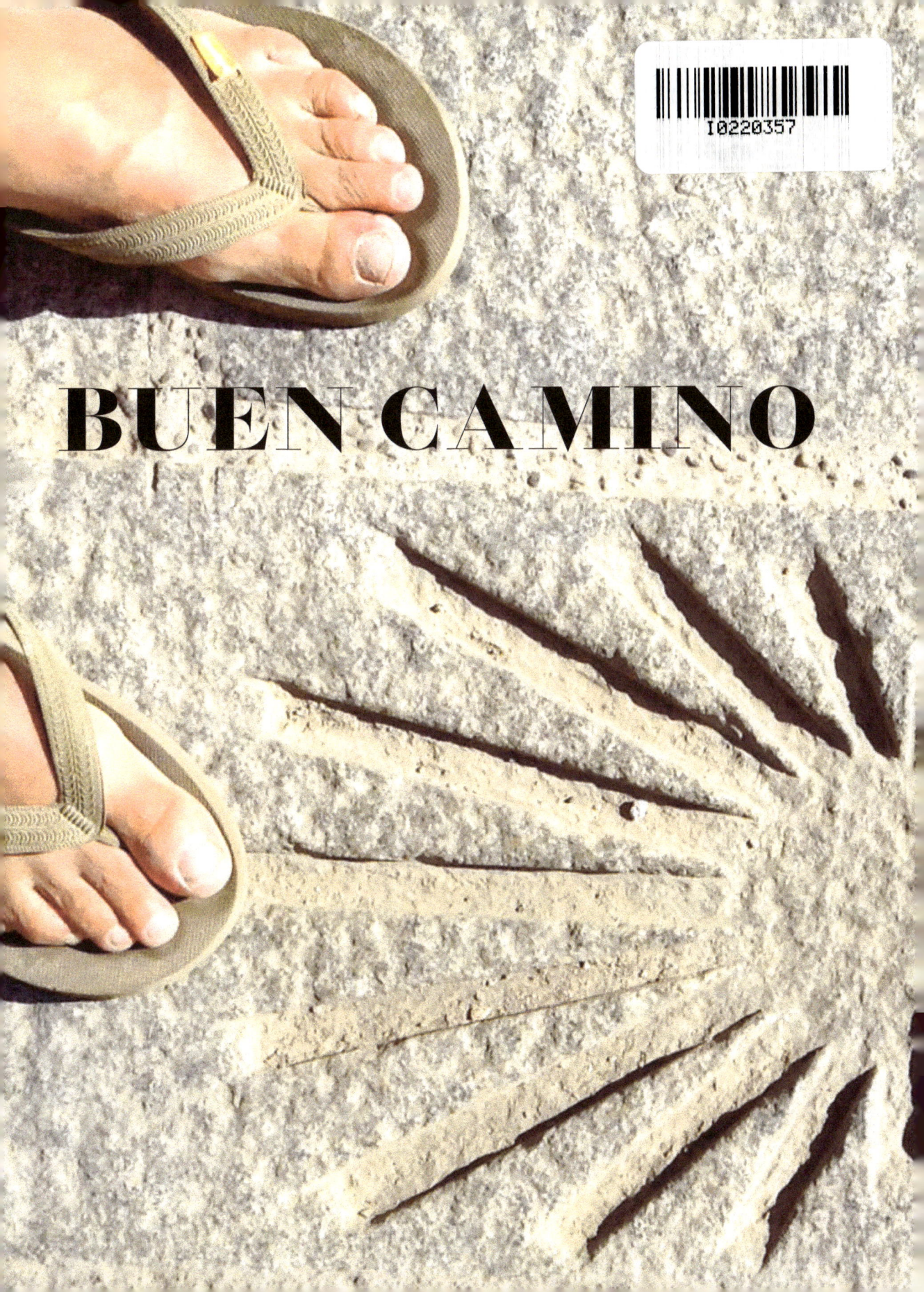

BUEN CAMINO

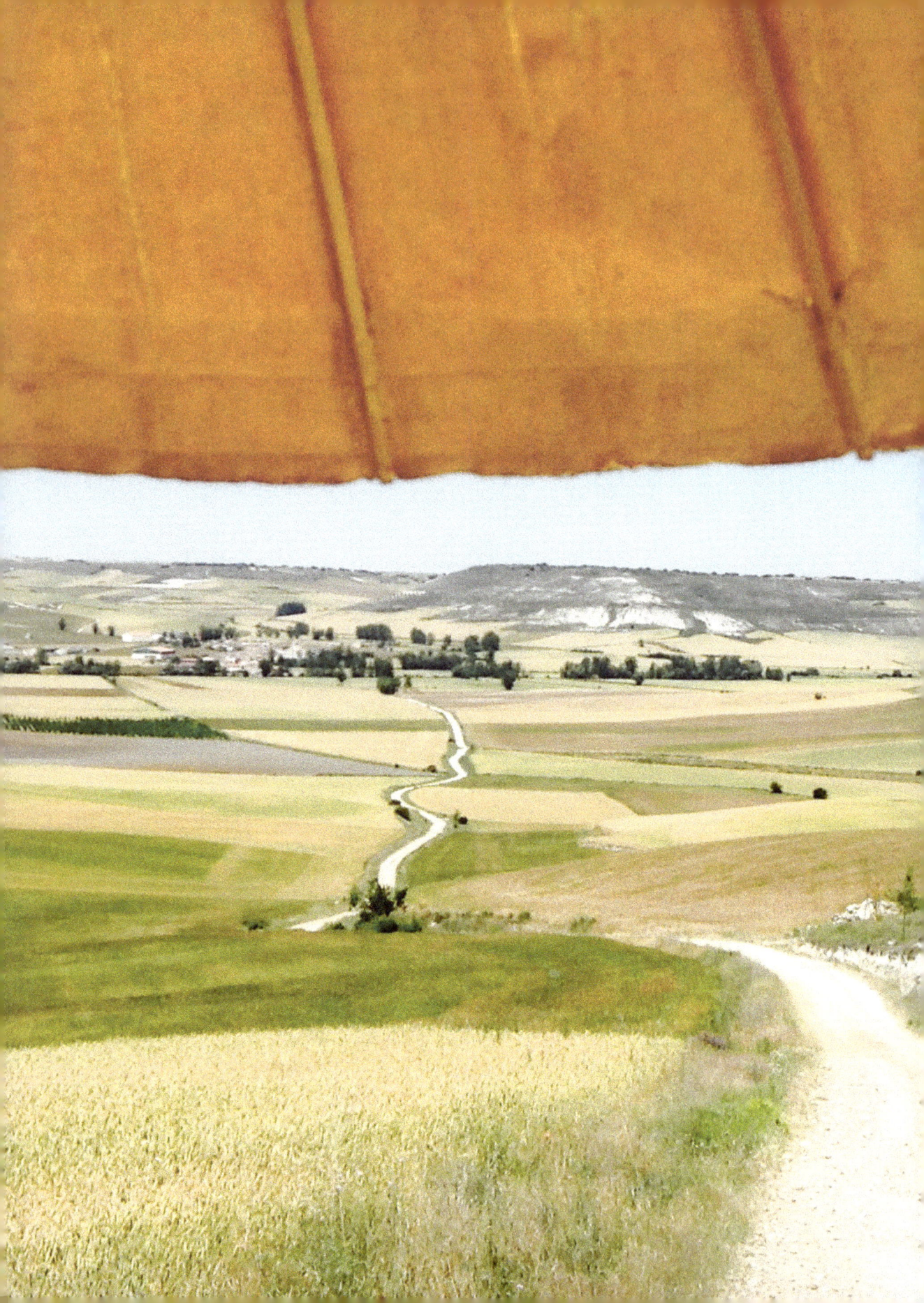

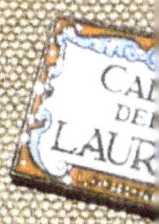

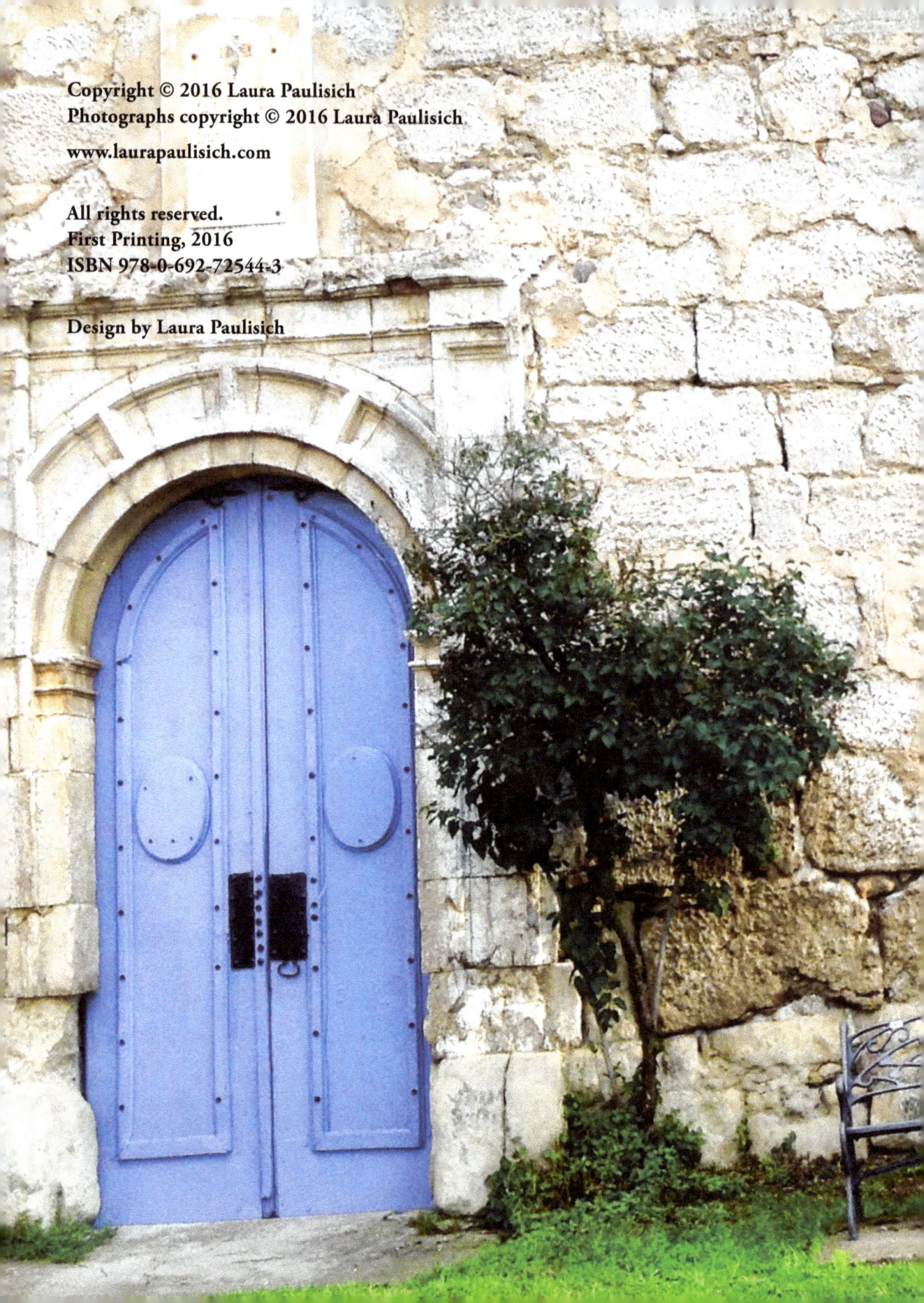

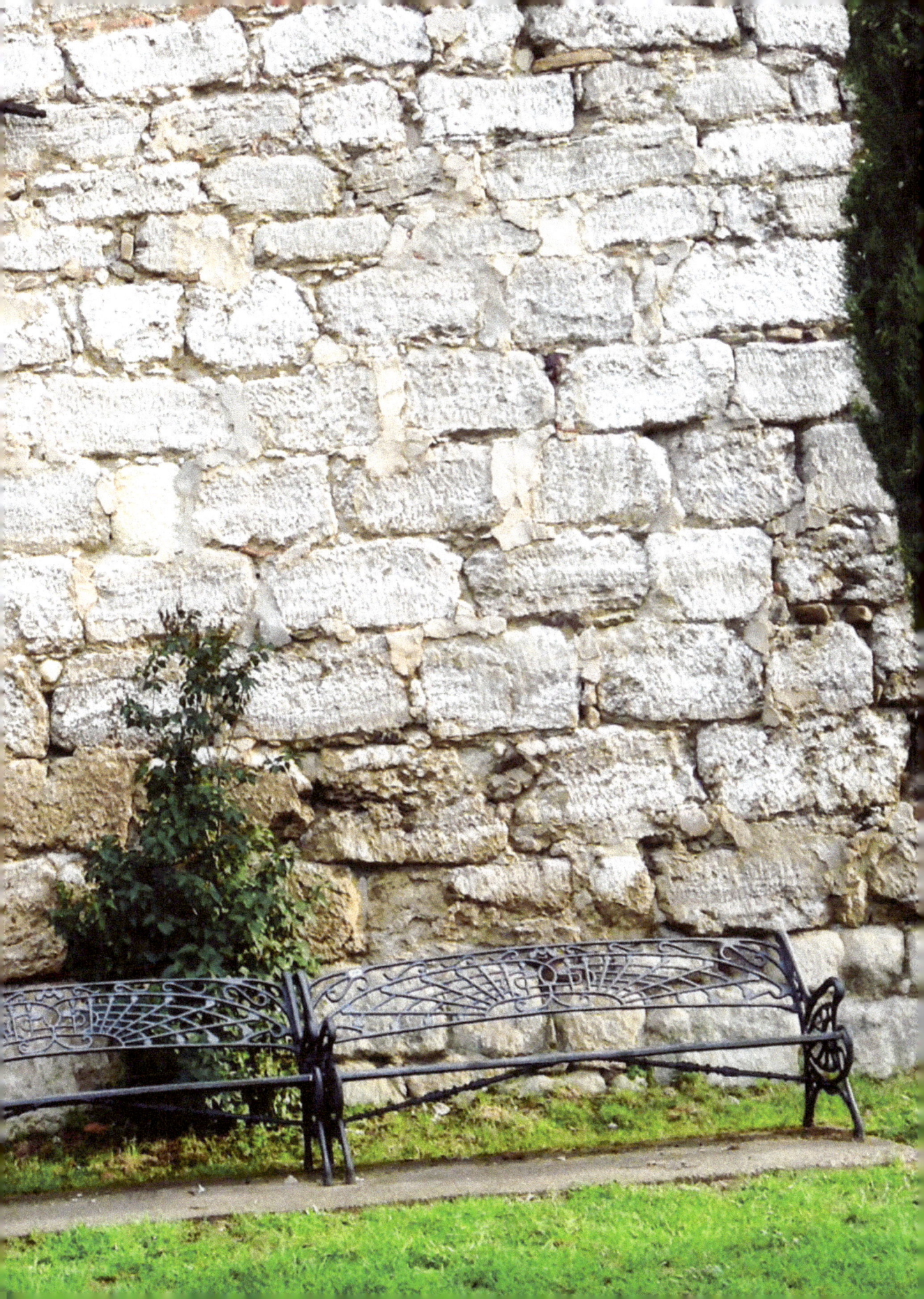

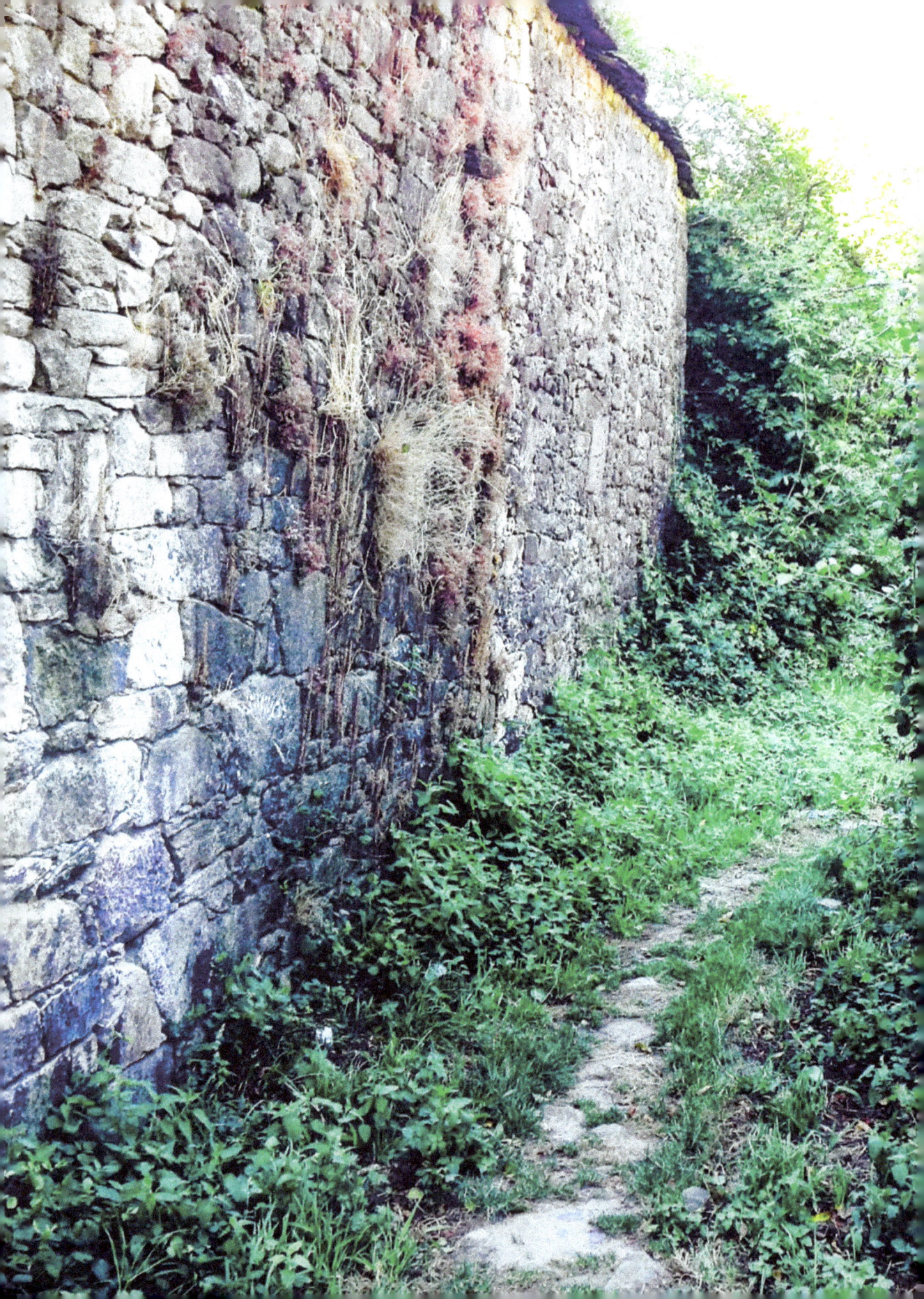

"Each of us limitless...
Each of us allow'd the eternal purports of the earth,
Each of us here as divinely as any is here."
-Walt Whitman *Leaves of Grass*

with grea

send God's

Laura on her p

May God protect

Fr. Gene Mo

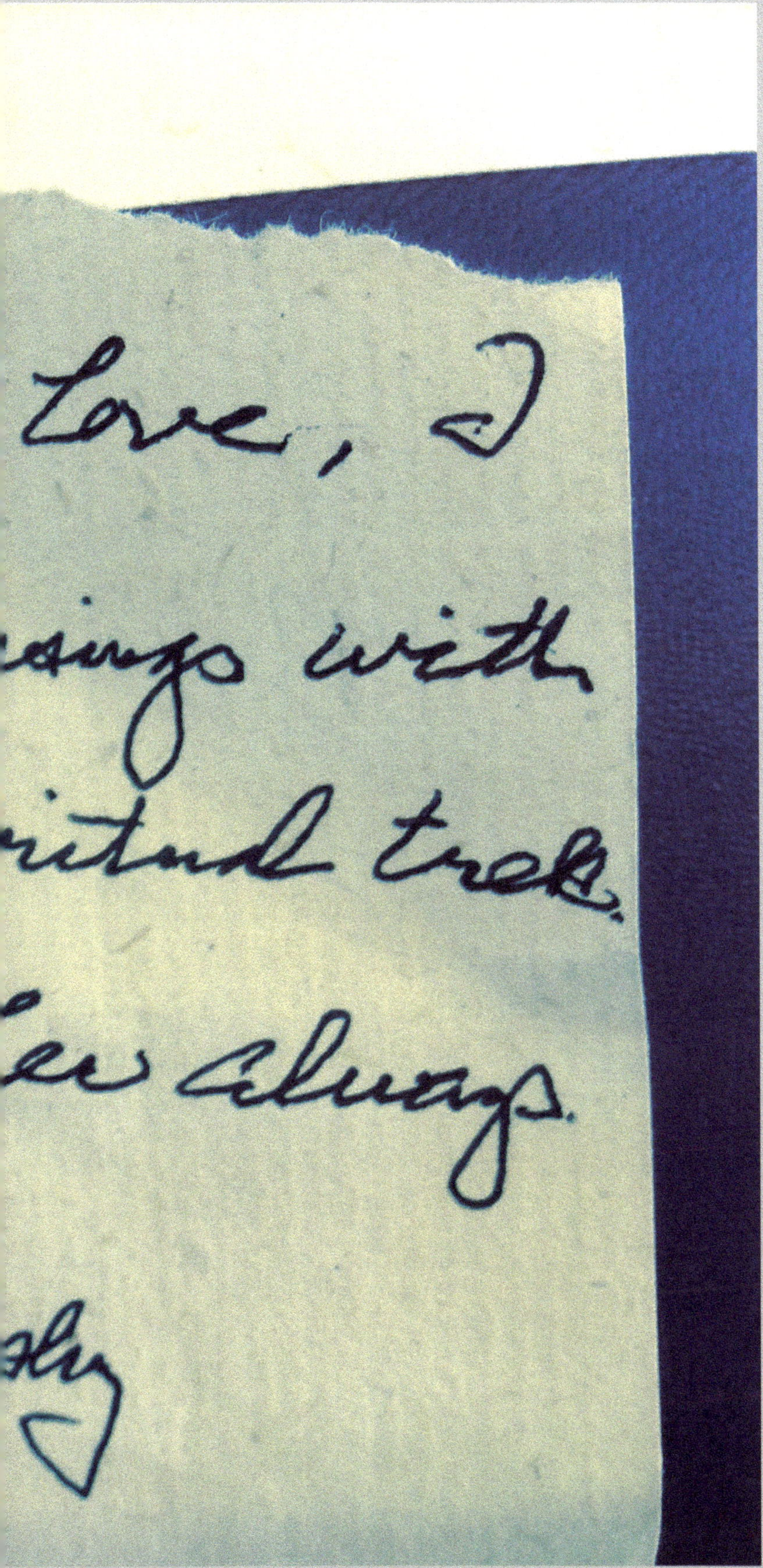

Dedication

To Jane & Gene
& MIRACLES

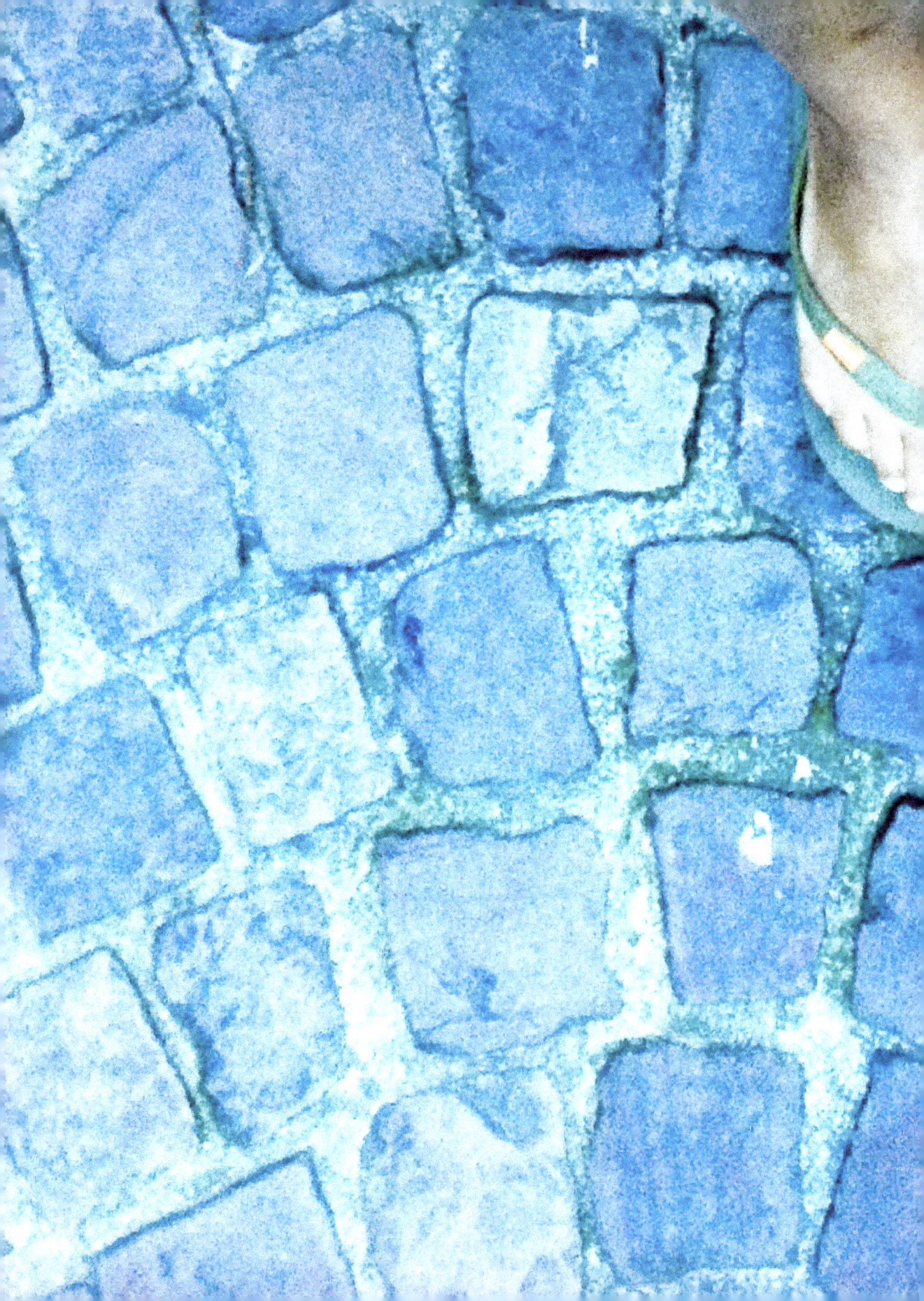

FOREWORD

Rarely do we have the opportunity to accompany such a deeply spiritual guide. We witness Laura experiencing a transformation along a 500 mile pilgrimage through Spain. Walking the distance in flip-flops, she brings us through small towns filled with wonderful and committed people who have assumed the role of "signposts," always anxious to help pilgrims avoid wrong turns.

Laura spent many days making her way along rocky paths and beautiful country lanes. A gifted storyteller, she brings to life the sights, sounds and smells of the hills and mountains of the Pyrenees and Spain.

Laura's story serves to guide us, like those guides along the Camino, gently indicating the path to spiritual growth and life fulfillment.

Fr. Gene Murphy

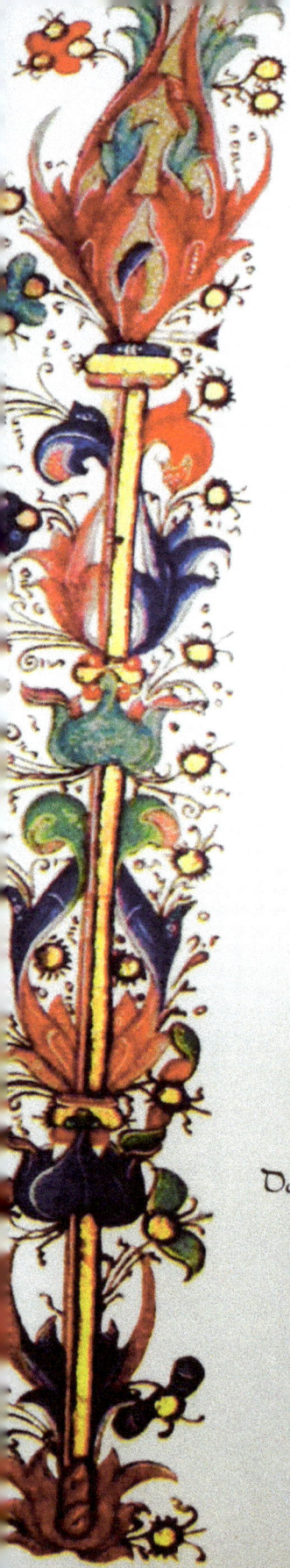

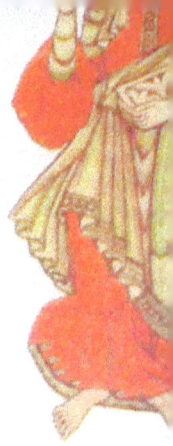

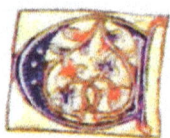

Capitulum huius Almae Apostolicae et Metropolitanae Ecclesiae Compostellanae, sigilli Altaris Beati Iacobi Apostoli custos, ut omnibus Fidelibus et Peregrinis ex toto terr Orbe, devotionis affectu vel voti causa, ad l SANCTI IACOBI, Apostoli Nostri, Hispani Patroni et Tutelaris convenientibus auther visitationis litteras expediat, omnibus et si praesentes inspecturis, notum facit: Dnam

Lauram Paulisich

hoc sacratissimum templum, perfecto Iti sive pedibus sive equitando post postrema cen milia metrorum, birota vero post ducenta, piet causa, devote visitasse. In quorum fidem praese litteras, sigillo ciusdem Sanctae Ecclesiae muni ei confert.

Datum Compostellae die 11 mensis Iulii anno Dni

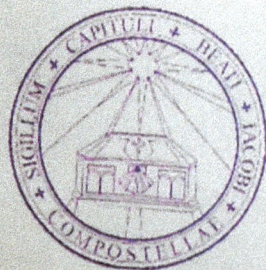

Segundo L Pérez López

NOTE TO READER

In life and on the Camino, many people wonder about and ask me about my habits: "How can you not eat after hiking 25 miles all day?!" "How are you progressing so quickly?" "How is your backpack so light?" "How do you always look so fresh and like this is effortless for you?" "You are NOT hiking in your flip-flops!" (even though they saw me hiking in my flip-flops!) "How do you not eat sugar/not drink alcohol/go to bed so early?"

My body is keto-adapted (it burns fat instead of sugar). I often go long periods of time without eating, without hunger and without thoughts of food. I have gained extreme mental clarity, equanimity and endurance. I usually only eat once a day in the morning. My diet is approximately 60-70% fat, 20-35% protein and 5-20% carbohydrate. I do not eat sugar, processed foods, drink coffee or alcohol.

I eat foods produced by nature, and I consider the diets of the animals/the conditions of the soil. I buy whole animals, eggs, raw butter and cheese from farmers. I render fat from those animals and make bone broth. I purchase herbs from a co-op or outdoor farmer's market. I order seafood and salmon online from independent fisheries. I buy coconut oil and olive oil that have been made using traditional methods.

I eat like royalty every day! I use traditional methods of cooking, unglazed clay cookware and the best ingredients the U.S.A. produces. My cholesterol test results are: cholesterol total: 247 (H); triglycerides: 24 (L); HDL cholesterol: 135; LDL cholesterol: 107; chol/hdl ratio: 1.83. I also sleep 9-10 hours every night. I don't use aspirin, over-the-counter medications or recreational drugs.

I avoid all chemicals as much as humanly possible! I wear natural clothing and shoes, wash my hair using only filtered water without shampoo, sleep on a natural rubber mattress with natural bedding and use essential oils to make homemade toothpaste, lotion, perfume, body/room spray, and cleaning solution. I use soapnuts to hand wash and line dry my clothing.

All of these "habits" have occurred gradually over time as I have learned more and more and have discovered the pure joy, happiness and freedom of living simply and treating my body and life impeccably! M I R A C L E ! !

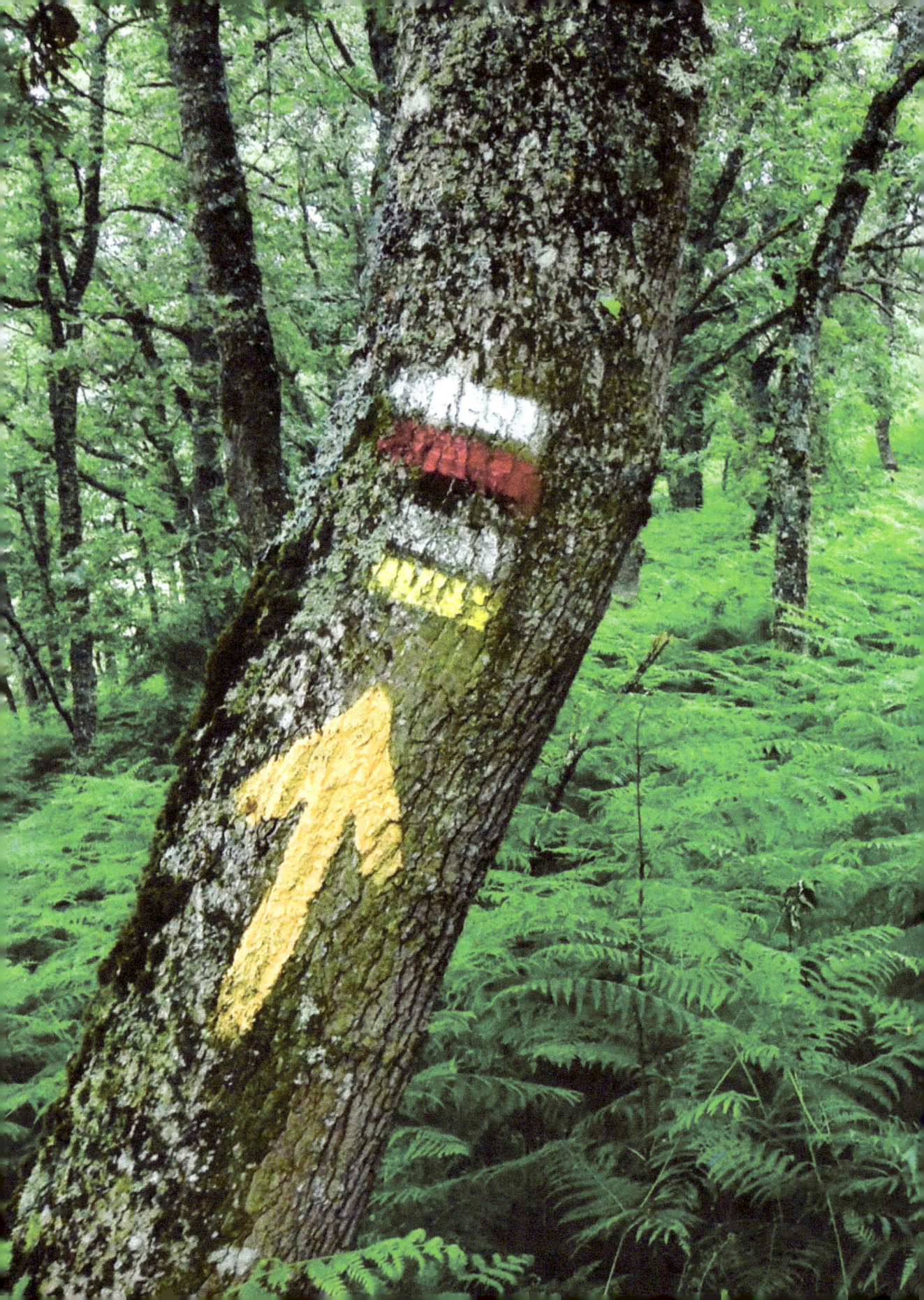

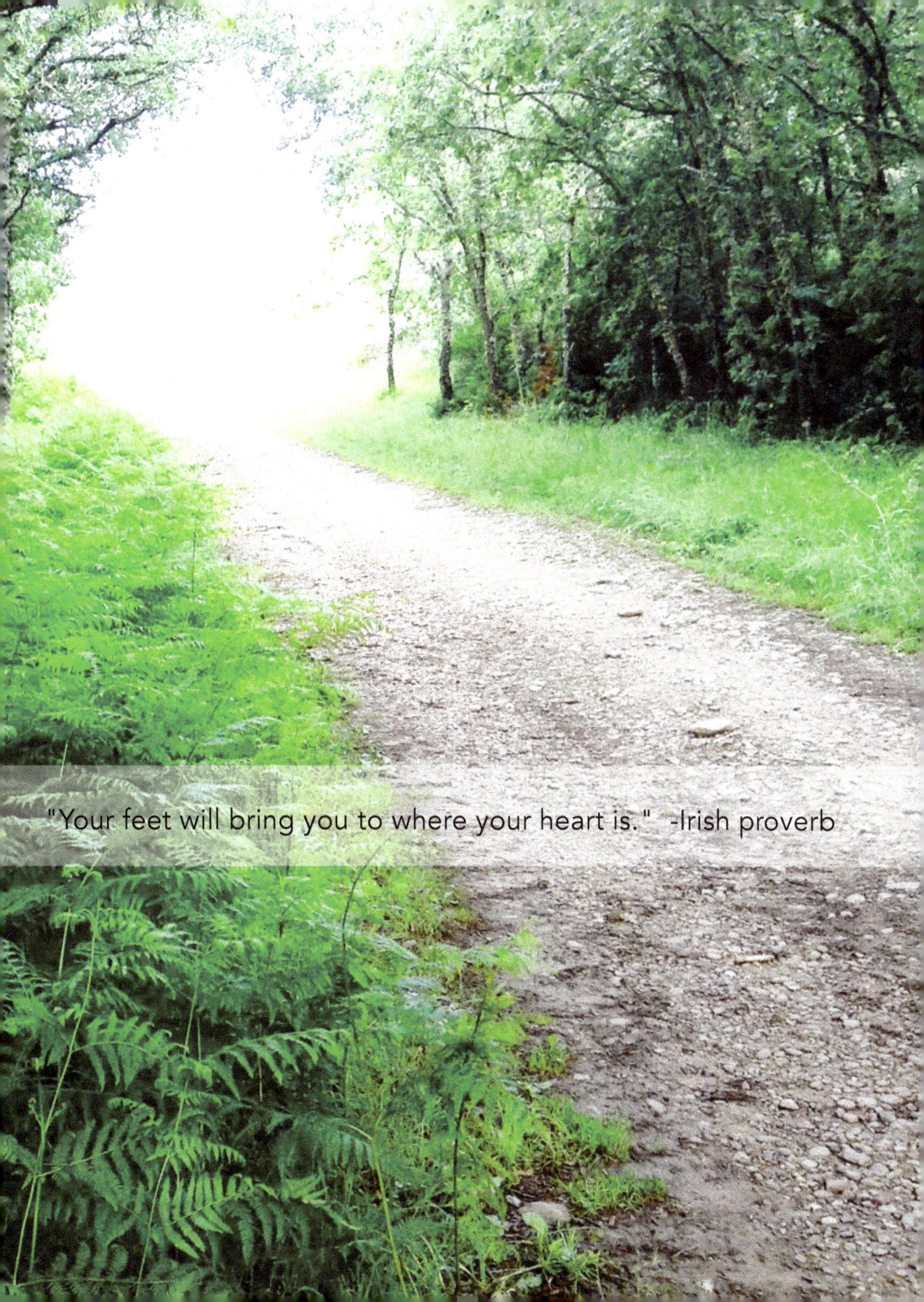

"Your feet will bring you to where your heart is." -Irish proverb

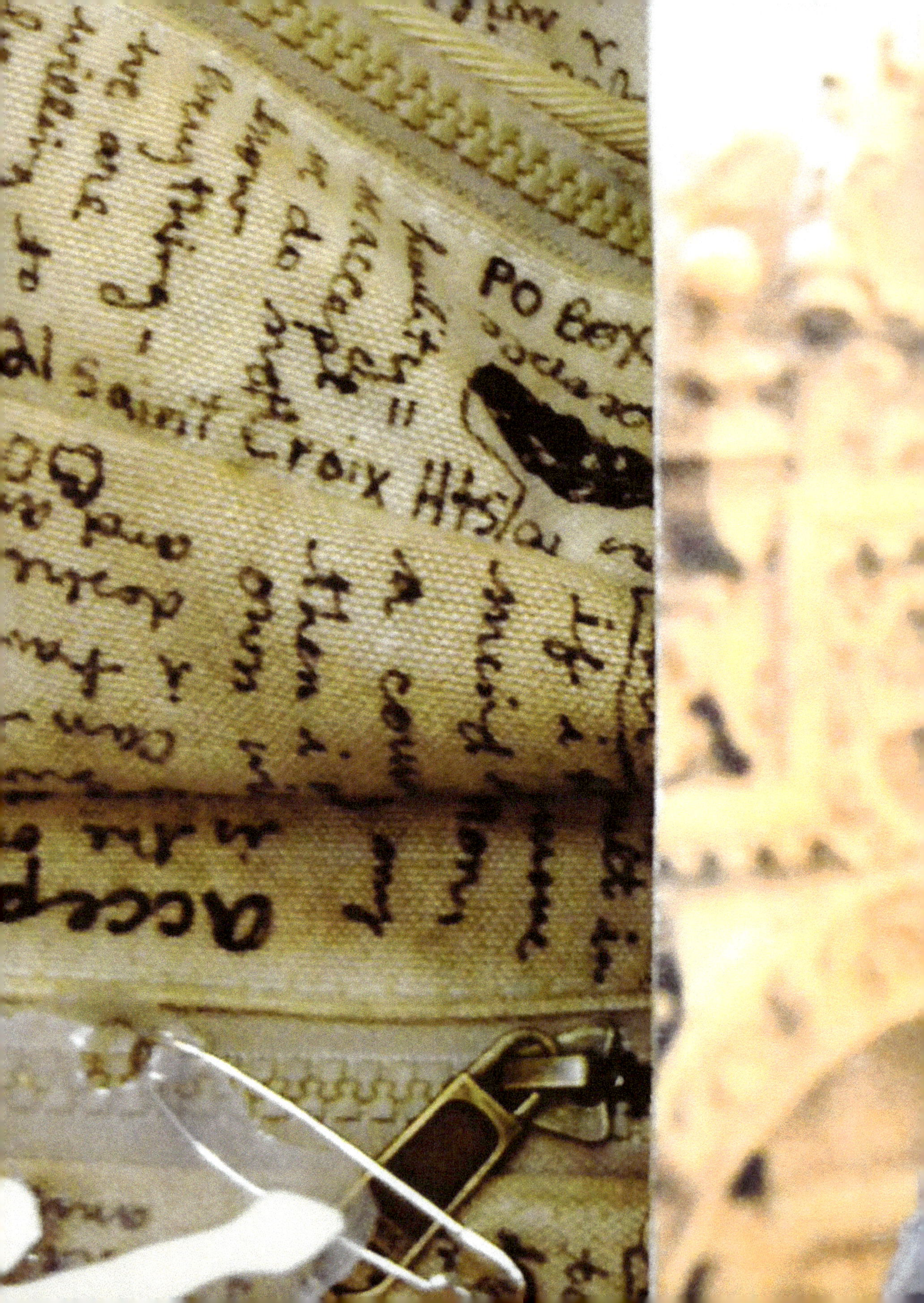
PO Box
Saint Croix Hts

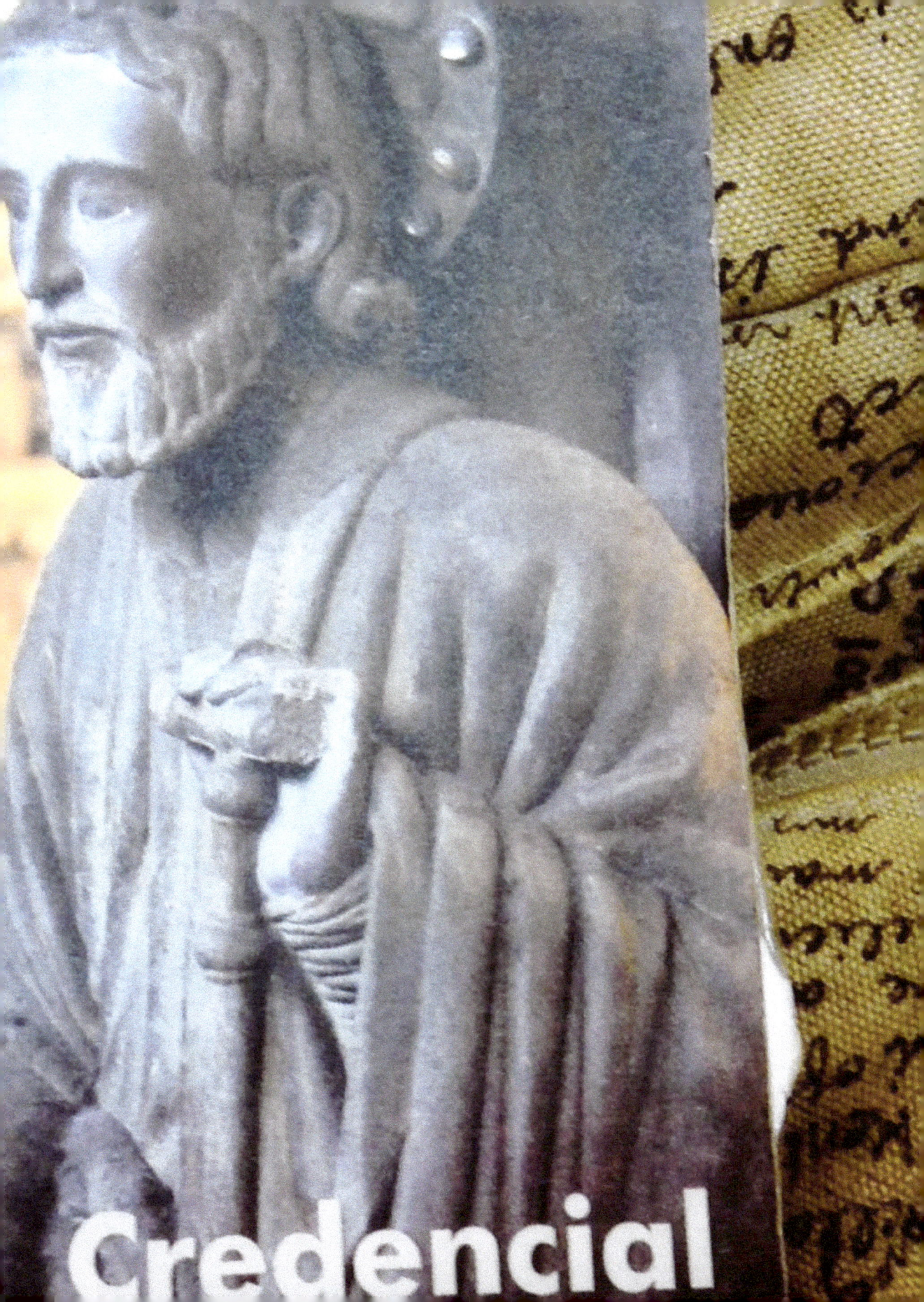

Credencial

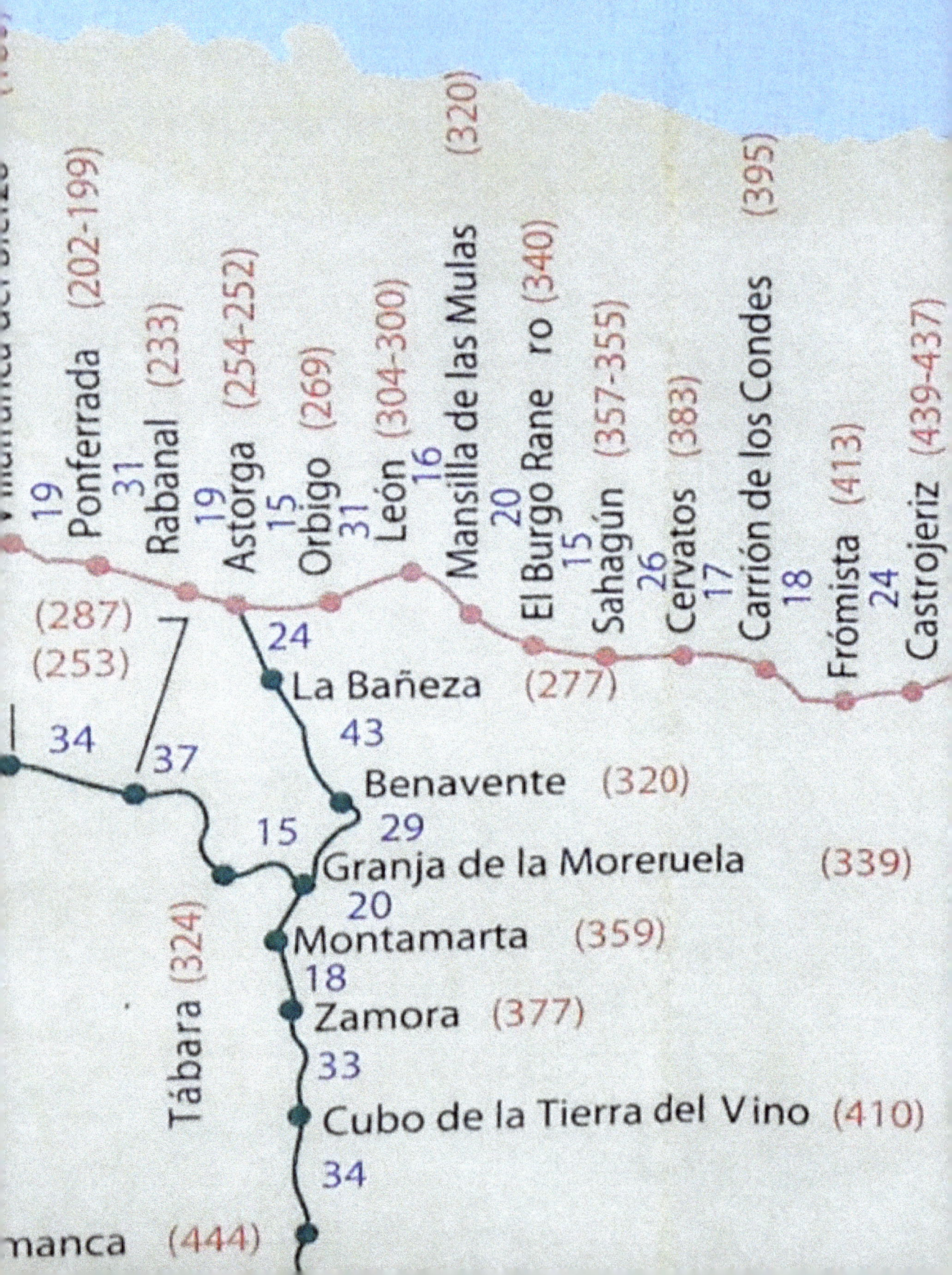

Villafranca del Bierzo (189)

Ponferrada (202-199)
19
Rabanal (233)
31
Astorga (254-252)
19
Orbigo (269)
15
León (304-300)
31
Mansilla de las Mulas (320)
16
El Burgo Ranero (340)
20
Sahagún (357-355)
15
Cervatos (383)
26
Carrión de los Condes (395)
17
Frómista (413)
18
Castrojeriz (439-437)
24

(287)
(253)

24

La Bañeza (277)

34

37

43

Benavente (320)

15

29

Granja de la Moreruela (339)

20

Montamarta (359)

18

Tábara (324)

Zamora (377)

33

Cubo de la Tierra del Vino (410)

34

Salamanca (444)

Camino
Francés

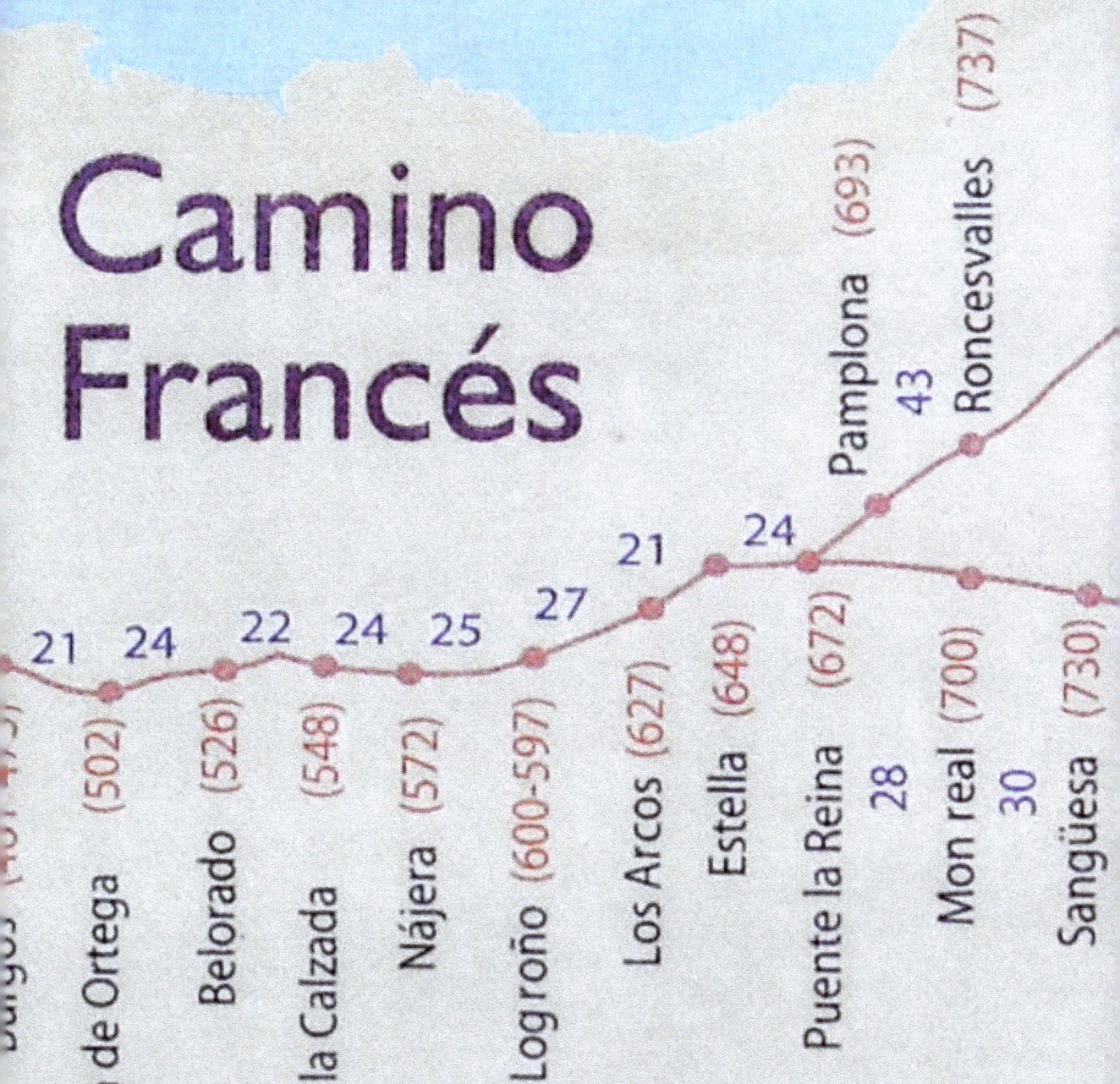

Roncesvalles (737)

Pamplona (693)

43

24

21

27

24

21

24

22

24

25

S. Juan de Ortega (502)

Belorado (526)

. Domingo de la Calzada (548)

Nájera (572)

Logroño (600-597)

Los Arcos (627)

Estella (648)

Puente la Reina (672)

28

Mon real (700)

30

Sangüesa (730)

Pa

Núcleo urbano
que cuenta
con refugio
para peregrinos

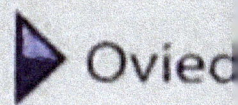

▶ Ovied

Pola de

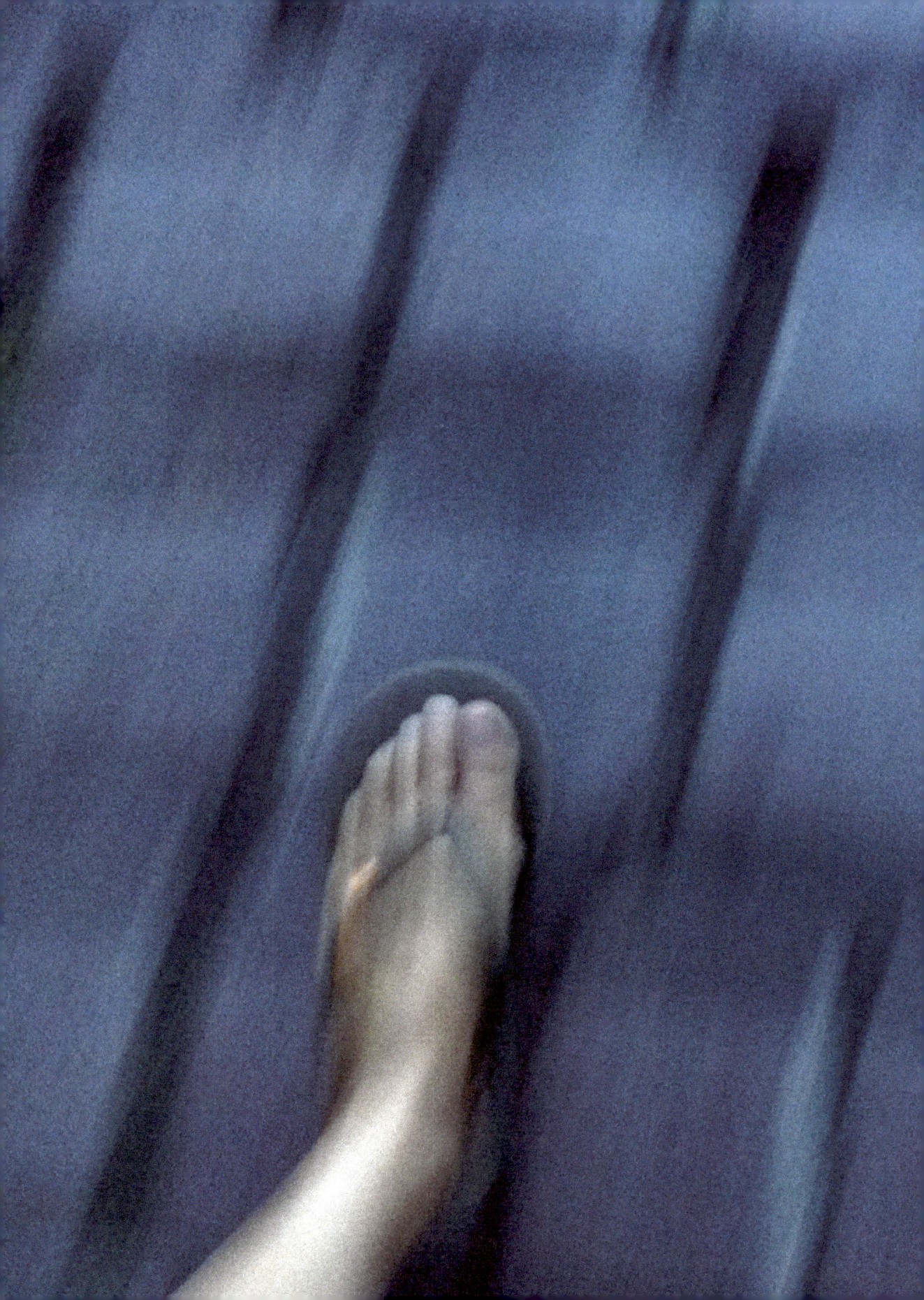

Starting point
Saint-Jean-Pied-de-Port, France

Ending point
Finisterre, Spain

Total miles
550 miles (plus additional detour miles)

Total days to walk across Spain
31 days (June 14 - July 14)

Shoes
natural rubber flip-flops (4 pairs)

Supplies
2 skirts (organic cotton/naturally dyed/zipper pouch)
2 tube tops/tube dresses (organic cotton/naturally dyed)
1 scarf/shawl/towel (organic silk)
1 tank top/dress (organic cotton/naturally dyed)
"rain gear": waterproof/sunproof parasol (leather oiled)
& 2 plastic garbage bags
1 wooden toothbrush with natural bristles
baking soda/sea salt/peppermint oil tooth powder
1 small glass spray bottle of bed bug/body spray/sleep
aromatherapy (lavender oil/tea tree oil/filtered water)
1 week supply of food (grass-fed, raw & aged cheese;
mountain grass-fed artisan chorizo &/or acorn-fed, semi-
wild pork; organic extra virgin olive oil)
money, passport, iPod

Objective
MIRACLES

Introduction

During the fall of 2014, I was searching online for volunteer opportunities. The Internet continually directed me to the website Meetup.com. I became intrigued and perused through all the interesting groups and categories. I discovered a group called Camino. I read the description (a pilgrimage across Spain) and immediately joined the group even though I had no money for travel. I intended to participate as observer by walking, listening and experiencing the Camino through others (if they let me!).

On January 1st 2015, I attended my first Camino Meetup. We went for a hike and "talked and walked Camino." I quickly learned that these people were some of the most genuine, generous, enthusiastic adventurers I had ever met! Everyone approached me encouraging me to not let a lack of money deter me from walking the Camino. I was buoyed and uplifted (and shocked!) by their encouragement and support. I instantly left a voice message for my mom with all of the exhilarating details of my encounter. A week later, she reported to me that my story inspired her to tell a friend and the two of them had decided to pay for me to walk the Camino. I was going to Spain! M I R A C L E ! !

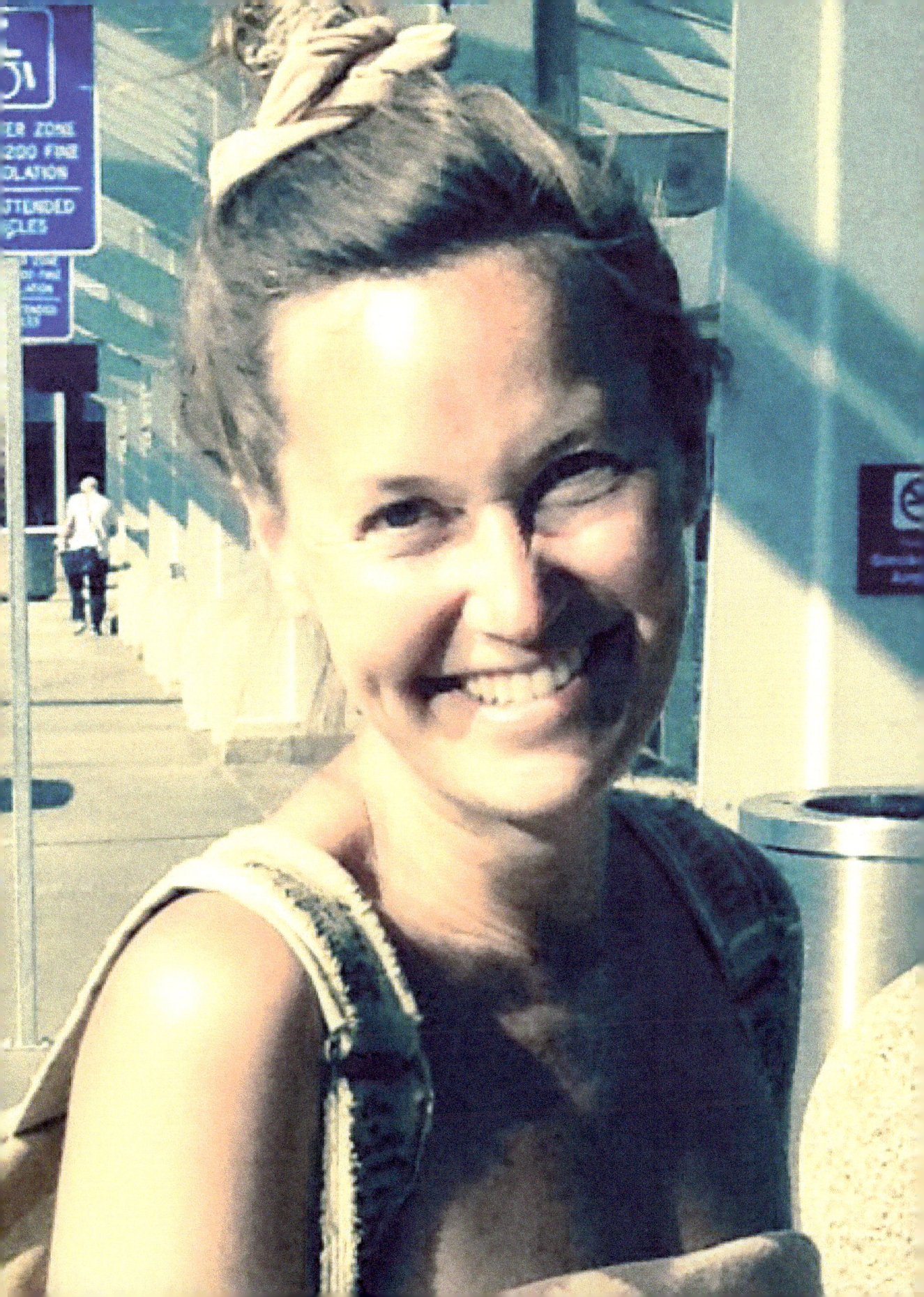

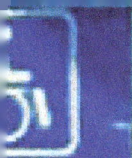

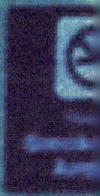

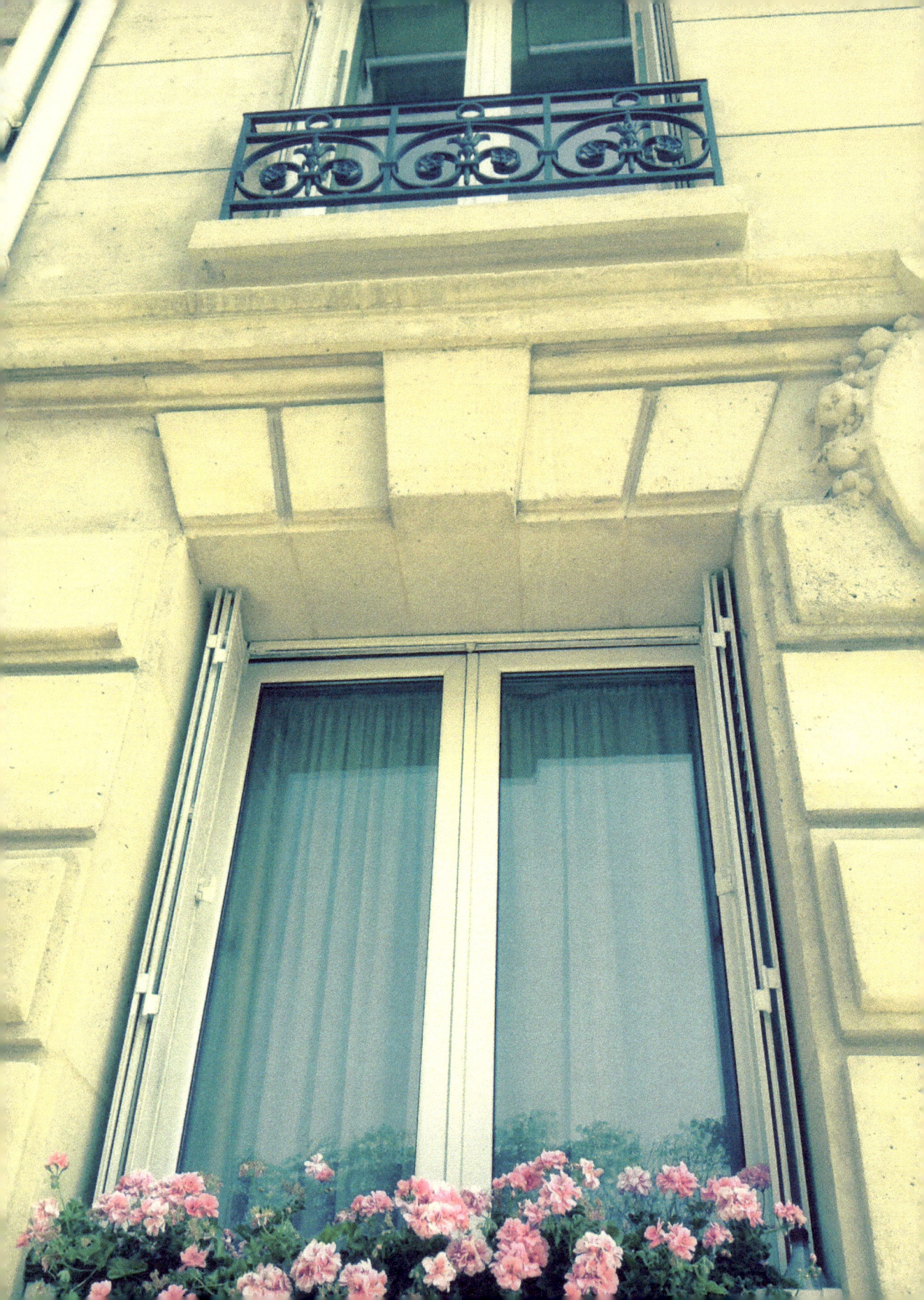

Contents

Camino de Santiago

Ierario Cultural Europeo

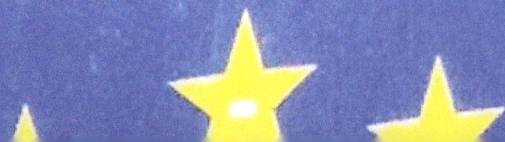

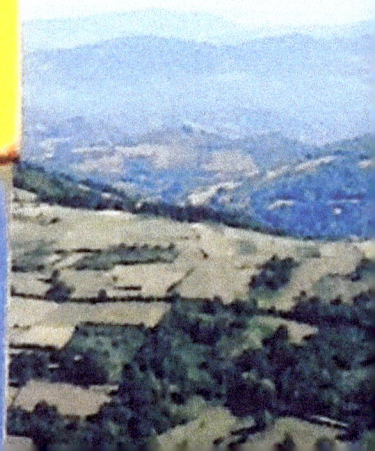

Begin

· ·

"All glory comes from daring to begin" -e.f. ware

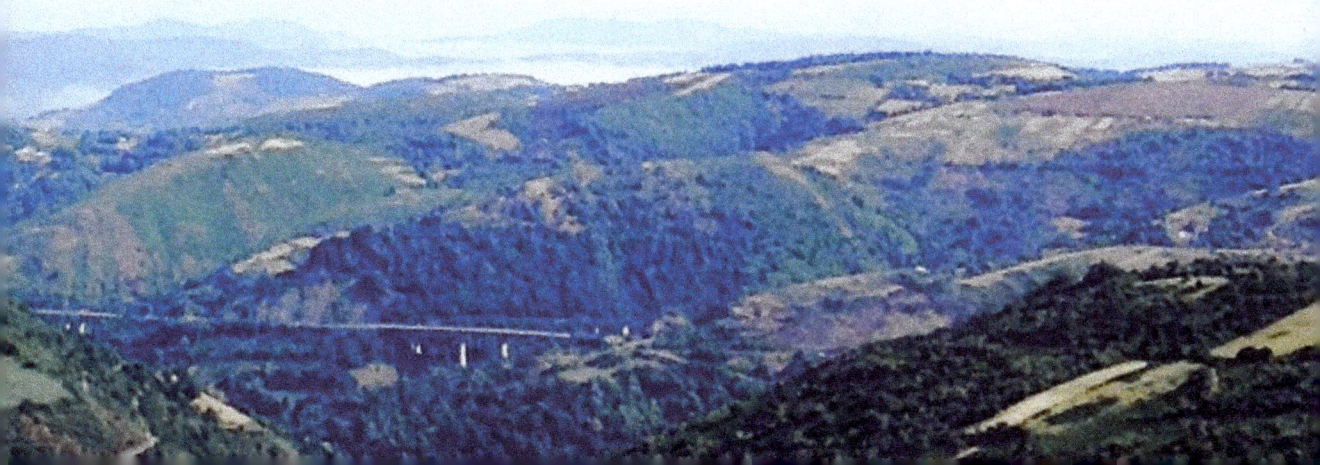

research

READ IMAGINE PONDER INQUIRE

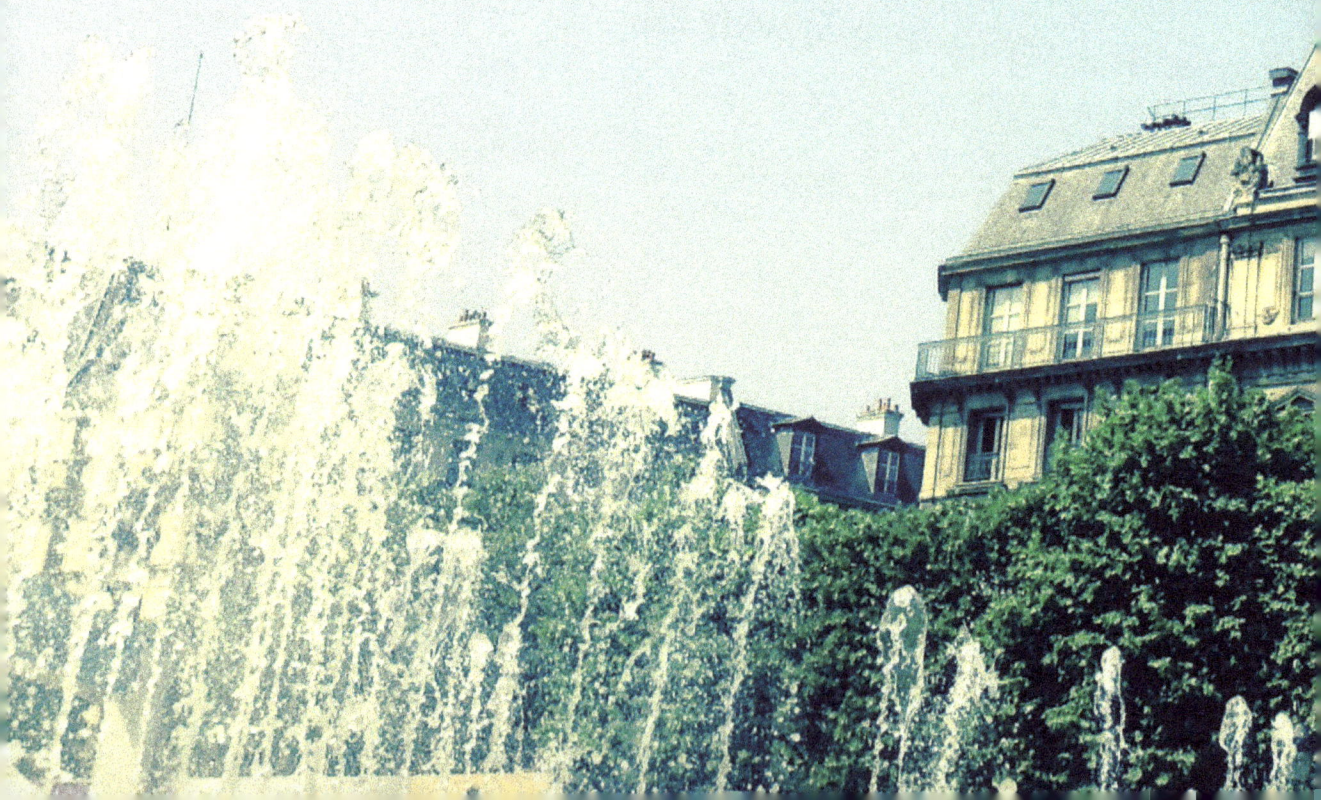

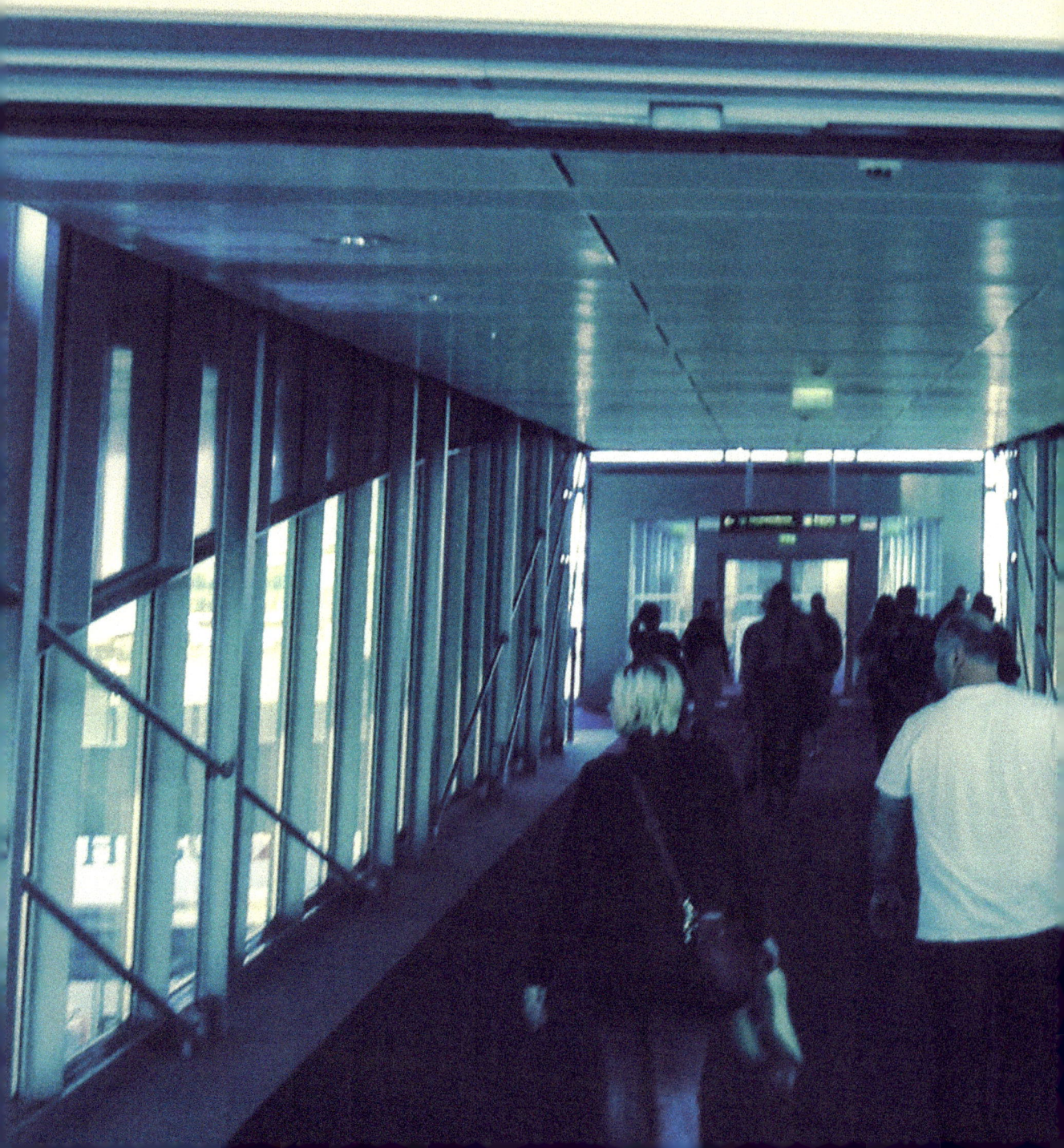

bienvenue à Pa

welcome to Paris / bienvenidos

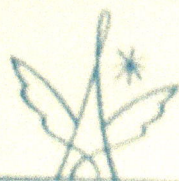

AÉROPORTS DE PARIS

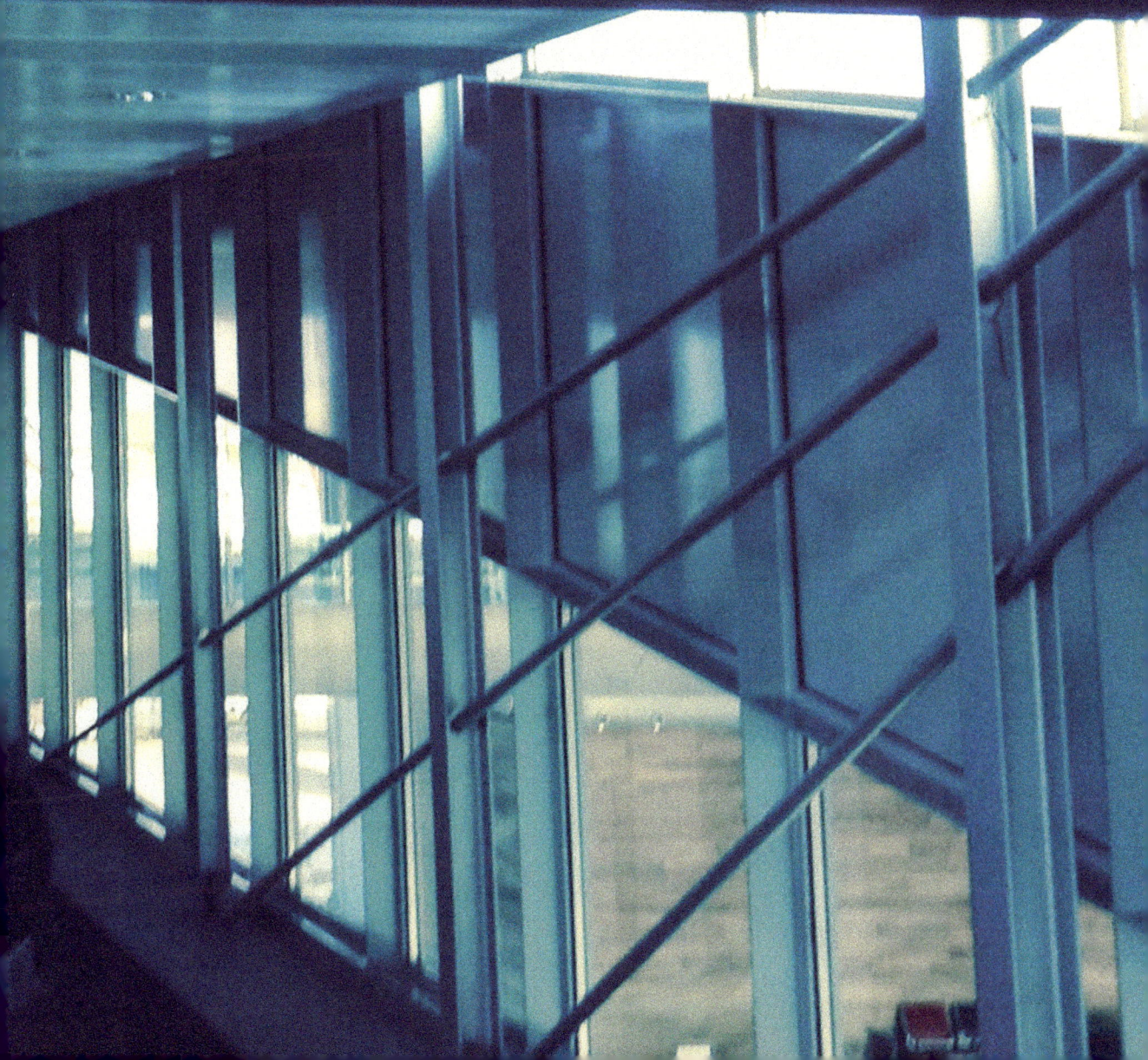

As soon as I learned I was going to walk the Camino, I ordered stacks of books from the library and began reading, searching, perusing and LEARNING everything about Spain, the Camino, traveling, Europe, food and hiking. I learned many pilgrims fly to Paris, take the train, then a bus to a popular starting point Saint-Jean-Pied-de-Port, France. This sounded like the most exciting plan! Flying to Paris! M I R A C L E ! !

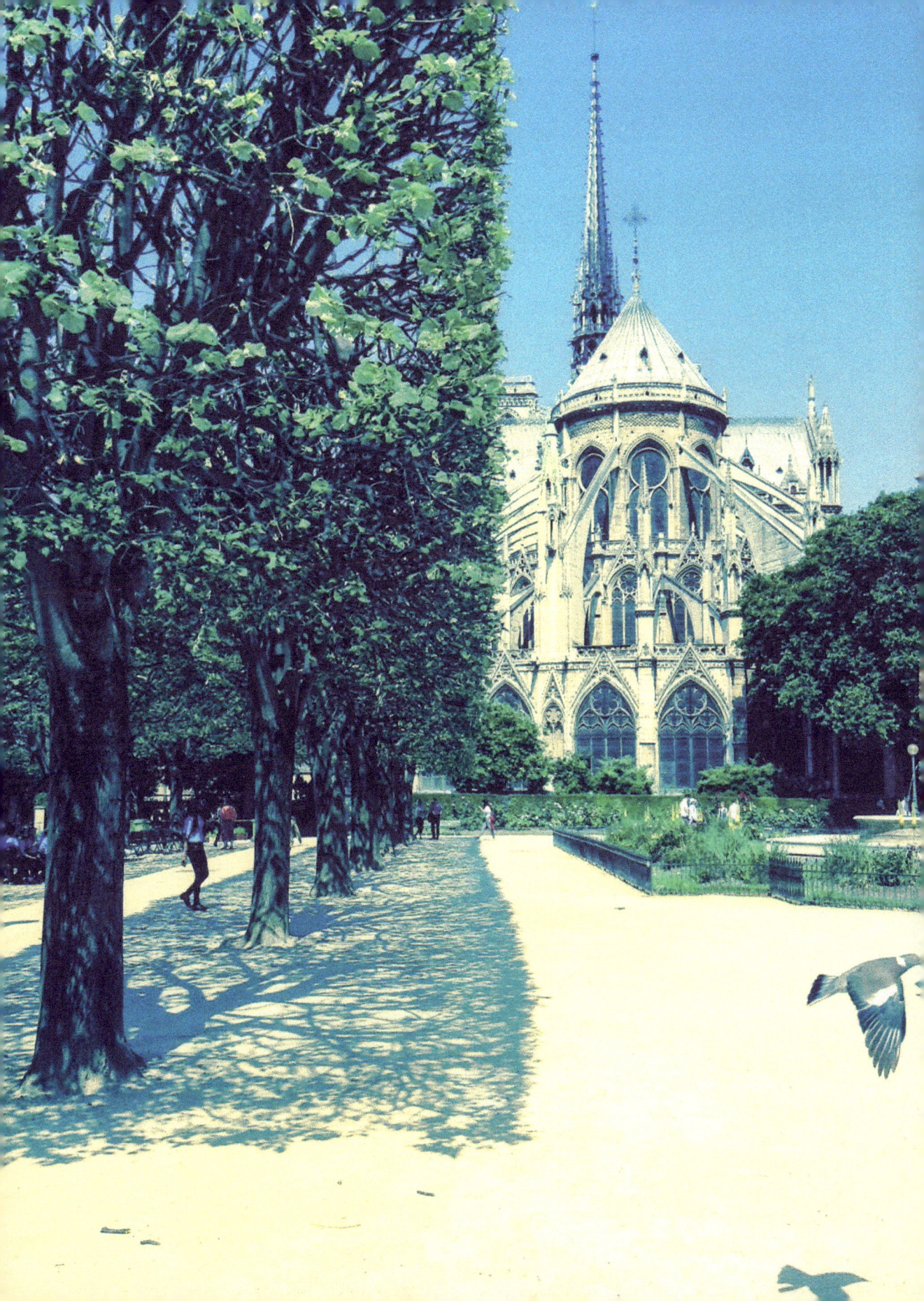

miracle miracle miracle miracle miracle miracle miracle miracle miracle miracle miracle miracle miracle miracle miracle mira

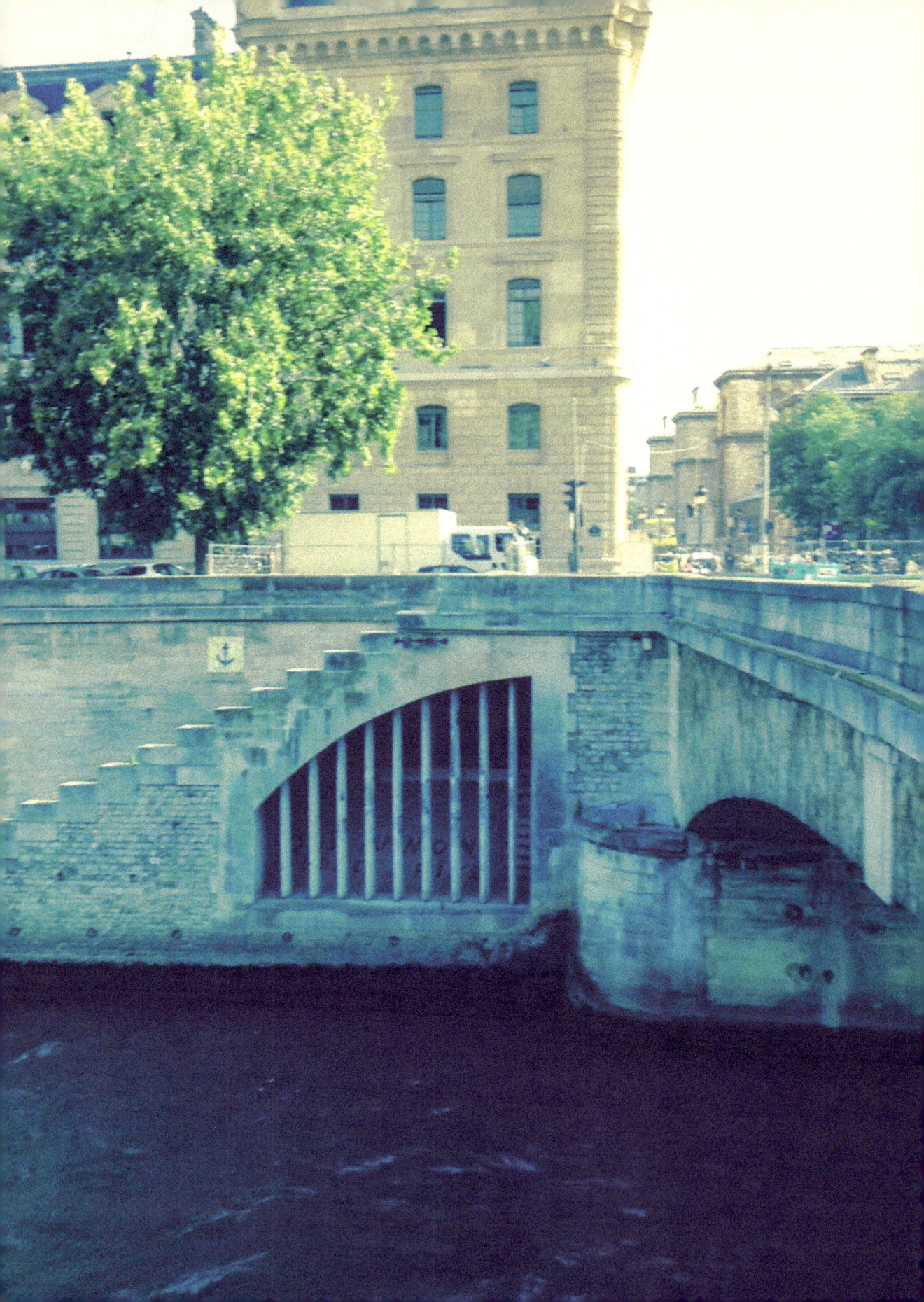

"if you seek beauty you will find it"
-bill cunningham

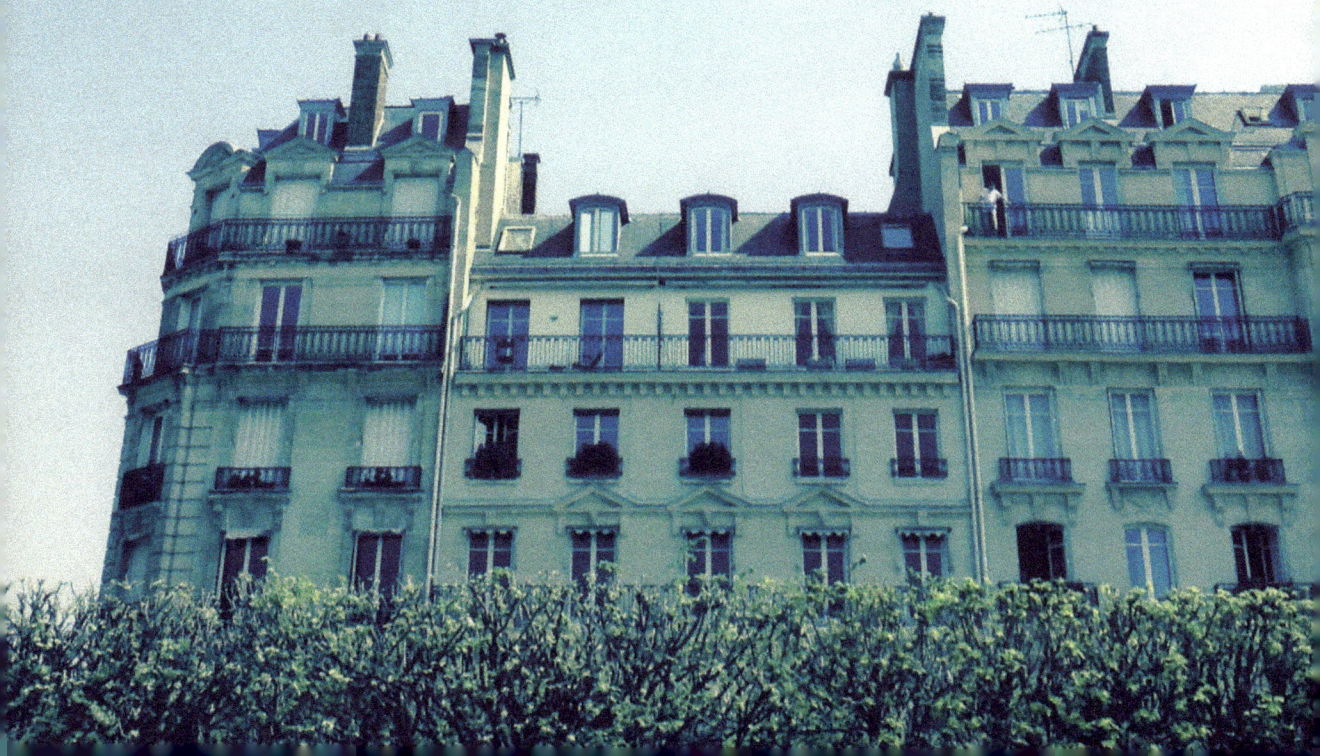

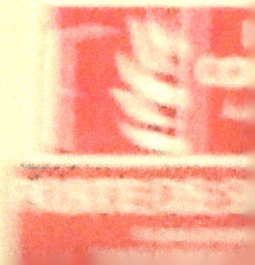

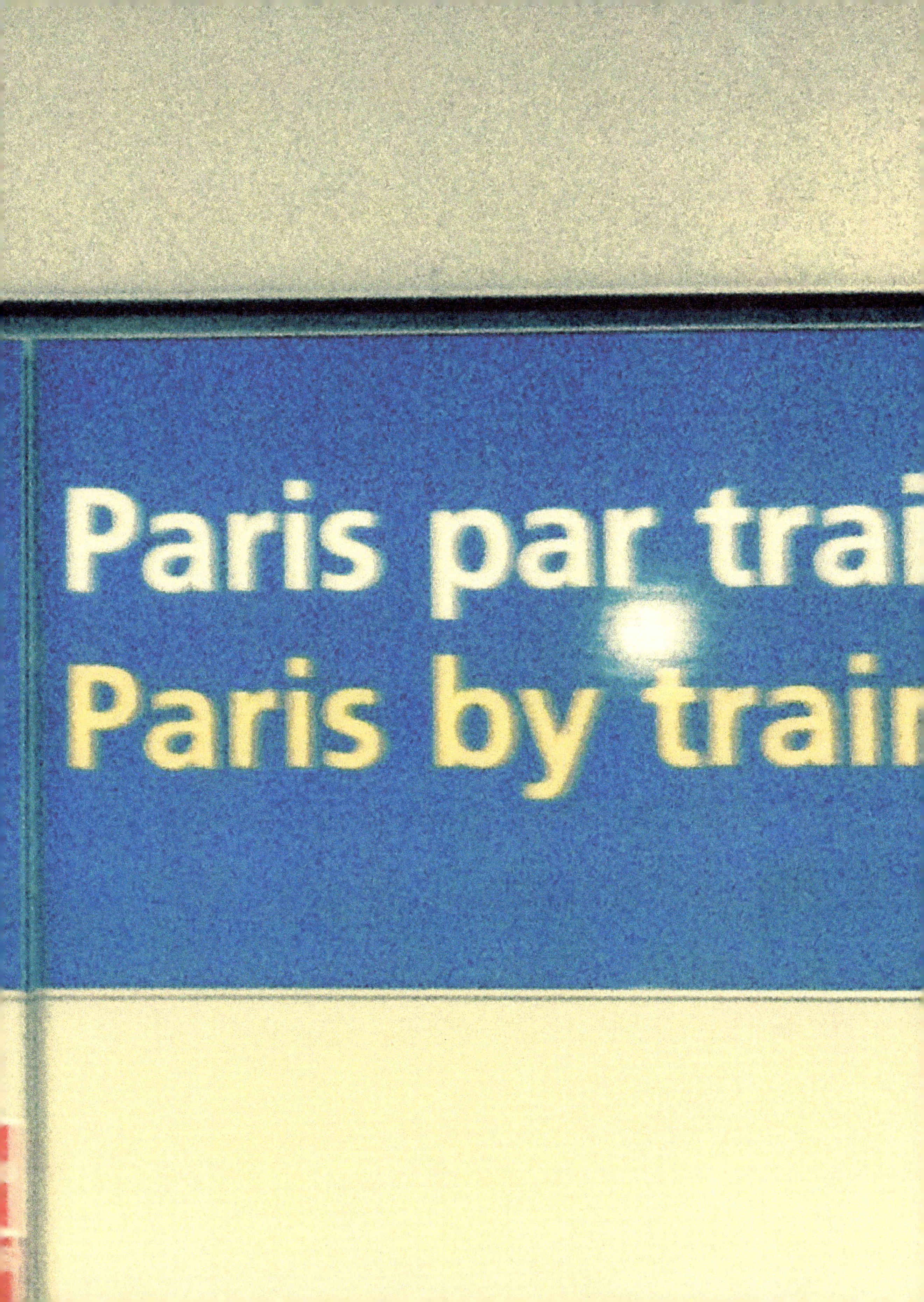

Paris par train

Paris by train

merci (**mair-see**) thank you

bonjour (**bohn-zhoor**) hello

au revoir (**o ruh-vwahr**) goodbye

Île de la Cité (**EEL duh lah see TAY**)

Seine (**SEHN**)

Louvre (**LOO-vruh**)

Bastille (**bah-STEE-yuh**)

Champs-Élysées (**SHAHN-zay-lee-ZAY**)

Haussmann (**ohss-MAHN**)

Charles de Gaulle (**sharl-duh-GOHL**)

Hôtel des Invalides (**oh-TELL-day-zan-vah-LEED**)

Sainte-Chapelle (**SANT-shah-PELL**)

Carnavalet (**car-nah-vah-LAY**)

Place de la Concorde(**PLAHSS-duh-lah-kawn-KOHRD**)

Montmartre (**mawn-MART-ruh**)

Pont Neuf (**pawn-noohf**)

Pont des Arts (**pawn-day-zahr**)

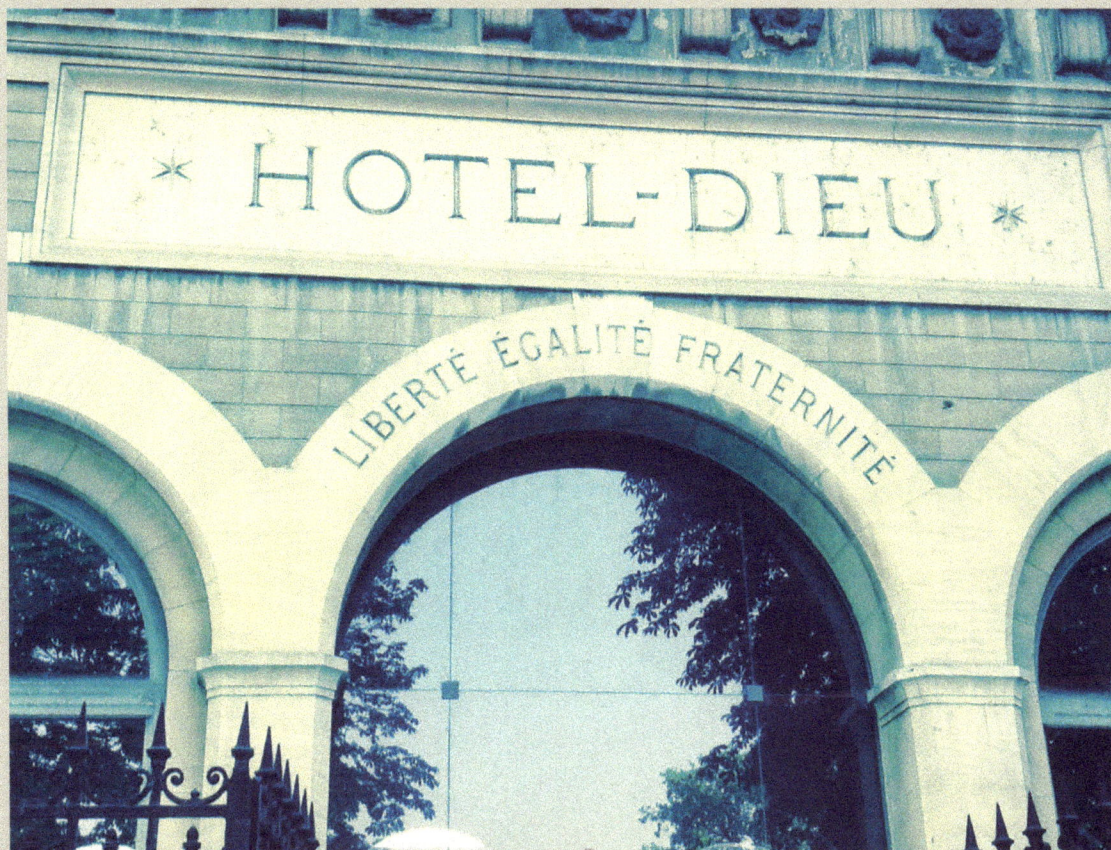

HÔTEL-DIEU

hospital and hotel
profits go to charity

Hôtel-Dieu Hospitel
1 Place du Parvis
Île de la Cité
Notre-Dame   75004
PARIS
+33 (0) 1 44 32 01 00
www.hotel-hospitel.fr

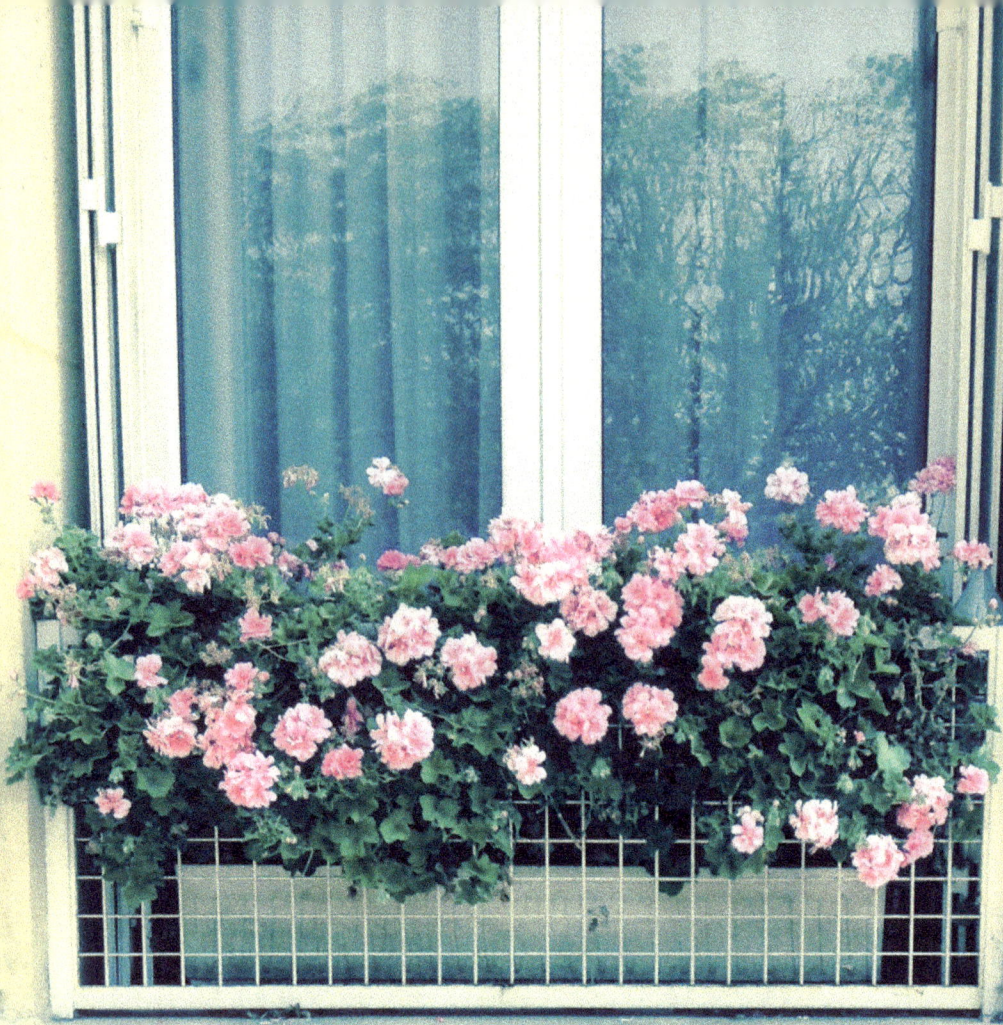

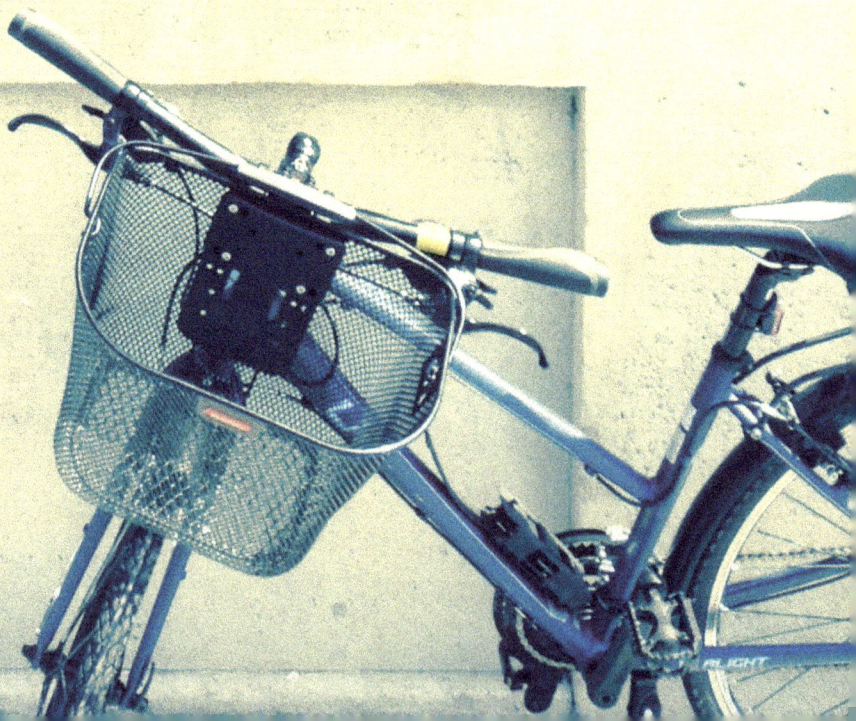

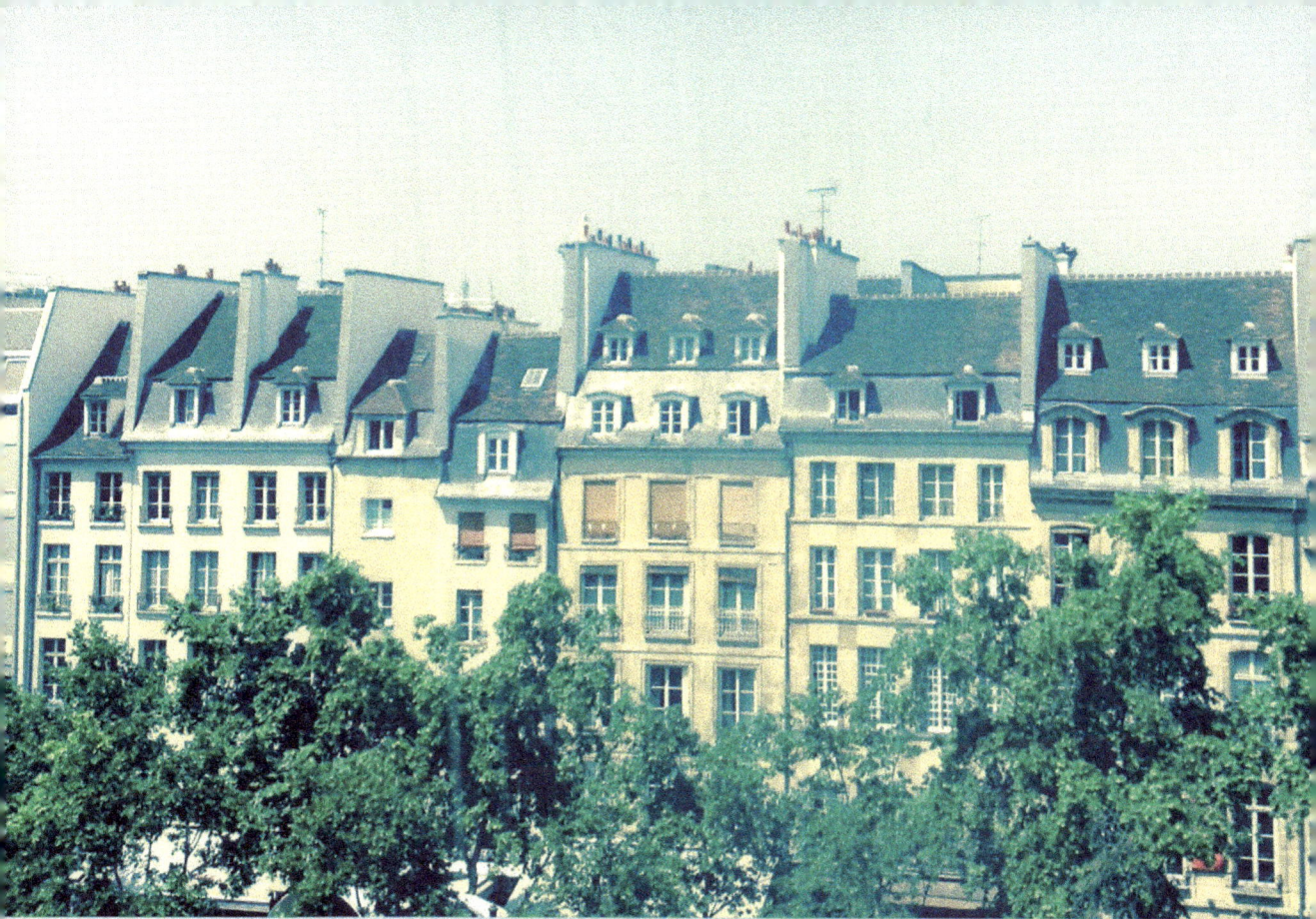

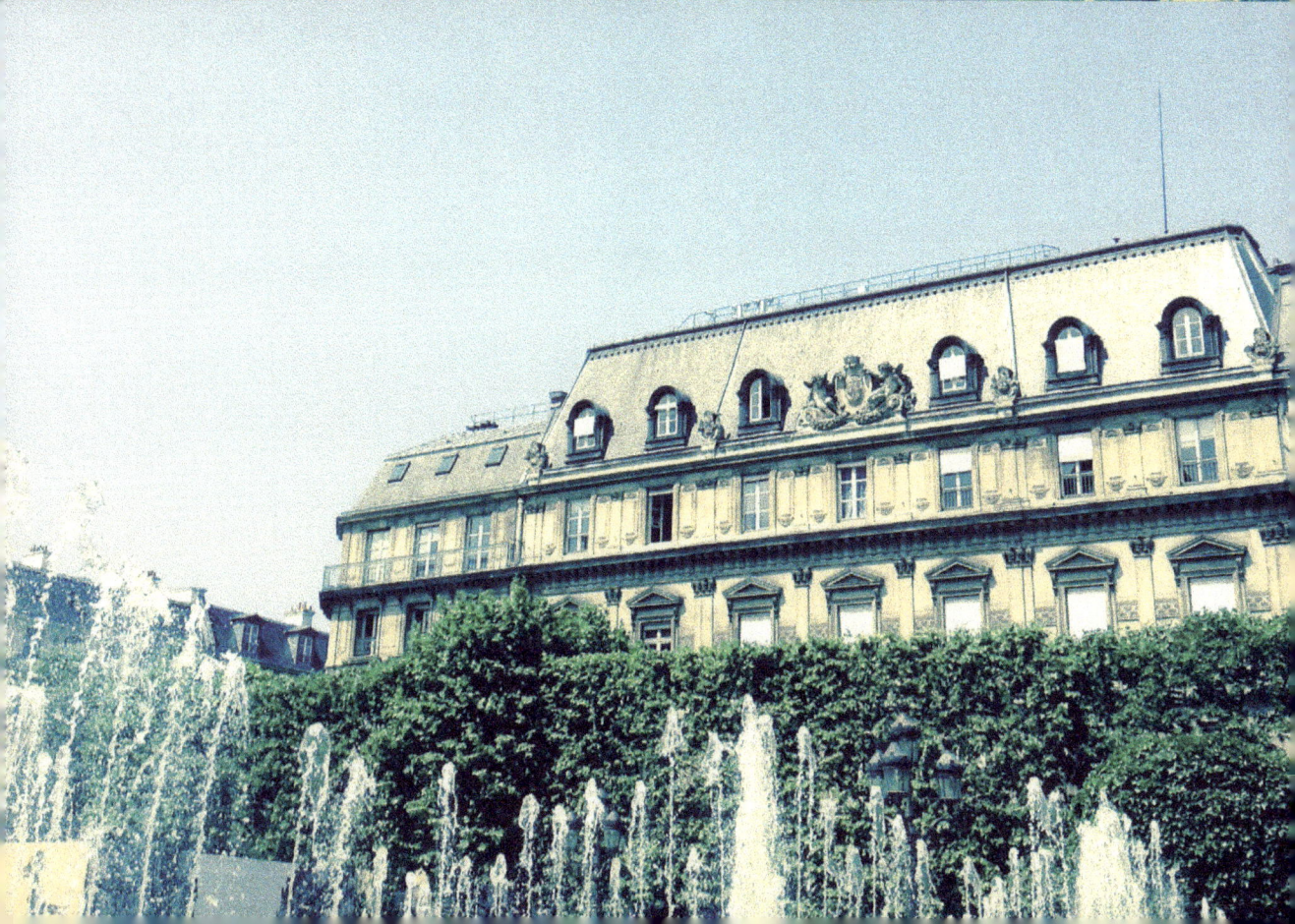

PARIS
48 hours

Day 1

1. Purchase **PARIS MUSEUM PASS** in airport

2. Take train to **NOTRE-DAME** (approximately 1 hour)

3. Check into the **HÔTEL-DIEU HOSPITEL** (139€)

4. Walk or **FLÂNER** (stroll aimlessly) to **LE MARAIS**

5. Purchase olive oil **A L'OLIVIER** (23, Rue de Rivoli Paris 4, alolivier.com)

6. Purchase cheese **FROMAGERIE DUBOIS** (97-99 rue Saint Antoine Paris 4)

7. Visit **VICTOR HUGO HOUSE**, **CITY HALL**, **CENTRE POMPIDOU**

8. Visit **SHAKESPEARE & CO** bookstore (37 rue de la Bûcherie)

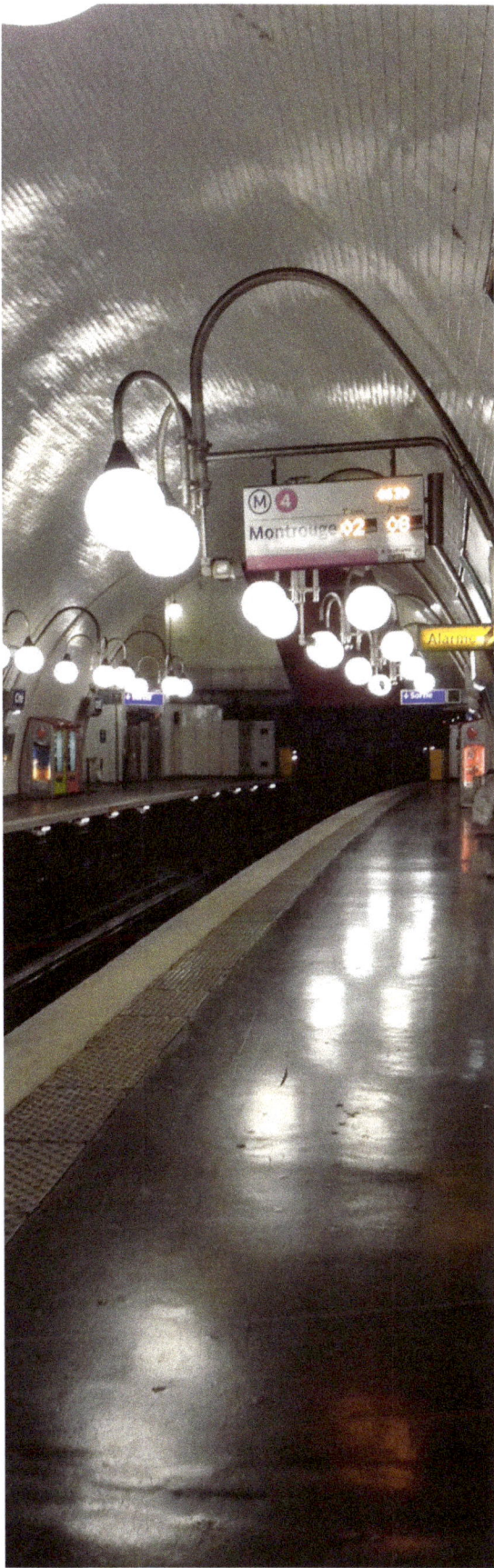

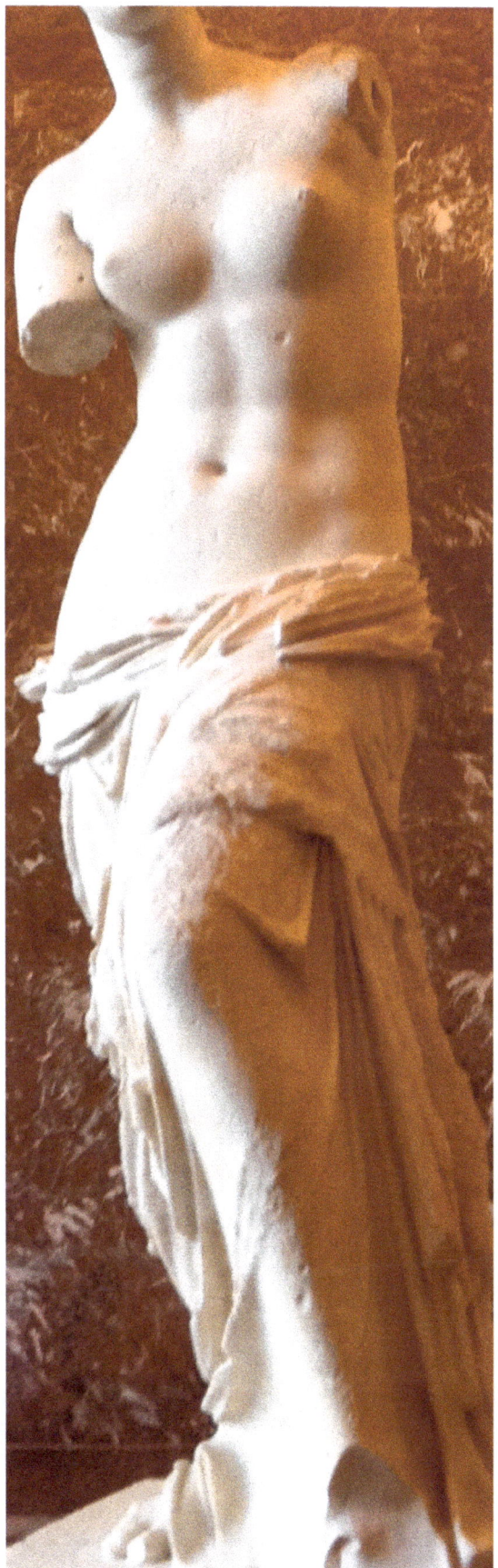

Day 2

1. Explore **NOTRE-DAME** 7:00am (no lines, empty & magical)

2. Rent **VÉLIB'** bicycle outside Notre-Dame for endless miles of exploring

3. Cross **PONT DES ARTS** ("love locks" bridge over the Seine)

4. Visit **MUSÉE DU LOUVRE** 9:00am (fastest access, Venus de Milo, Mona Lisa, Napoleon III Apartments)

5. Ride down **RUE DE RIVOLI**

6. **MUSÉE DES ARTS DÉCORATIFS**

7. Ride through **JARDIN DES TUILERIES, PLACE DE LA CONCORDE, CHAMPS-ÉLYSÉES, ARC DE TRIOMPHE, AVENUE MONTAIGNE**

8. Visit **PALAIS GALLIERA** (fashion museum, Jeanne Lanvin exhibition)

9. Visit **MUSÉE DE L'ARMÉE (TOMBEAU DE NAPOLÉON),MUSÉE RODIN** (The Thinker, The Kiss), **EIFFEL TOWER, MUSÉE DE L'ORANGERIE** (Monet's Water Lilies), **MUSÉE D'ORSAY, Café de Flore, La Grande Epicerie**

Favorites: Palais Galliera, Pont des Arts, Flaner Le Marais, velib.com, Paris Museum Pass, Pompidou, Musée de l'Orangerie, Tombeau de Napoléon, Musée Rodin

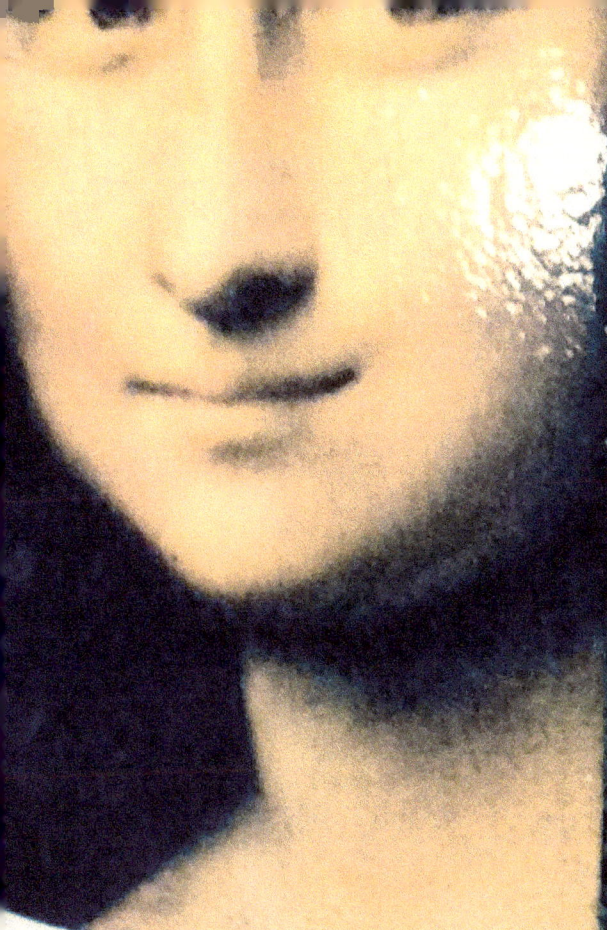

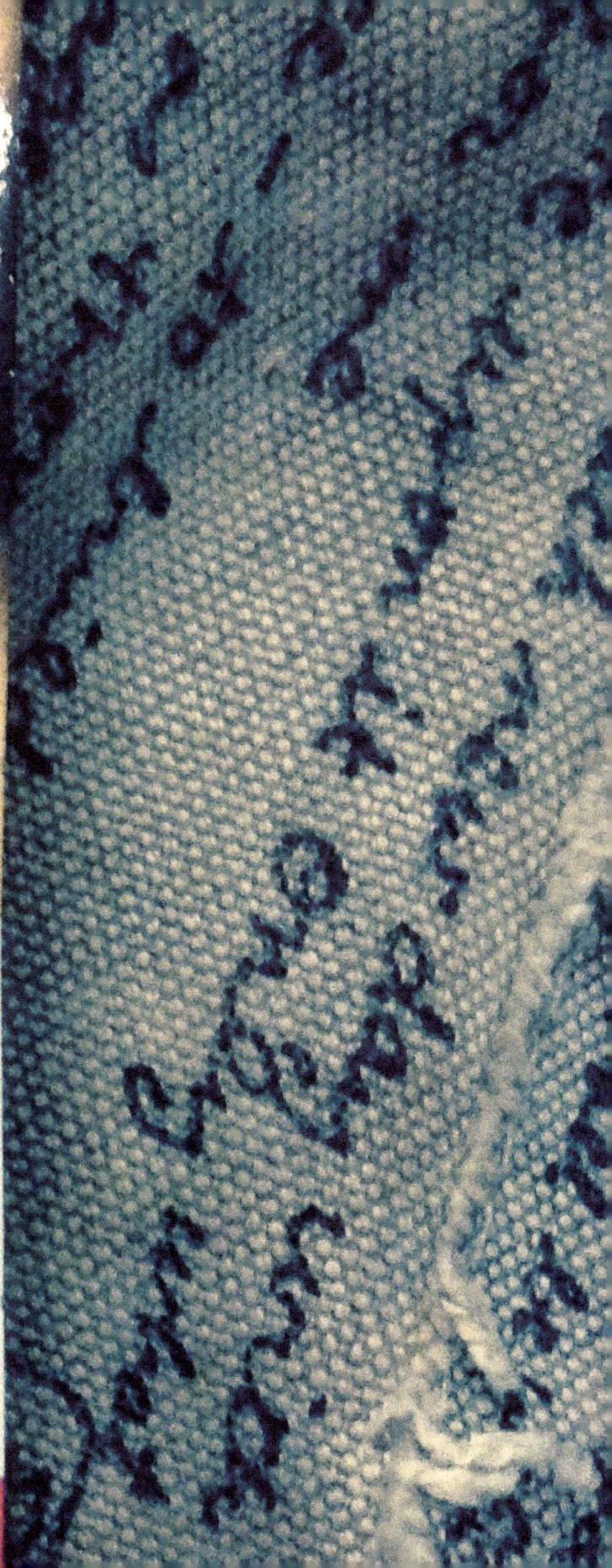

PARIS

SEUM

PASS

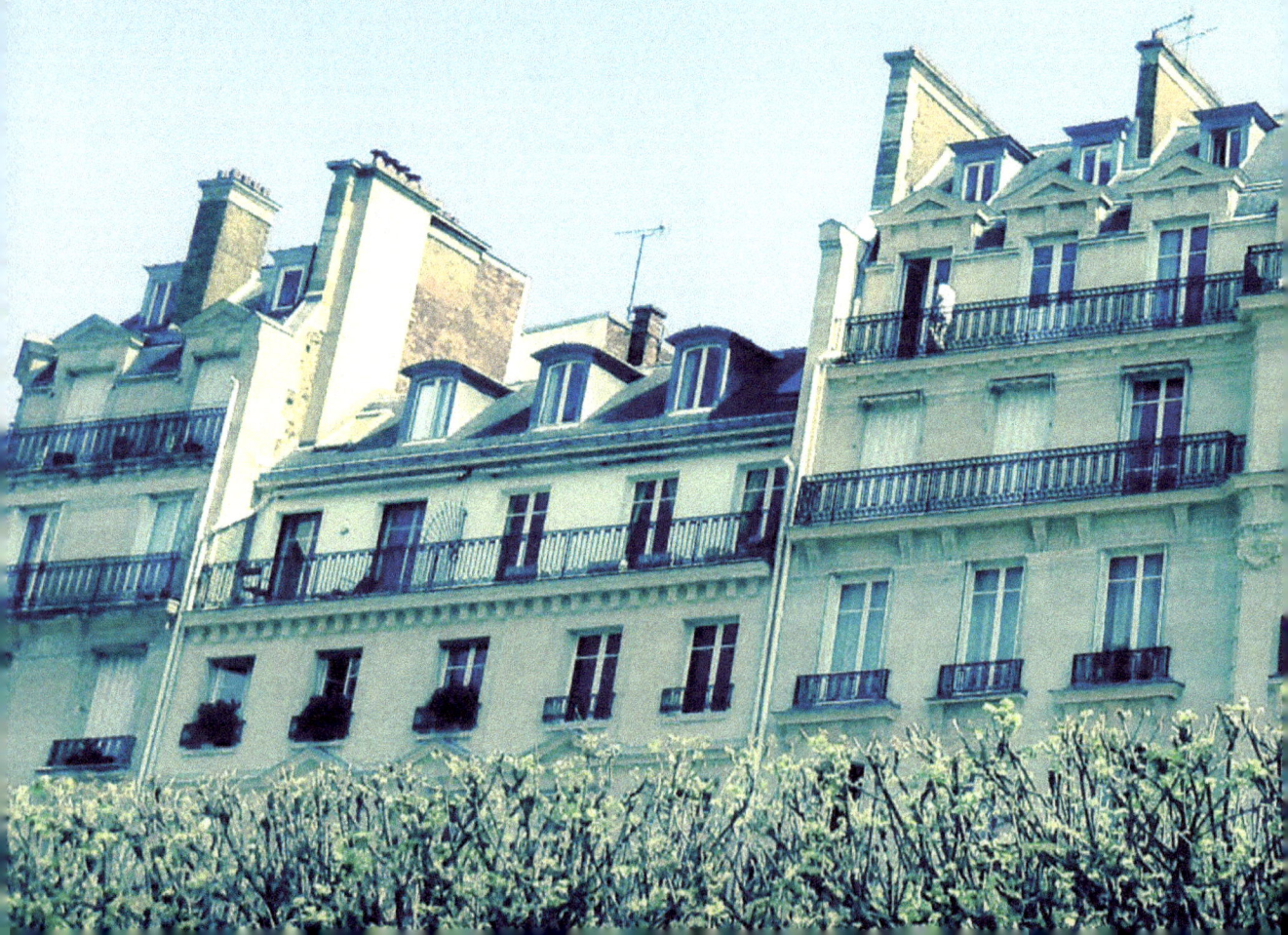

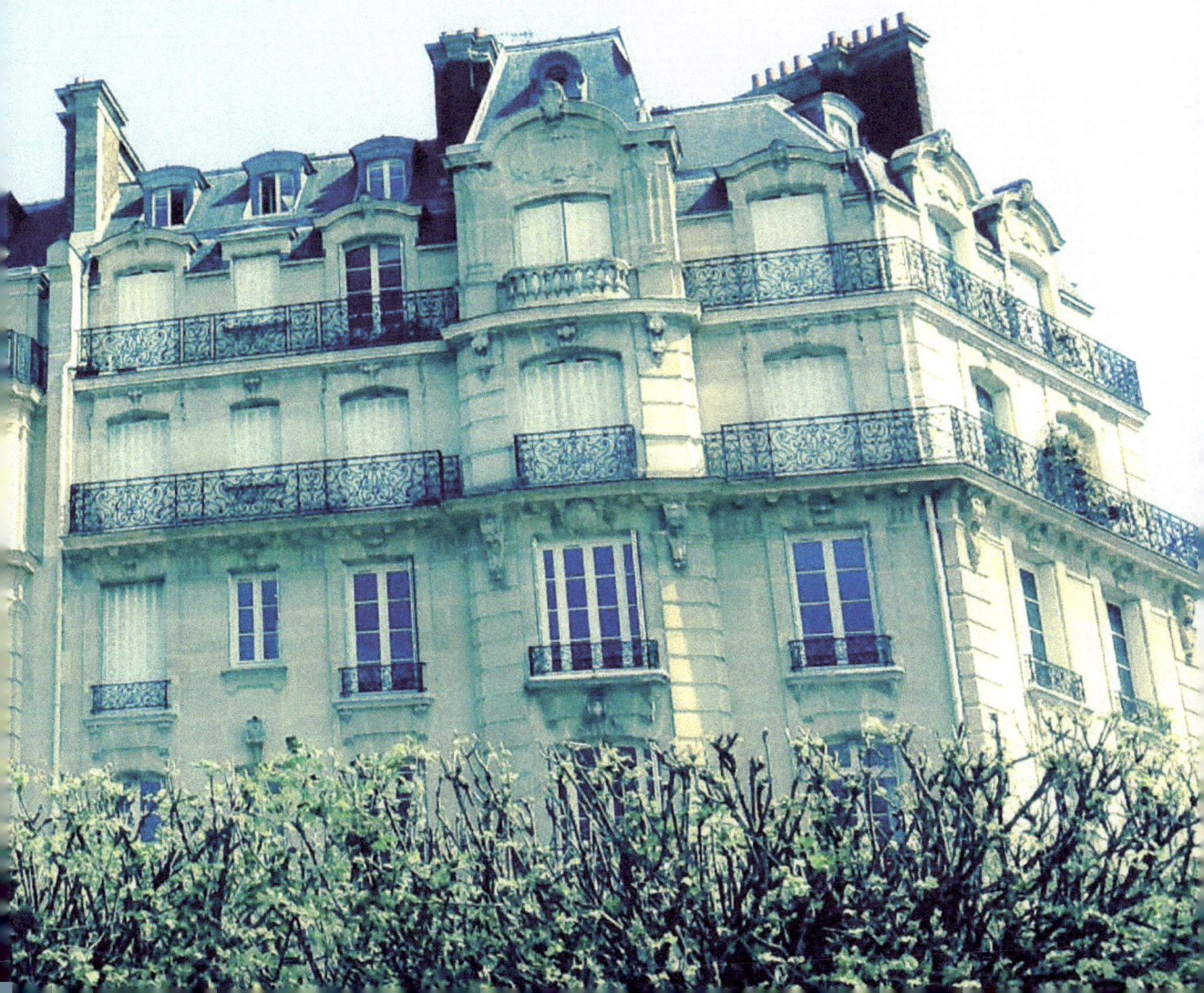

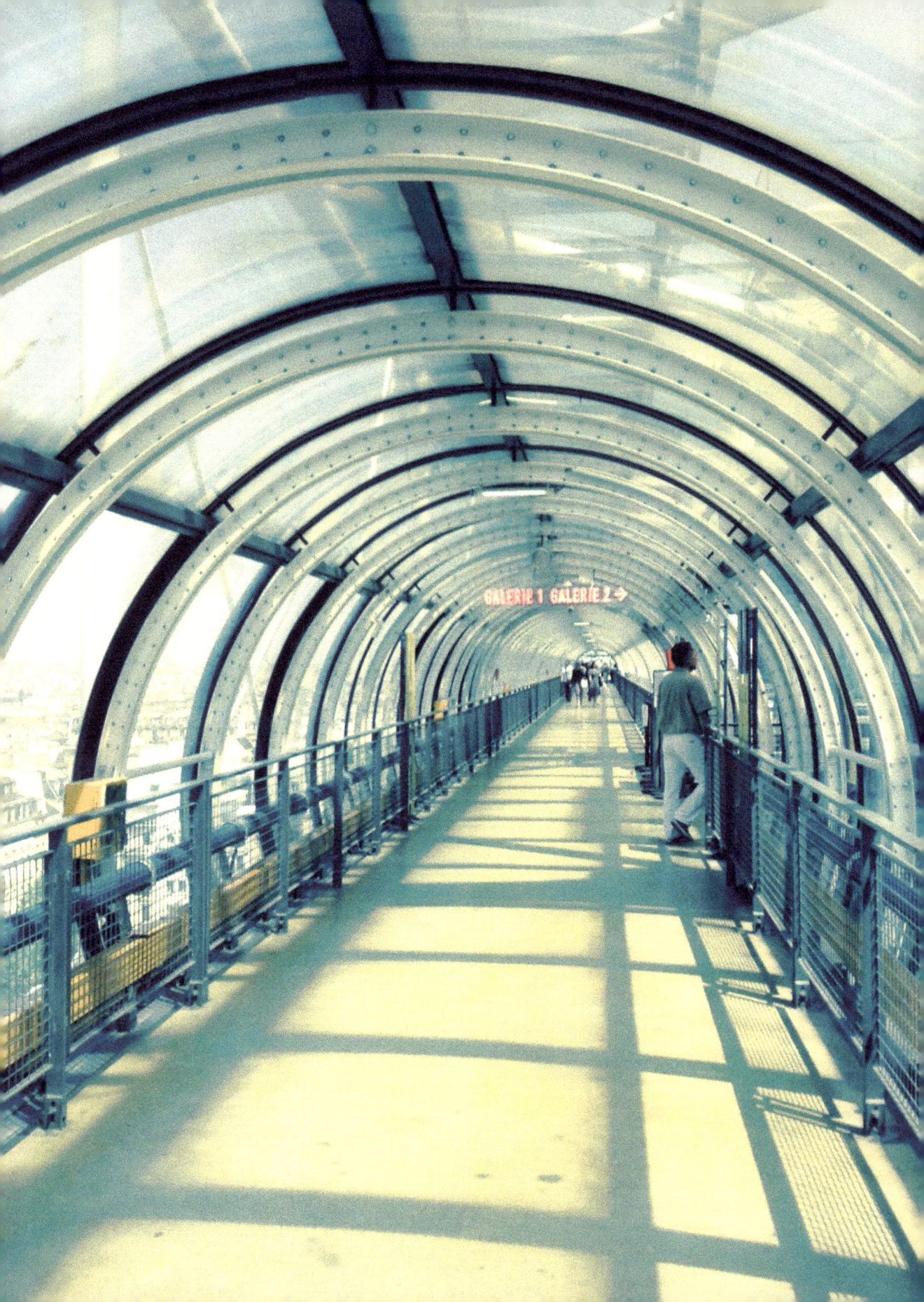

GALERIE 1 GALERIE 2 →

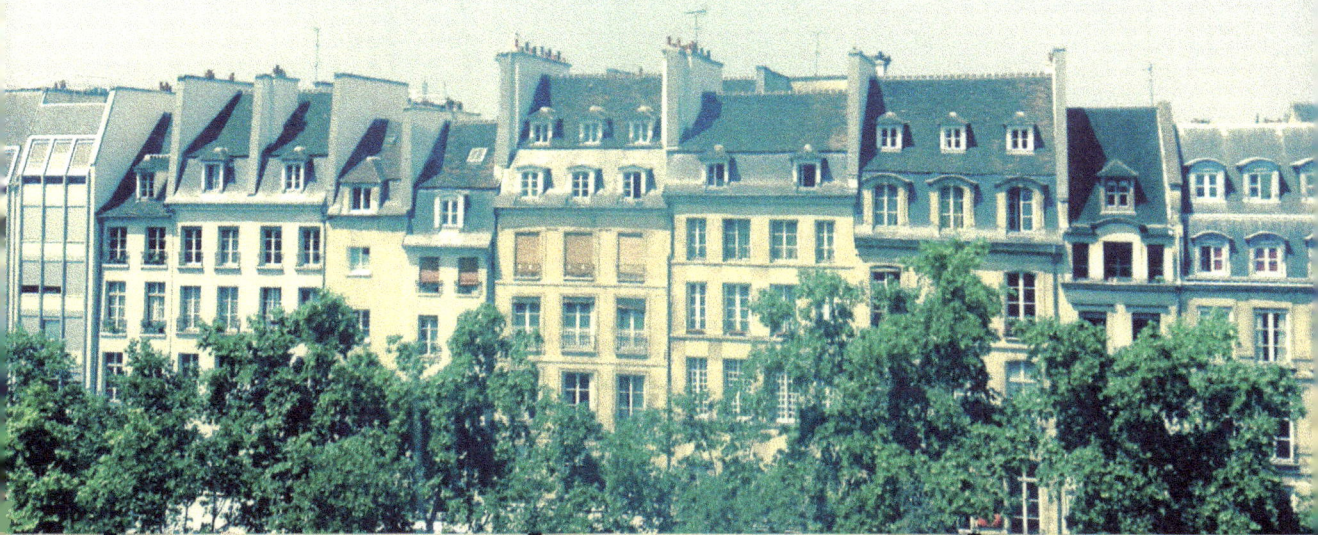

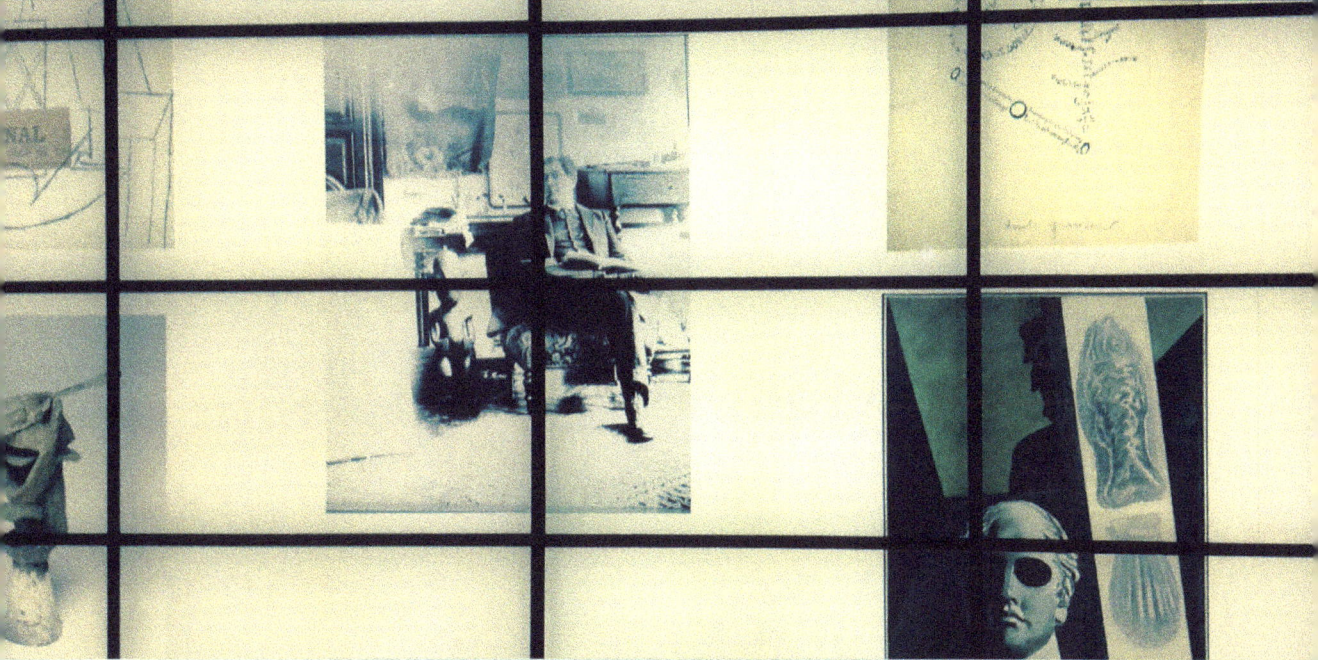

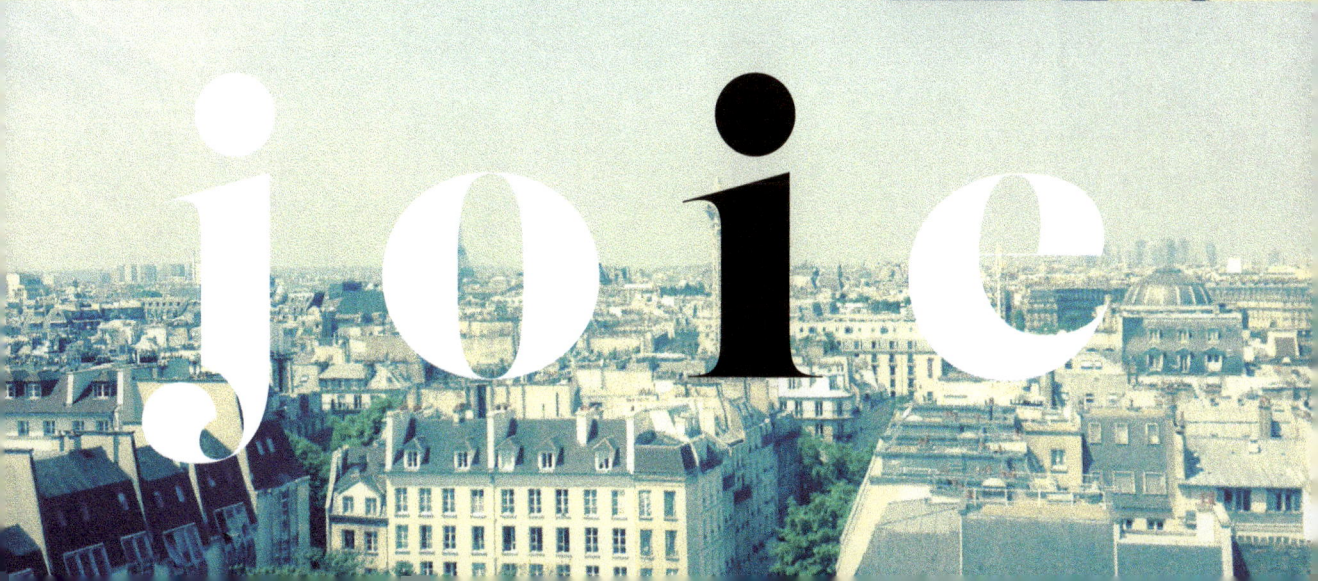

joie

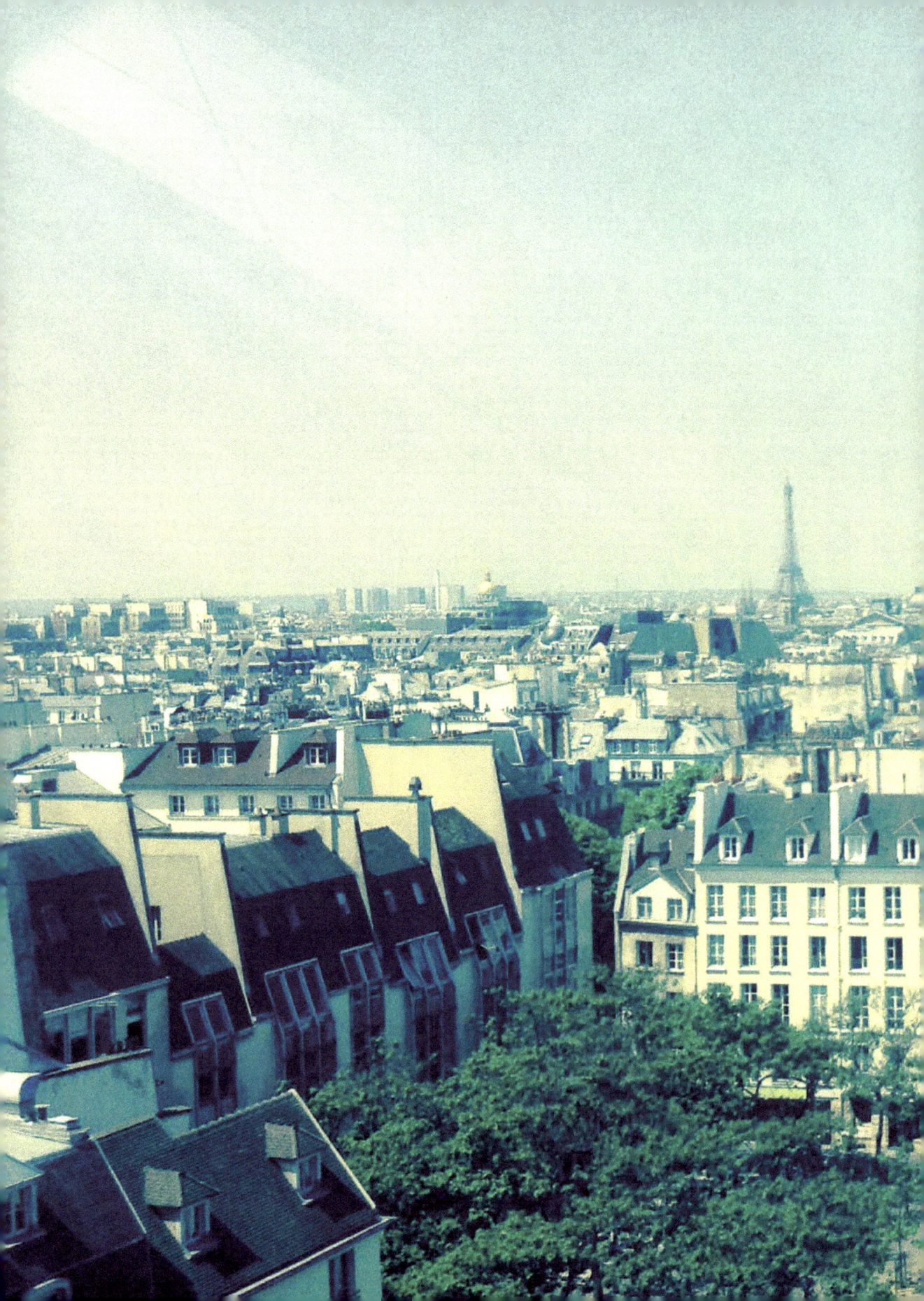

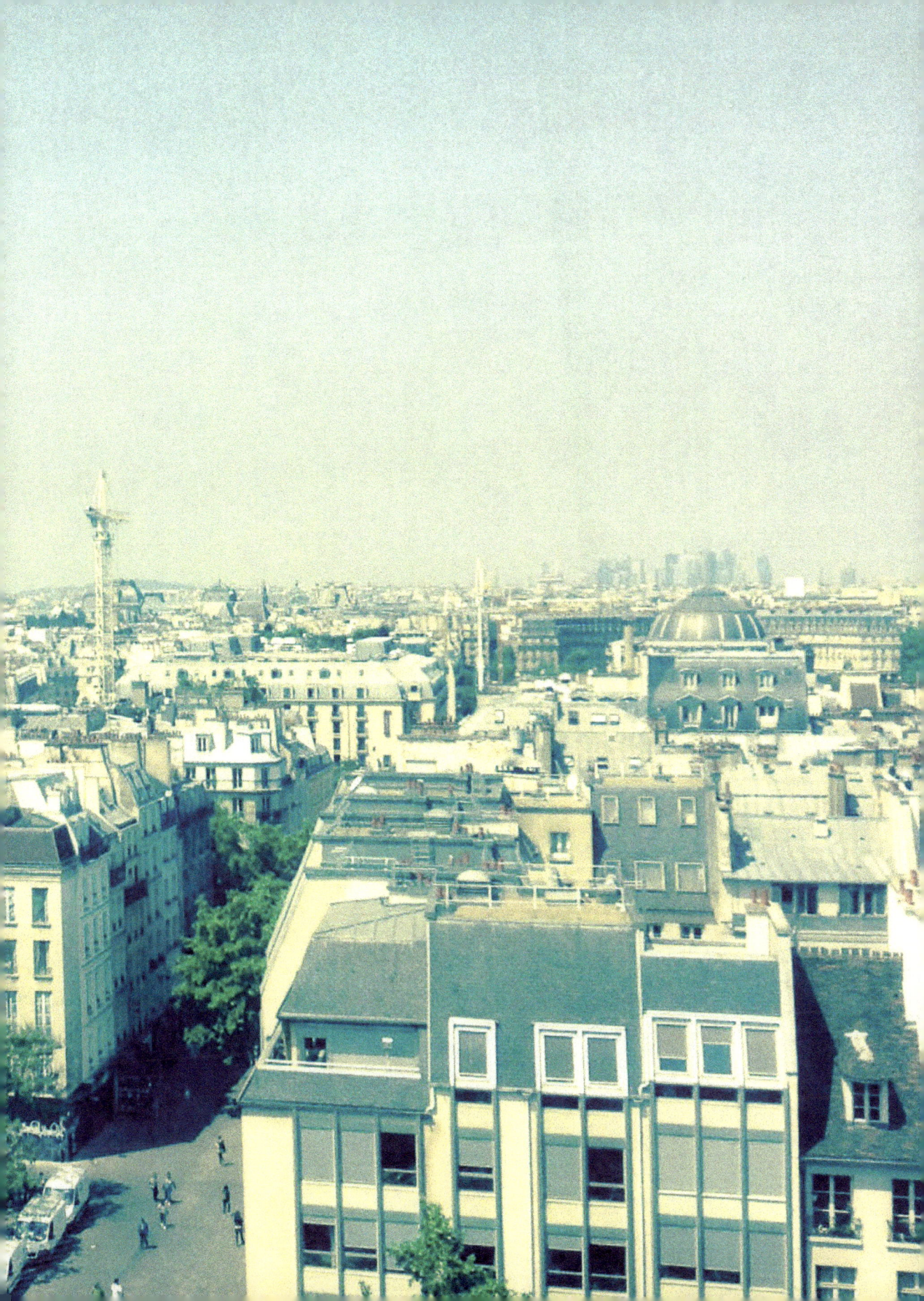

Saint-Jean-Pied-de-Port (starting point)

Day 3

1. 7:00am-12:30pm iDTGV train
Paris to Bayonne, France €59.90 (www.sncf.com)

2. 3:30-5:00pm SNCF bus
to Saint-Jean-Pied-de-Port, France €10 (SNCF window)

3. Check into albergue
(€18 prepaid online)

4. Register with the Pilgrim's Office
(39 rue de la Citadelle)
receive passport & scallop shell

5. Purchase Ibérico de bellota
(100% acorn-fed, semi-wild pig)
(rue de la Citadelle)

6. Ask directions to find Camino in the morning,
talk to roommate, shower, dress for next day,
pack backpack and sleep

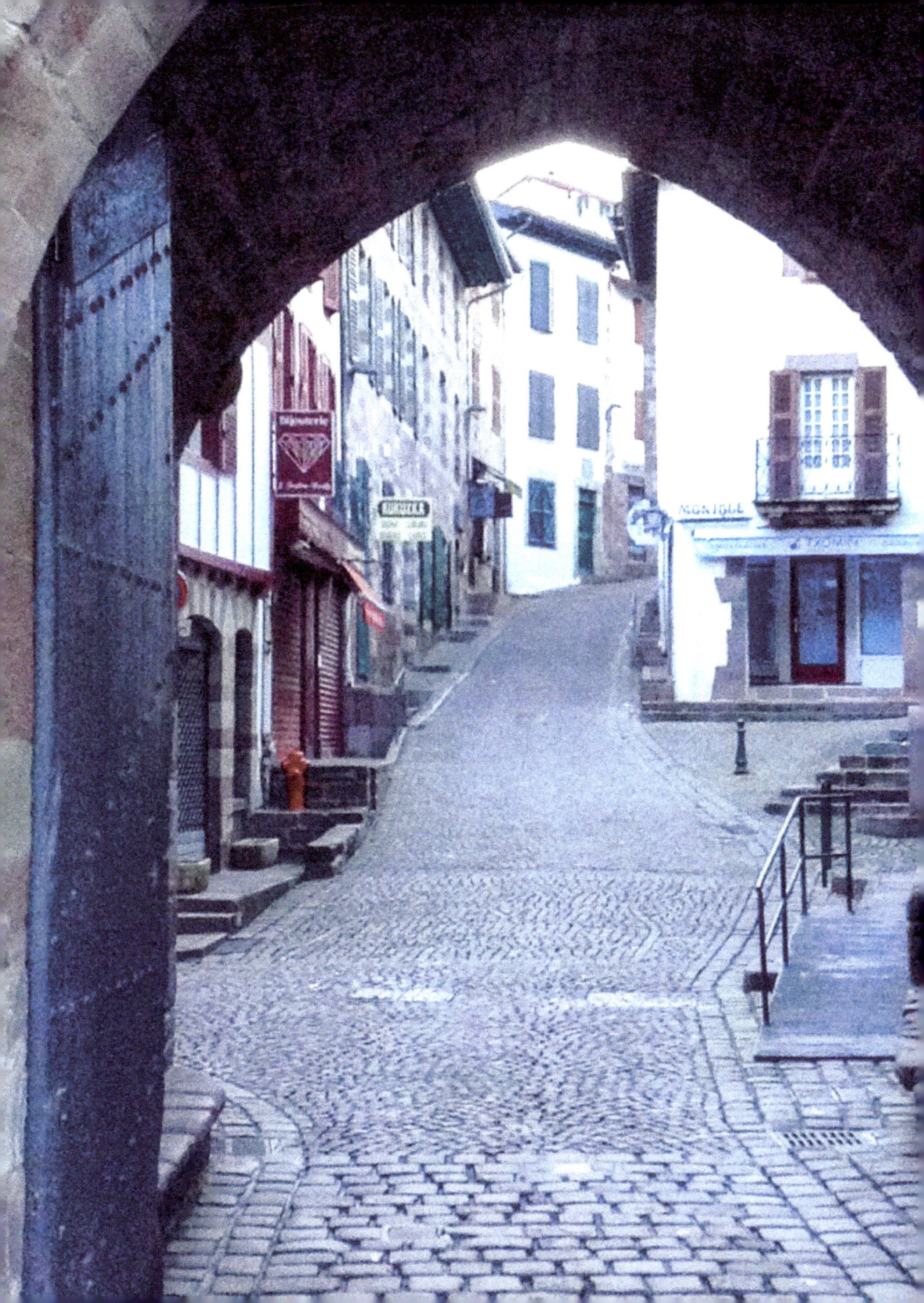

ROUTE
NAPOLEON

Alt 183 m

HONTO - Huntto

REFUGE D'ORISSON
Orisson aterpea

GR65 Voie du Puy

COL DE BENTARTE
Bentarteko lepoa

RONCEVEAUX - Orreaga

STAGE 1

1. 6:00am tiptoe out of room & albergue; start walking
2. arrows work! follow arrows
3. climbing begins immediately
4. 9:00am eat while walking
5. continue to climb and walk all day
6. 4:00pm Roncesvalles (€15 prepaid online; effortless arrival)
7. shower, wash clothes in sink & line dry overnight; go to bed early; fall asleep fast and hard; sleep throughout the entire night in a large room with hundreds of people! MIRACLE!

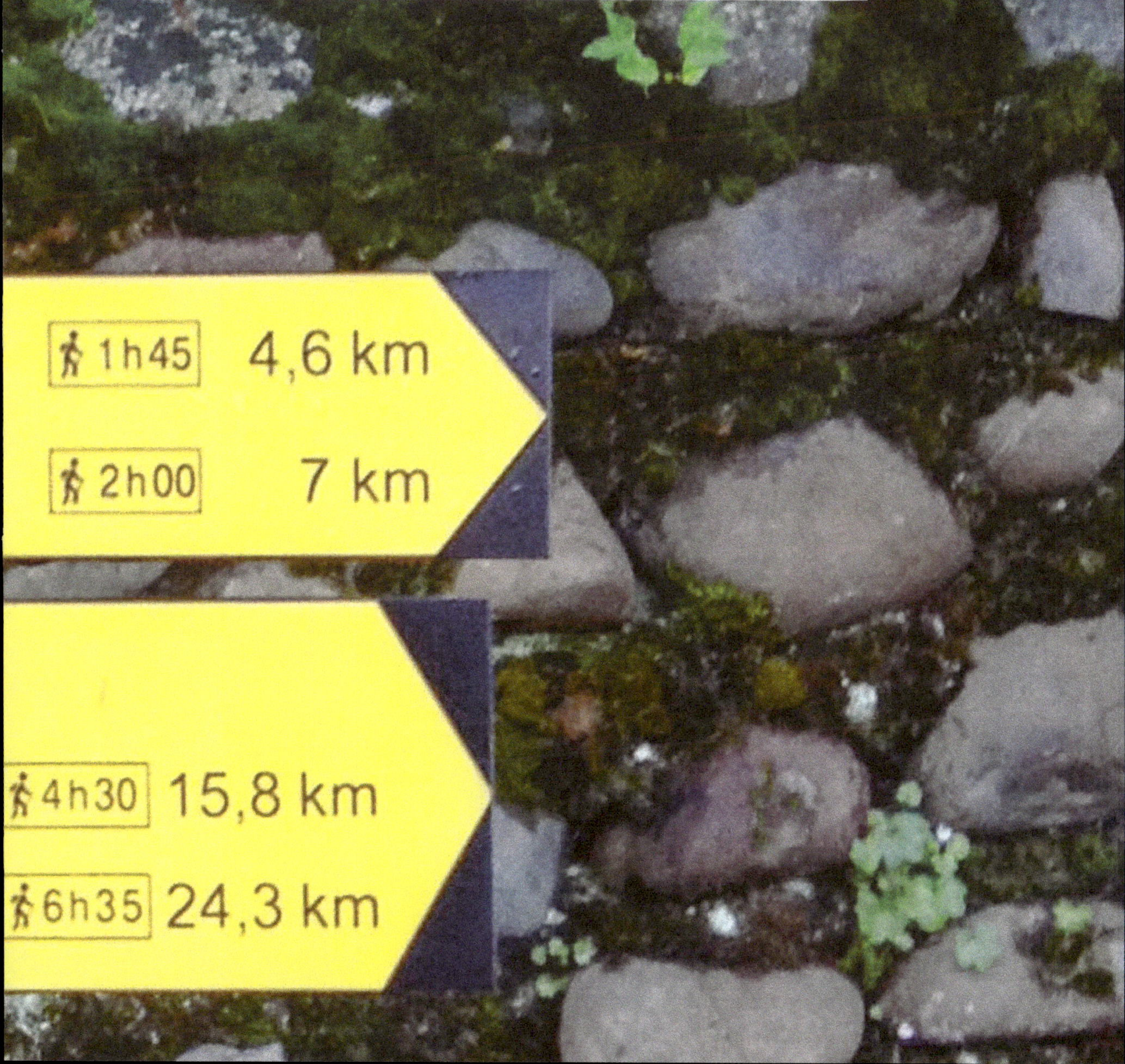

🚶 1h45   4,6 km

🚶 2h00   7 km

🚶 4h30   15,8 km

🚶 6h35   24,3 km

I must admit that Stage 1 research may have caused some stress. There was so much written from so many different sources that said this was the most difficult section. I was sure that I wanted to take Route Napoléon (said to have been traveled by Napoléon but not verified as true) because of its stunning scenery and possible significant history depicted in the readings. It is a more challenging route because of the continuous climbing, the unpredictable weather and the lack of albergues/shelter. Once committed to the route, you just have to keep going and hope for the best. I did not know what to expect. I also was uncertain during my months of training whether I would be adequately prepared.

I was so happy to arrive to Roncesvalles without any problems. All went well, and I even arrived early to miss the downpour! The vistas were unlike any others. The adrenaline of the excitement and the thrill of achievement were well worth it. I was also delighted to experience real mountain shepherds who let me help them! I made lifelong friends along the way on day one and uplifting forever memories.

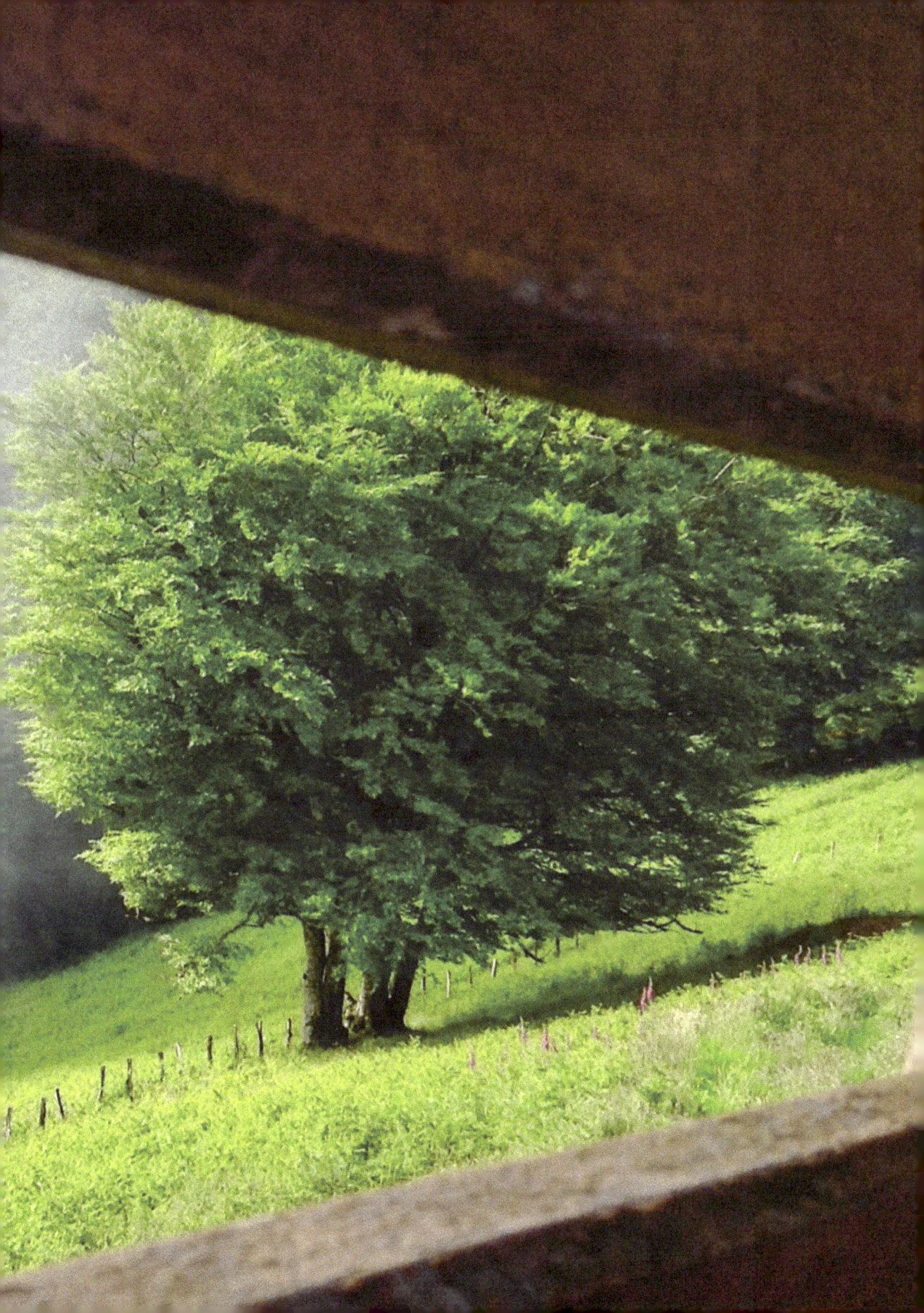

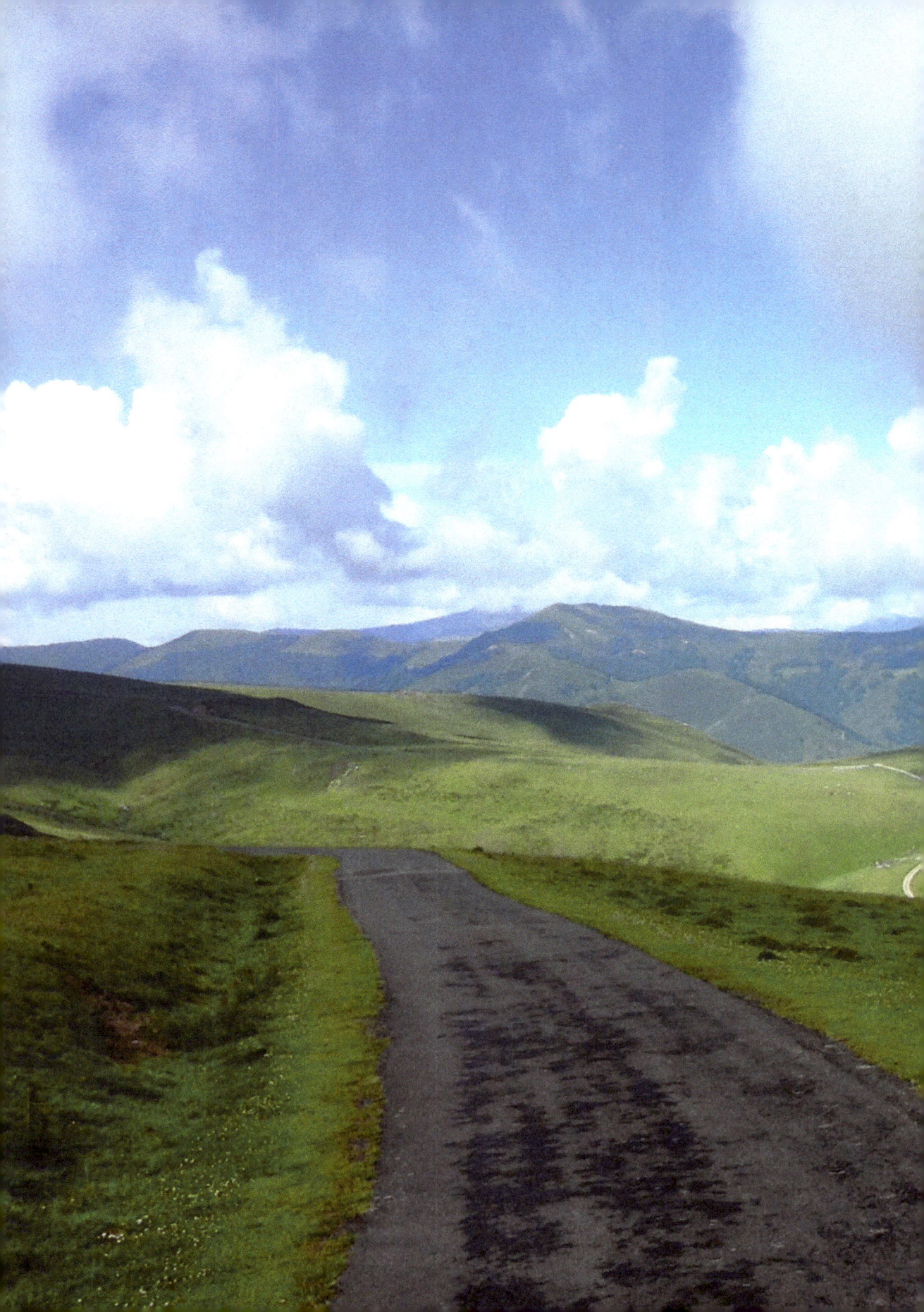

"There is no better designer than nature."
-Alexander McQueen

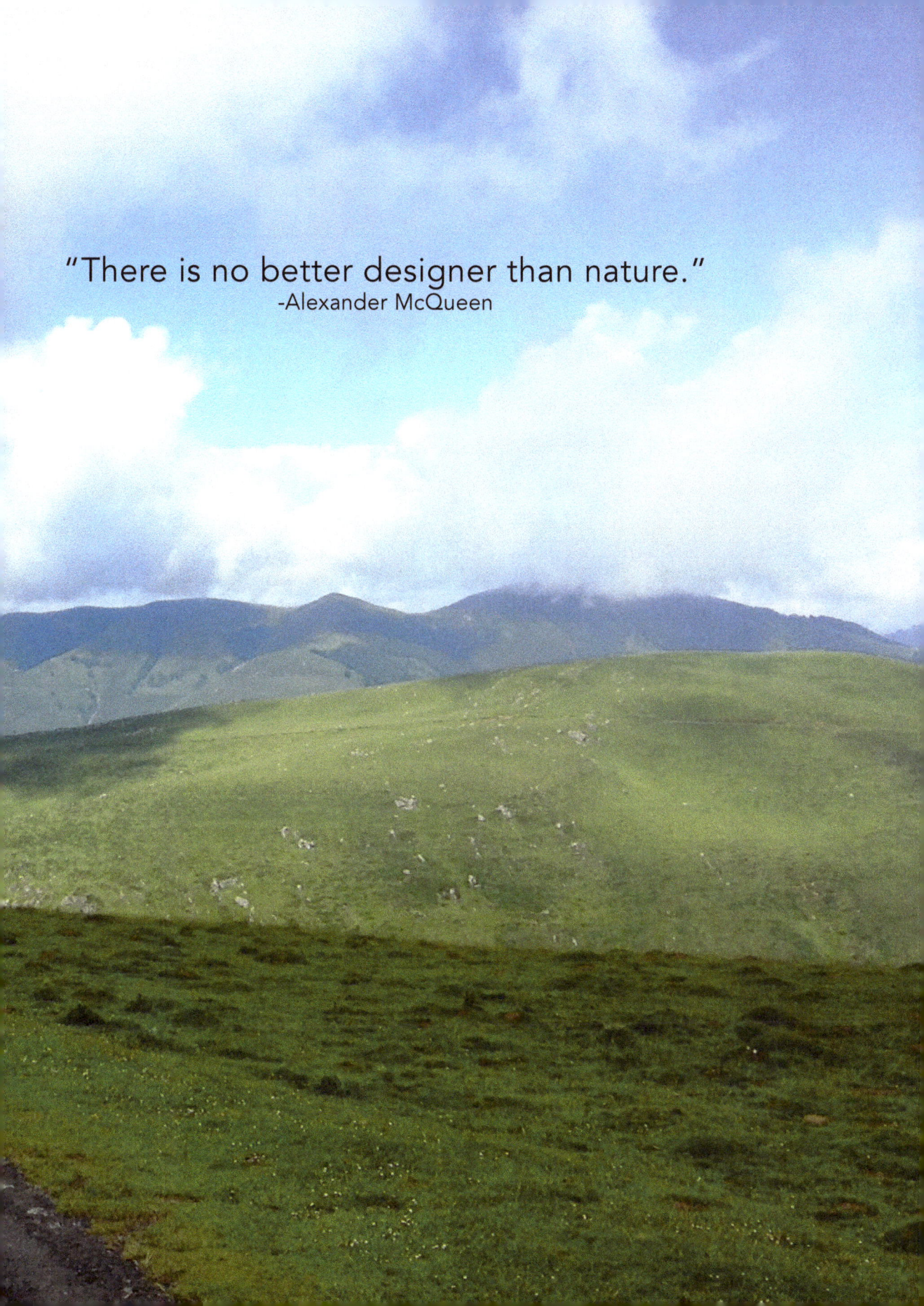

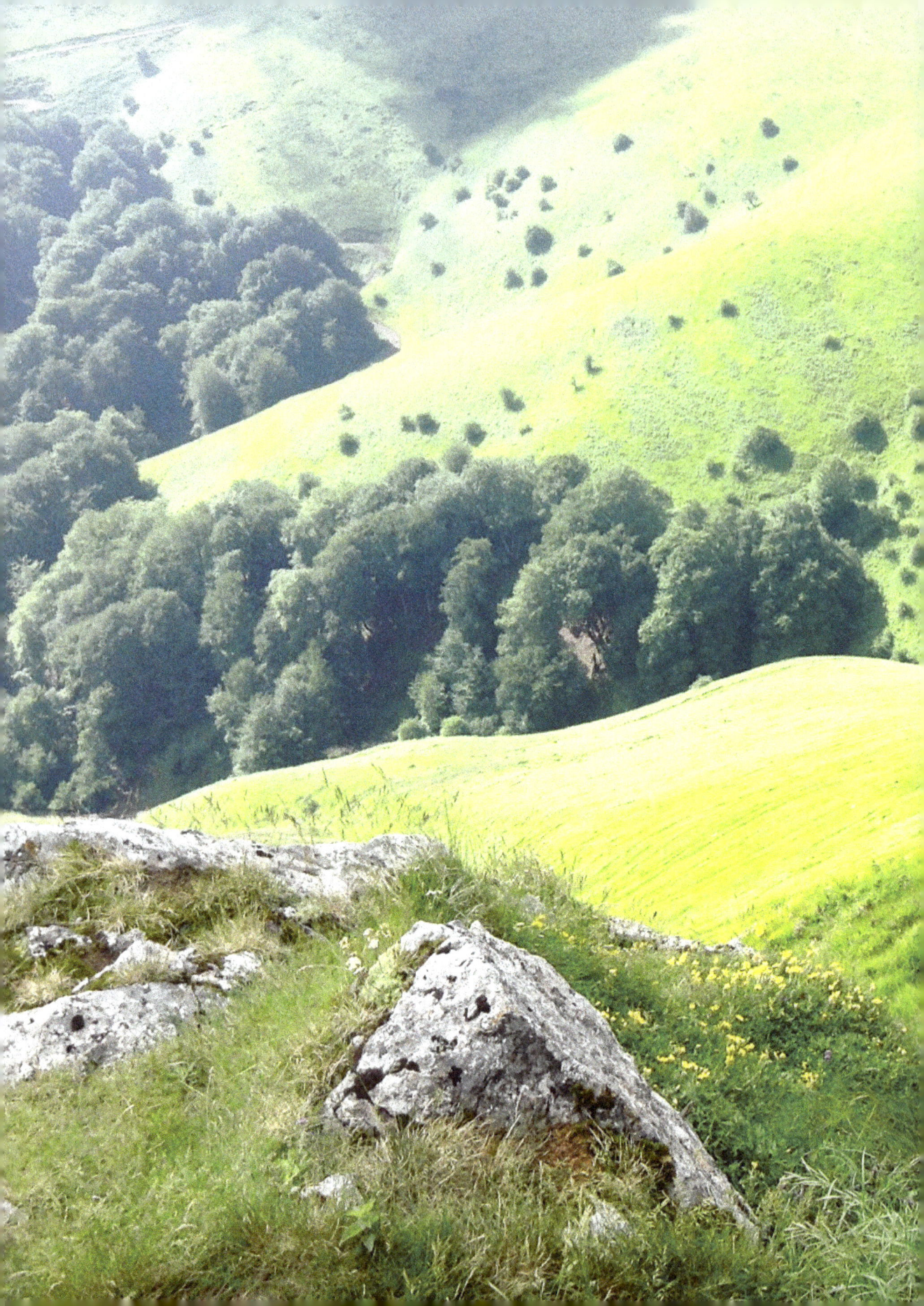

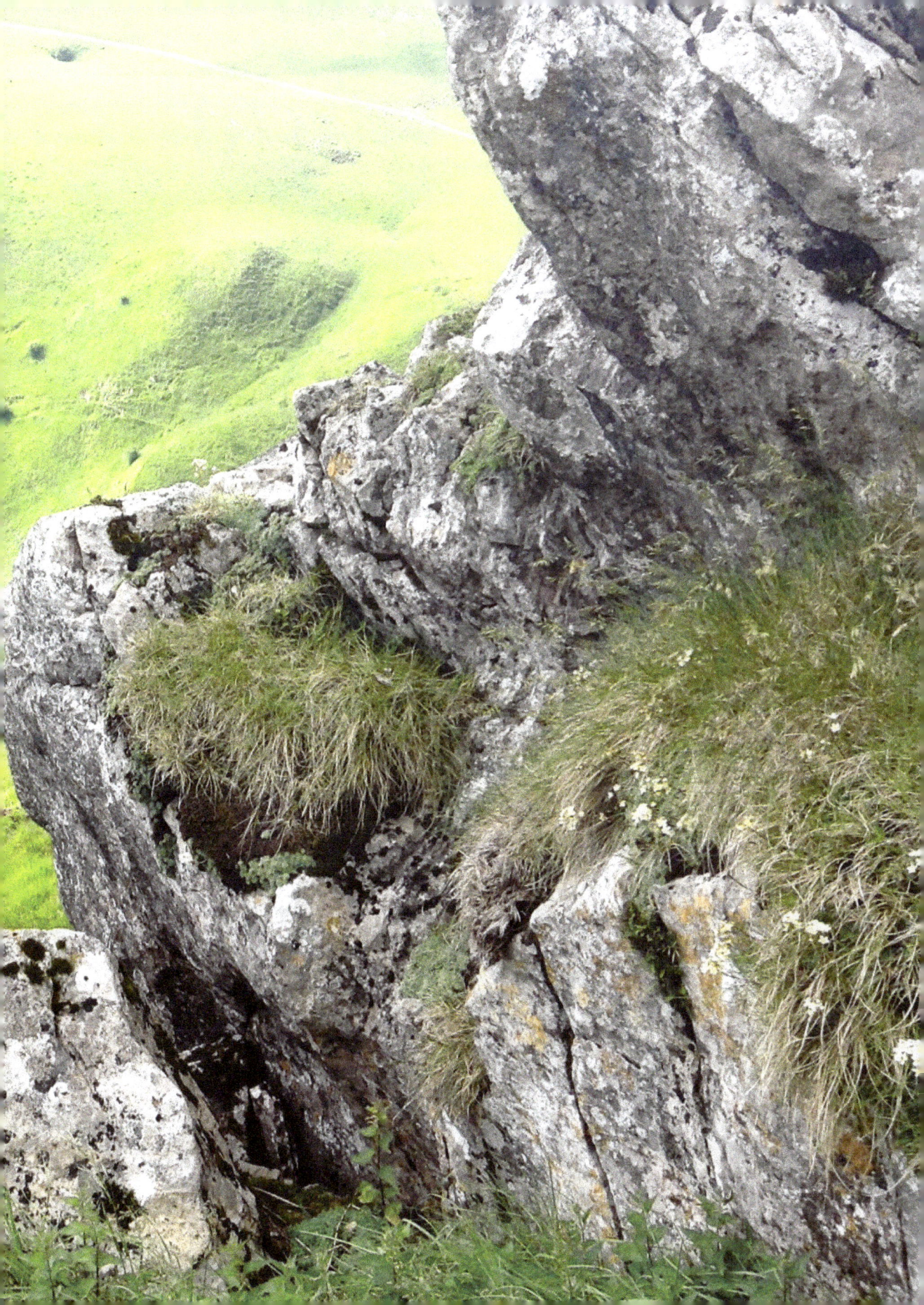

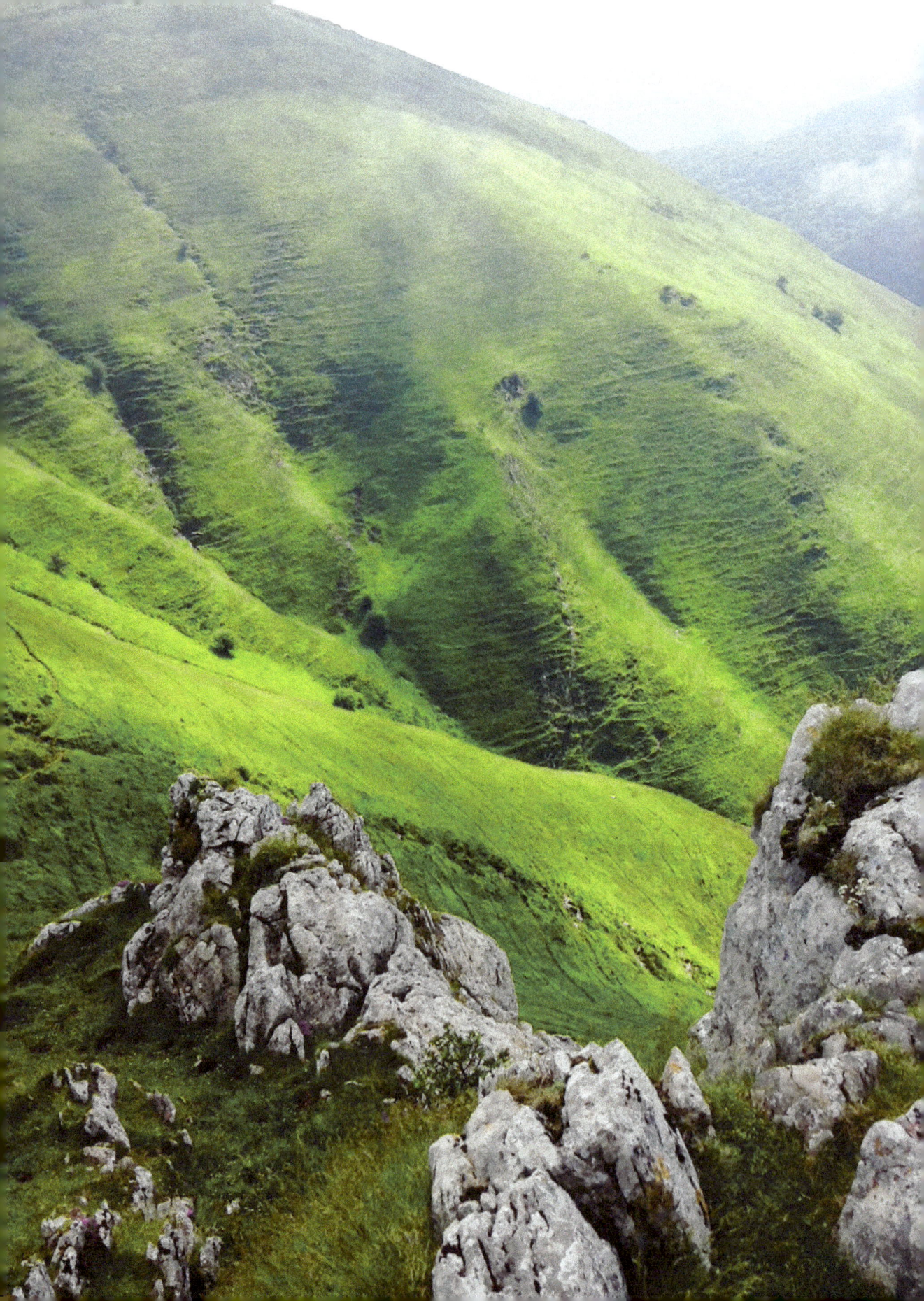

After reading several books and websites about the Camino, I started making plans. Sleep was most important, so I started planning the route and hiking miles based on albergues with a small number of beds in each room. Also, I wanted to hike completely across Spain from the border to the coast. I was excited to be in Paris, so I wanted some time there but also felt an urgency to get started hiking before the Camino holiday crowds in July and August.

I had noted a few albergues and towns from the reading research that I really didn't want to miss and also closely studied a book (*A Village to Village Guide to Hiking the Camino de Santiago* by Anna Dintaman and David Landis) that showed elevations and a fast/regular/slow schedule for walking. It took a lot of planning, replanning and recalculating but then magically a route started to form.

As I was researching online and starting to contact albergues and to make reservations, I discovered the website www.urcamino.com. This became my favorite source for finding albergues. I looked at detailed pictures, read reviews and all contact information and direct links were included there in one place. It was heavenly! I usually chose an albergue based on the rating system, location to accommodate daily miles and the sleeping arrangements. Sometimes I changed the whole route and plan if I discovered an alluring comment about a town and/or albergue. It worked really well, because I was so happy staying in every albergue and every town. The only "problem" I ever encountered was not wanting to leave the beautiful places!

During the days and months of planning and researching, I wondered if I was supposed to just "wing it" and be a "drop-in" pilgrim (a pilgrim who just shows up and figures it out along the way). I was really torn about this even as I began walking the Camino. I discovered that although the spontaneity of not planning was alluring and exciting (and much easier during the preceding months!) I am so happy with how I did it. I loved having a destination each day and all I had to do was look at my ultralight, disposable notes with the date, name of town, miles to walk, and the albergue name/phone number/address. It proved to be "effortless"!

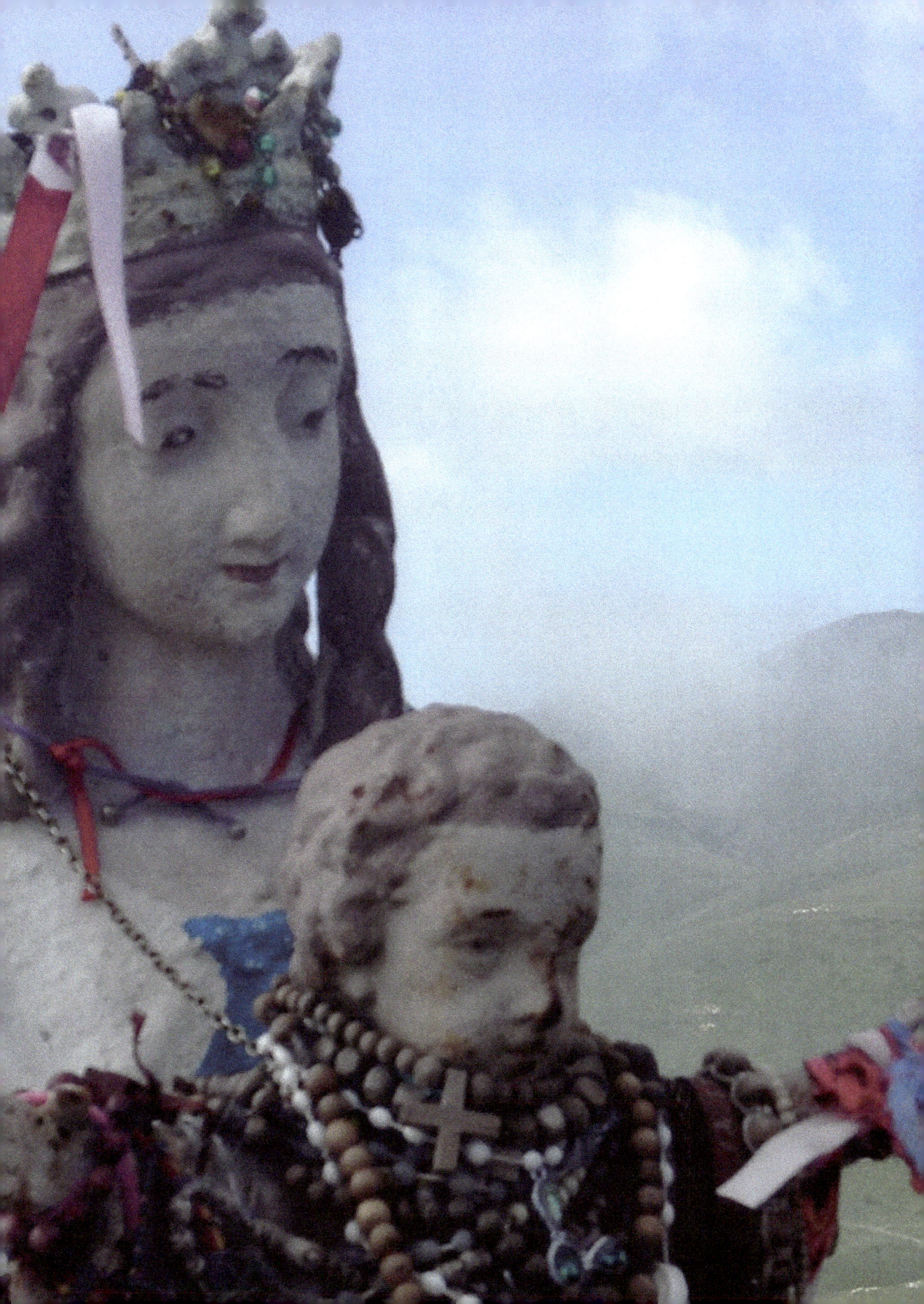

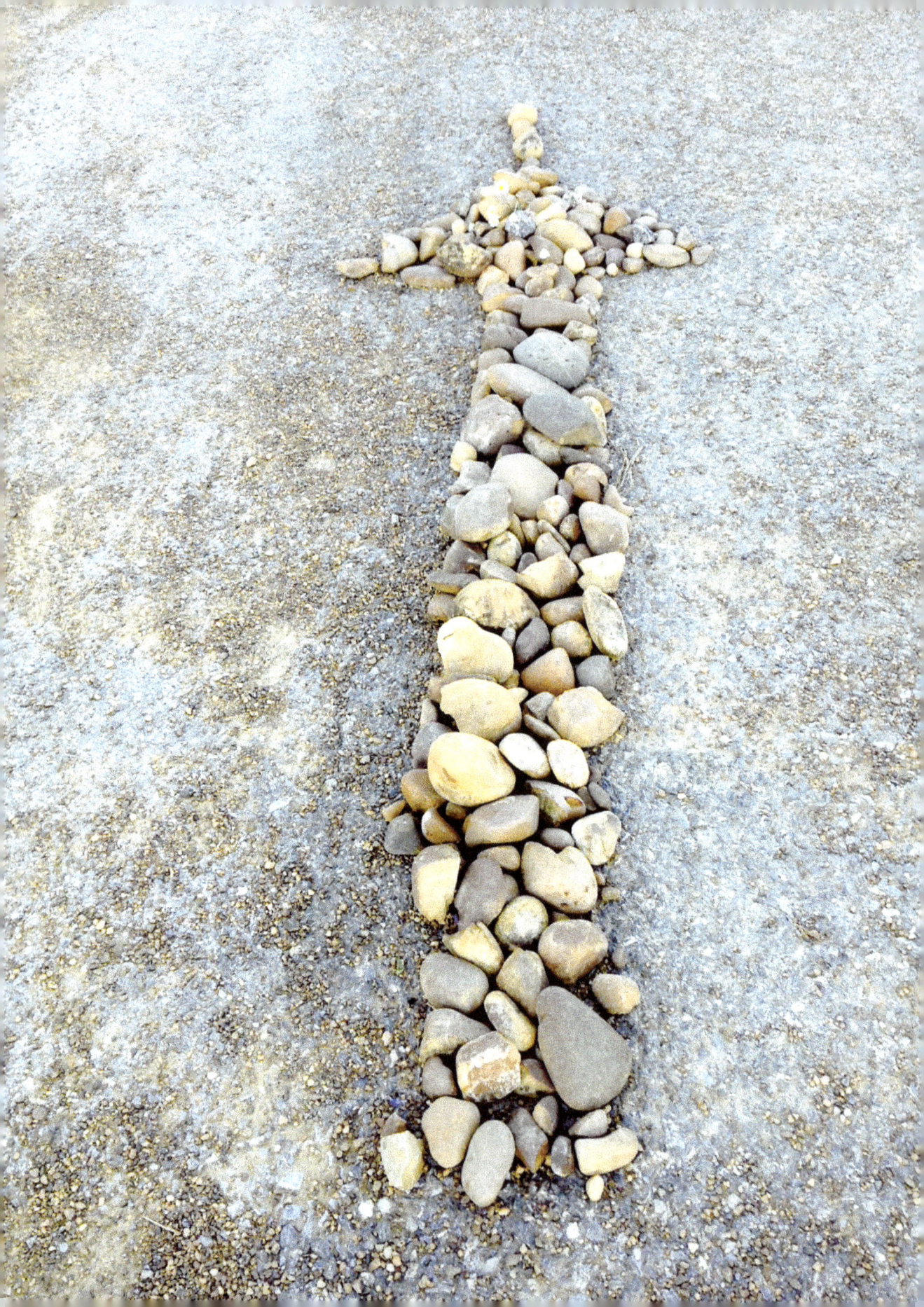

In addition to having a daily destination and uncumbersome notes to follow, I was totally free of daily stress about "where I was going to stay" or "how far I was going to walk." For me, these questions clutter my mind, spirit and ultimately my existence/experience. When cluttered, I lose my way and accomplish little. Instead, I experienced total freedom to enjoy every minute of walking, meeting people and seeing the unending beauty of Spain. I was 100% present for the Camino! It was the most fulfilling, uplifting feeling of freedom and joy to experience the Camino in its utmost divinity. M I R A C L E !

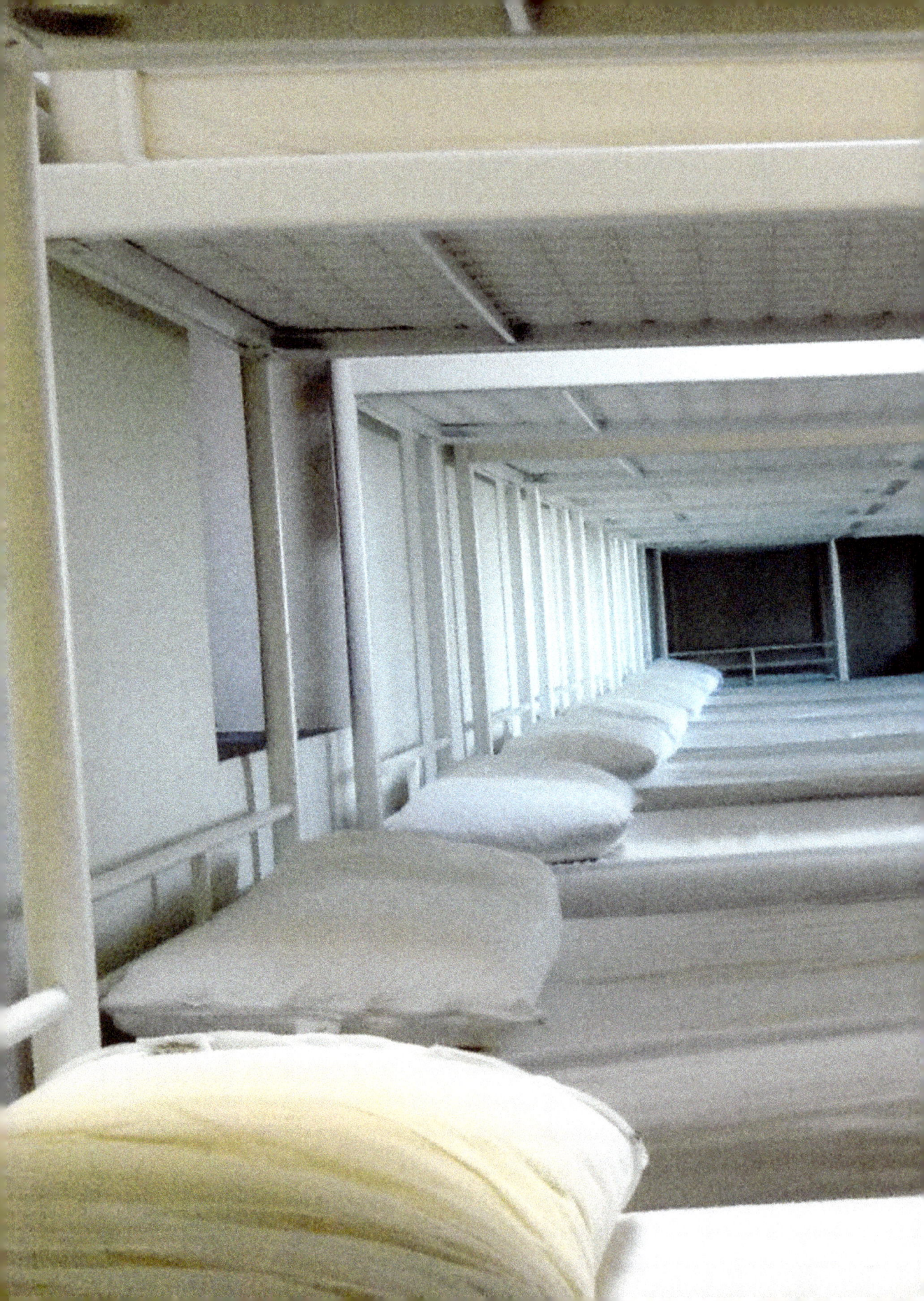

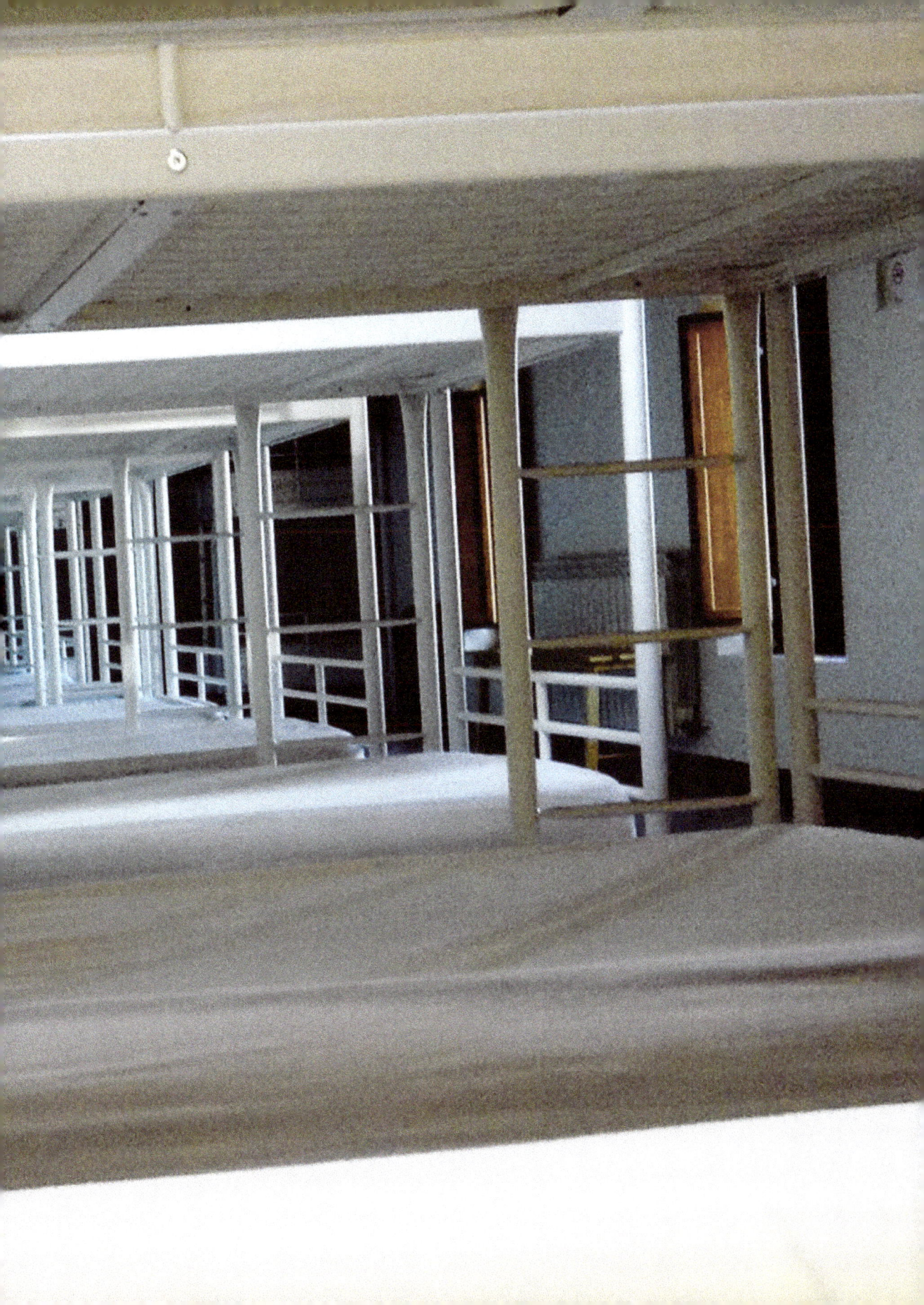

READING LIST

A Village to Village Guide to Hiking the Camino de Santiago: Camino Francés: St.-Jean-Santiago-Finisterre Anna Dintaman

A Pilgrim's Guide to the Camino Finisterre & Camino de Santiago Maps John Brierley

Camino Lingo Reinette Voa

Walking the Camino de Santiago Bethan Davies

Your Camino-A Lightfoot Guide to Practical Preparation for a Pilgrimage Sylvia Nilsen

Preparedness Guide for the Camino de Santiago: Learn Exactly What to Pack, Why You Need it, & How it Will Help You Reach Santiago Matthew Arnold Toy

Fodor's Paris 2015

Lonely Planet French Phrasebook

The Traveling Professor's Guide to Paris Prof. Stephen C Solosky

Lonely Planet's Best Ever Travel Tips Tom Hall

Seven Tips to Make the Most of the Camino de Santiago Cheri Powell

Trail Tested: A Thru-Hiker's Guide to Ultralight Hiking and Backpacking Justin Lichter

Spain: Recipes & Traditions from the Verdant Hills of the Basque Country to the Coastal Waters of Andalucía Jeff Koehler

Culture Shock! Spain: A Survival Guide to Customs & Etiquette Marie Louise Graff

Powerful Paleo Superfoods Heather Connell

Keto Clarity Jimmy Moore

Cholesterol Clarity Jimmy Moore

A Moveable Feast Ernest Hemingway

Paris Boulangerie-Patisserie L Dannenberg

Art & Paris: Impressionists & Post Impressionists: The Ultimate Guide to Artists, Paintings & Places in Paris & Normandy

Paris Portraits Renoir to Chanel: Walks on the Right Bank Mary Ellen Jordan Haight

Paris Walks

Walking Paris: Thirty Original Walks in & Around Paris Gilles Desmons

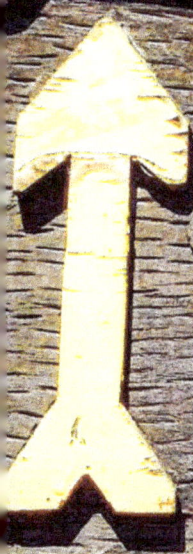

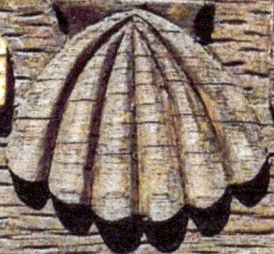

CAMINO DE SANTIAGO

"that thou art happy, thou owest to God;
that thou continuest such, thou owest to thyself"
-John Milton *Paradise Lost*

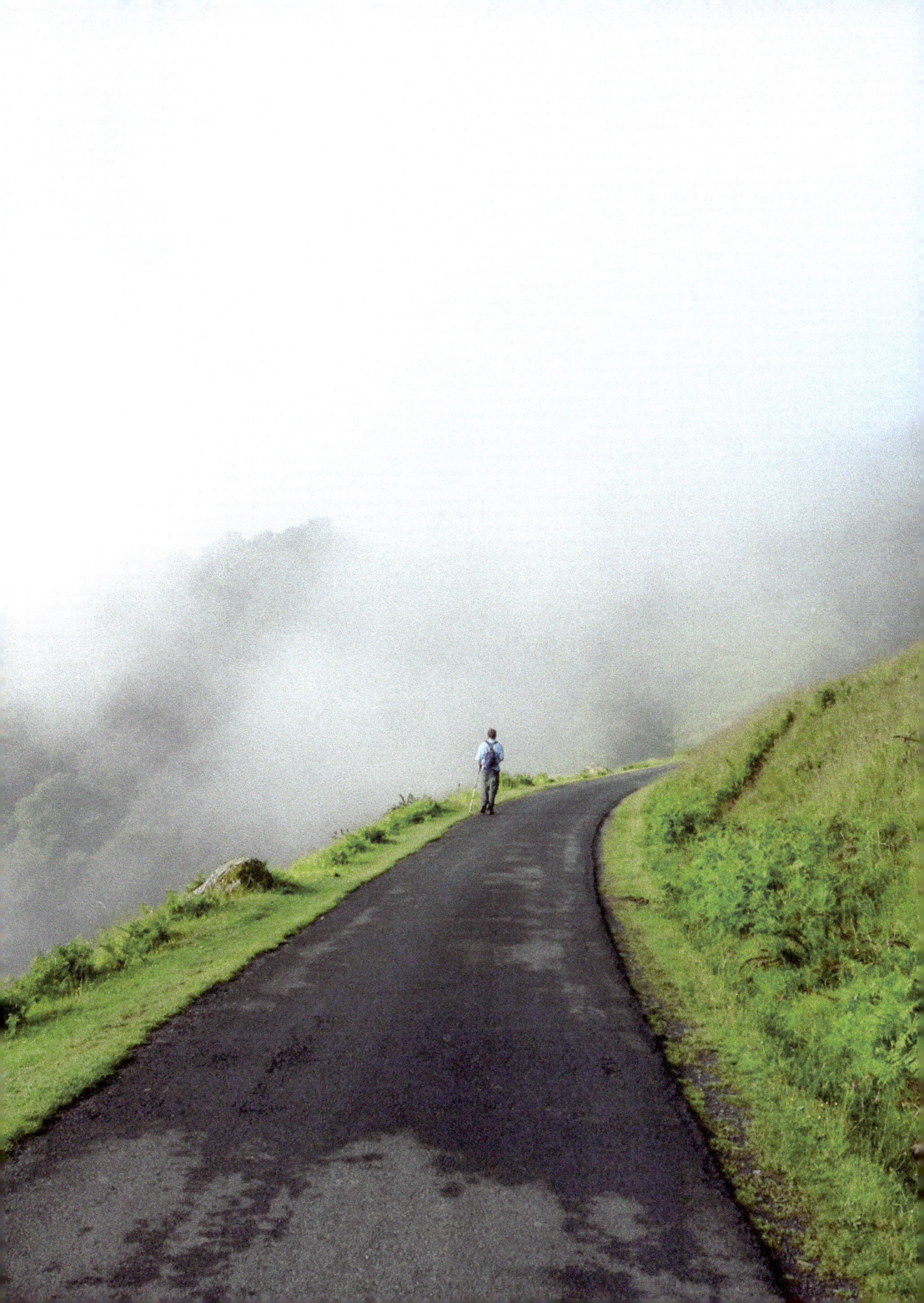

PEREGRINO

preparation
WALK CLIMB SLEEP REPEAT

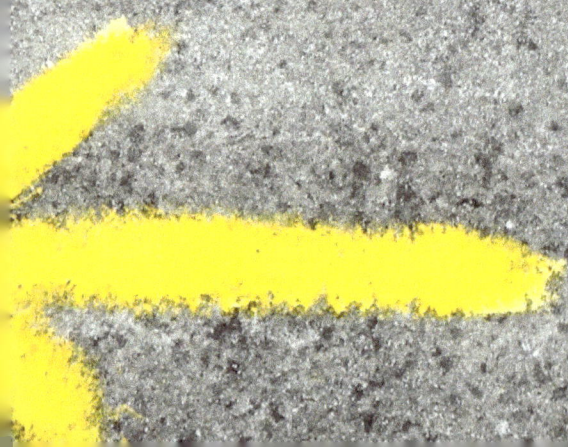

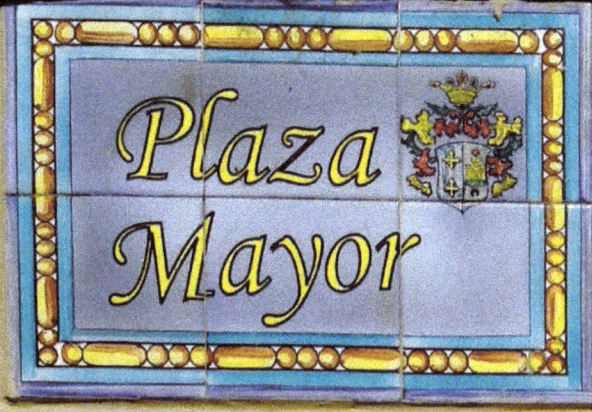

Plaza
Mayor

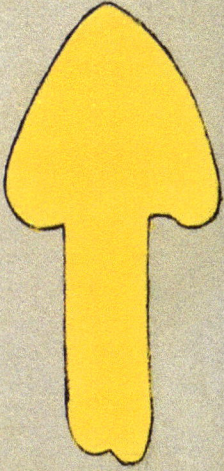

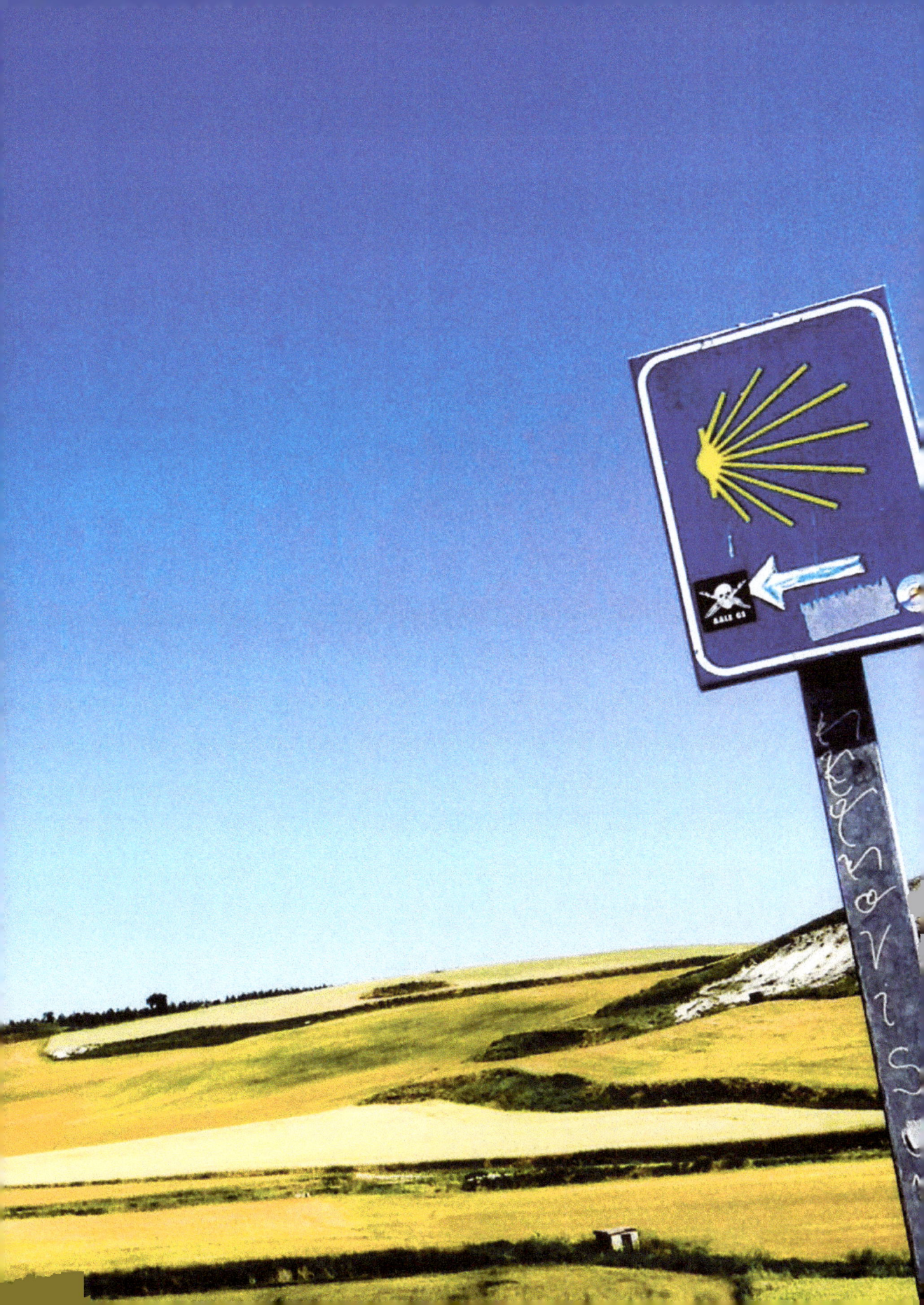

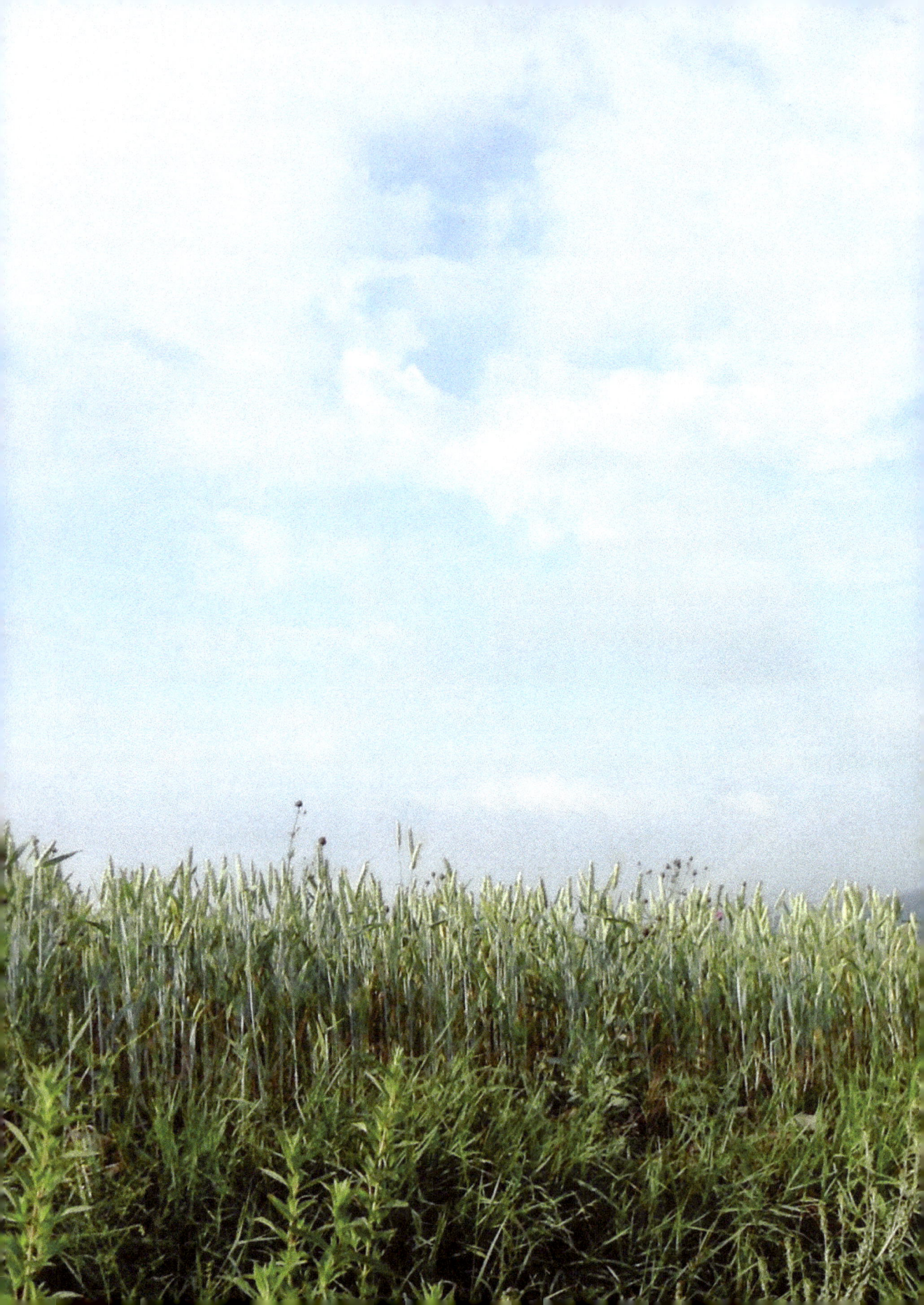

Adequate preparation on the Camino and in life requires me to be well rested by almost always sleeping 9-10 hours every night, keeping properly fueled by eating nutrient-dense real food and maintaining equanimity throughout life by consciously choosing enriching material to enter my mind (nature, art, literature, fashion, architecture, music). If I am well rested and properly fueled every day, it seems effortless to live in the moment being cheerful, polite, friendly, respectful, responsible, loving, happy, joyous, free, grateful, focused and ready to serve the world as best as possible! By choosing a path that is chemical free and impeccably healthy, I also am available to "input" all the truth, beauty and joy the world has to offer.

In life and on the Camino, I am continually amazed by the unending beauty of nature and its inhabitants. I fall deeply in love each and every day with all the world's creatures and all the world's manifestations. I am so grateful for finding a path of real sleep, real nutrition, real joy. As I walked the Camino, I was over-whelmed with love and gratitude for every sign, arrow, fountain, trash receptacle, bed, wide path, rest area, blanket and person.

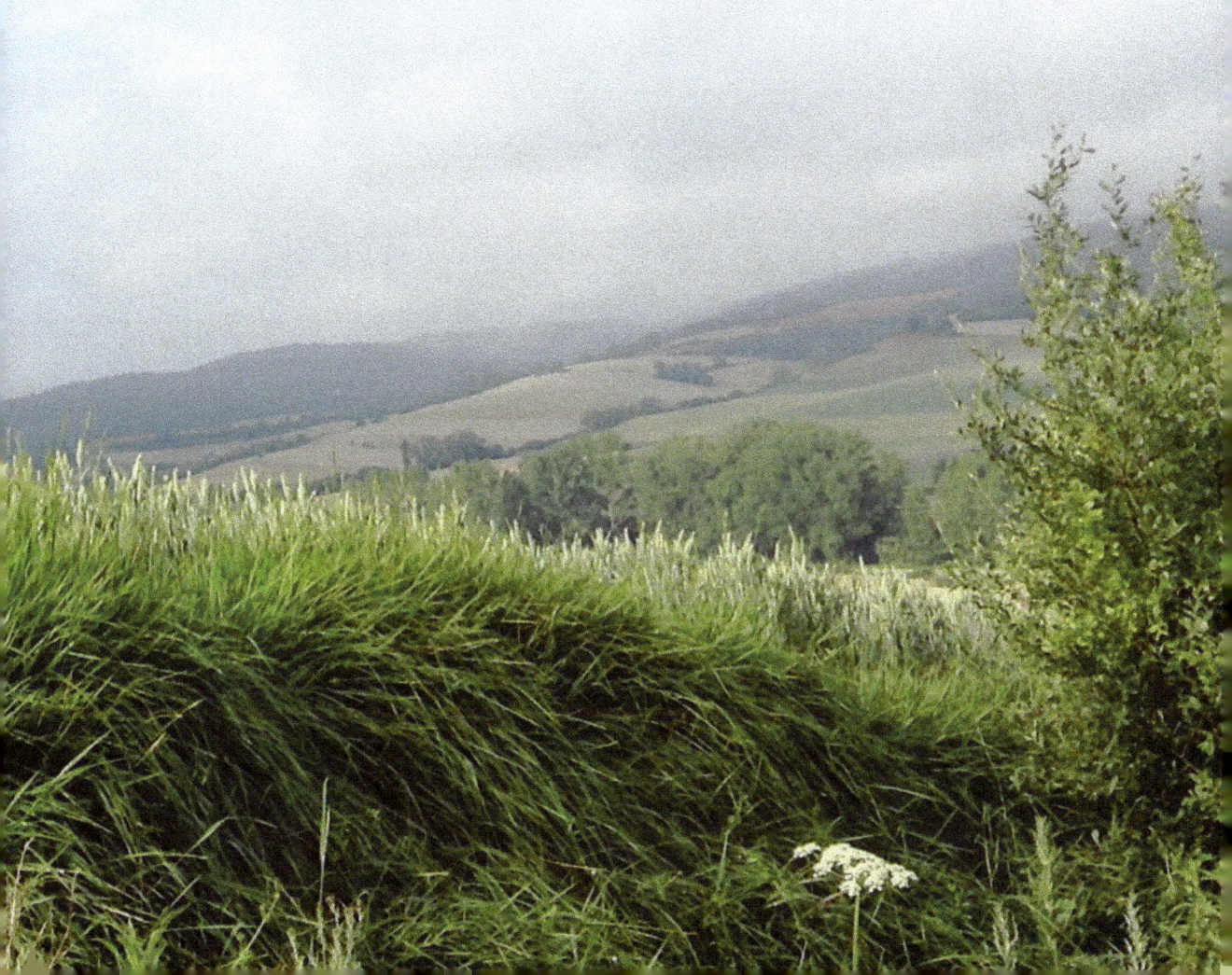

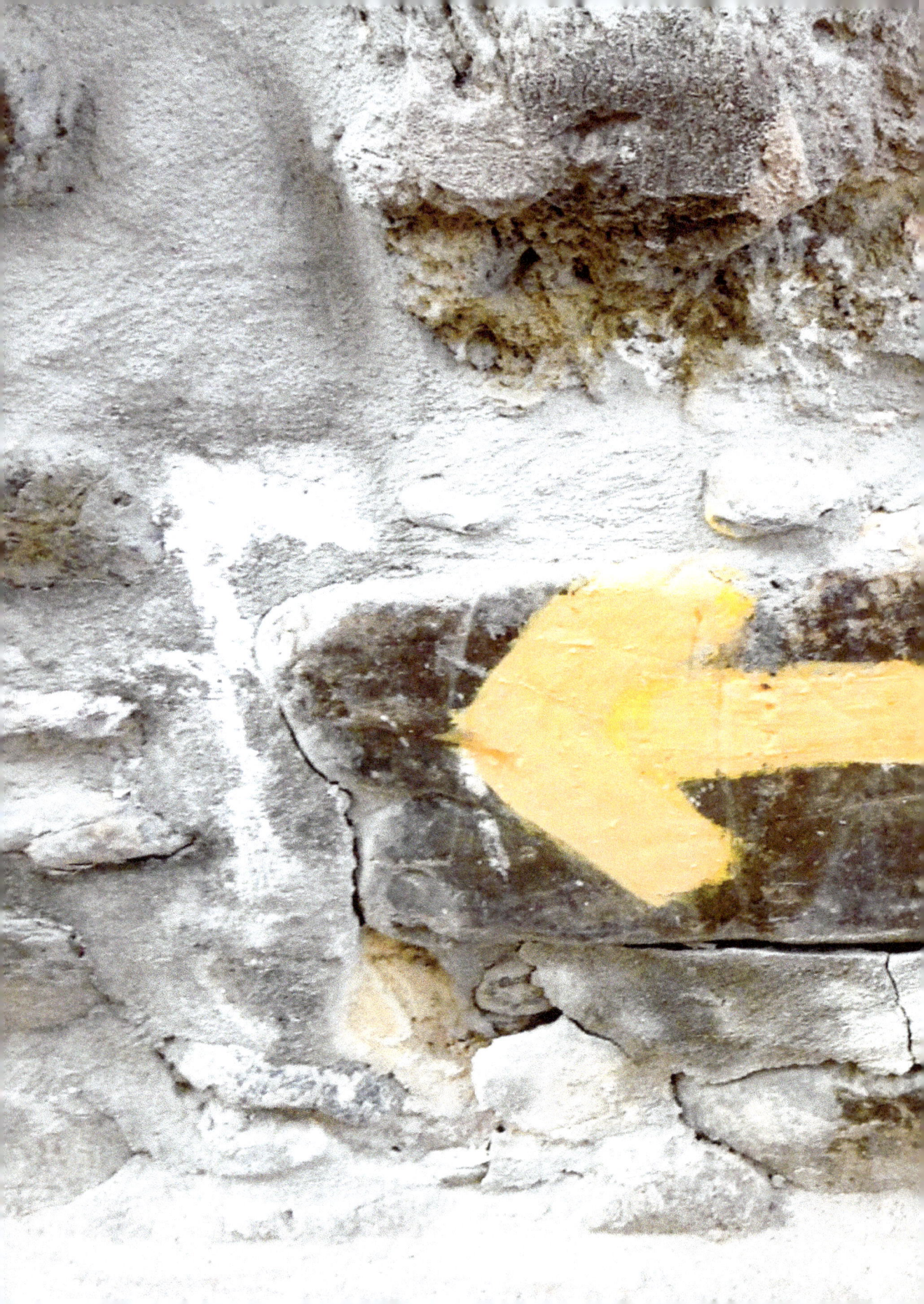

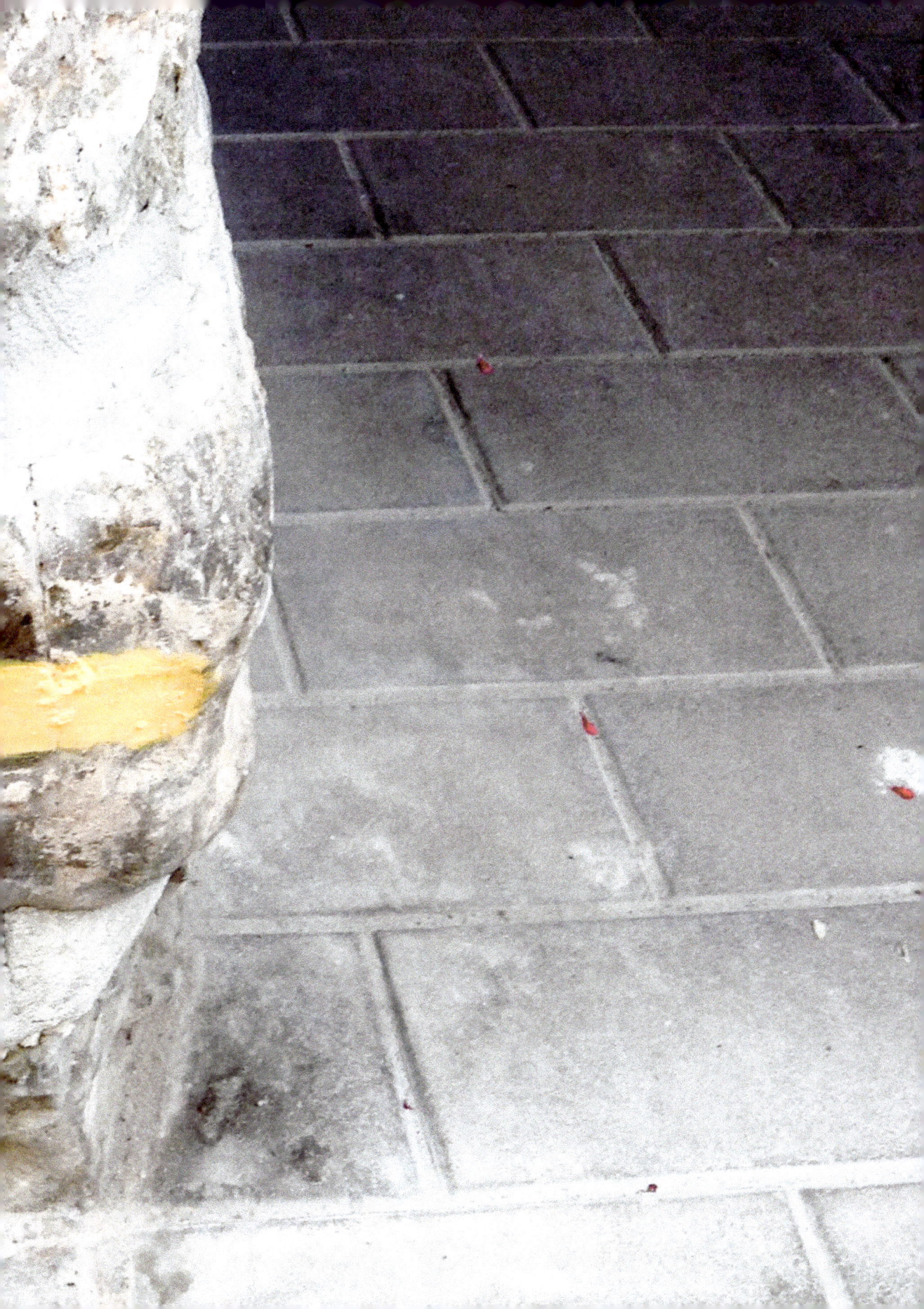

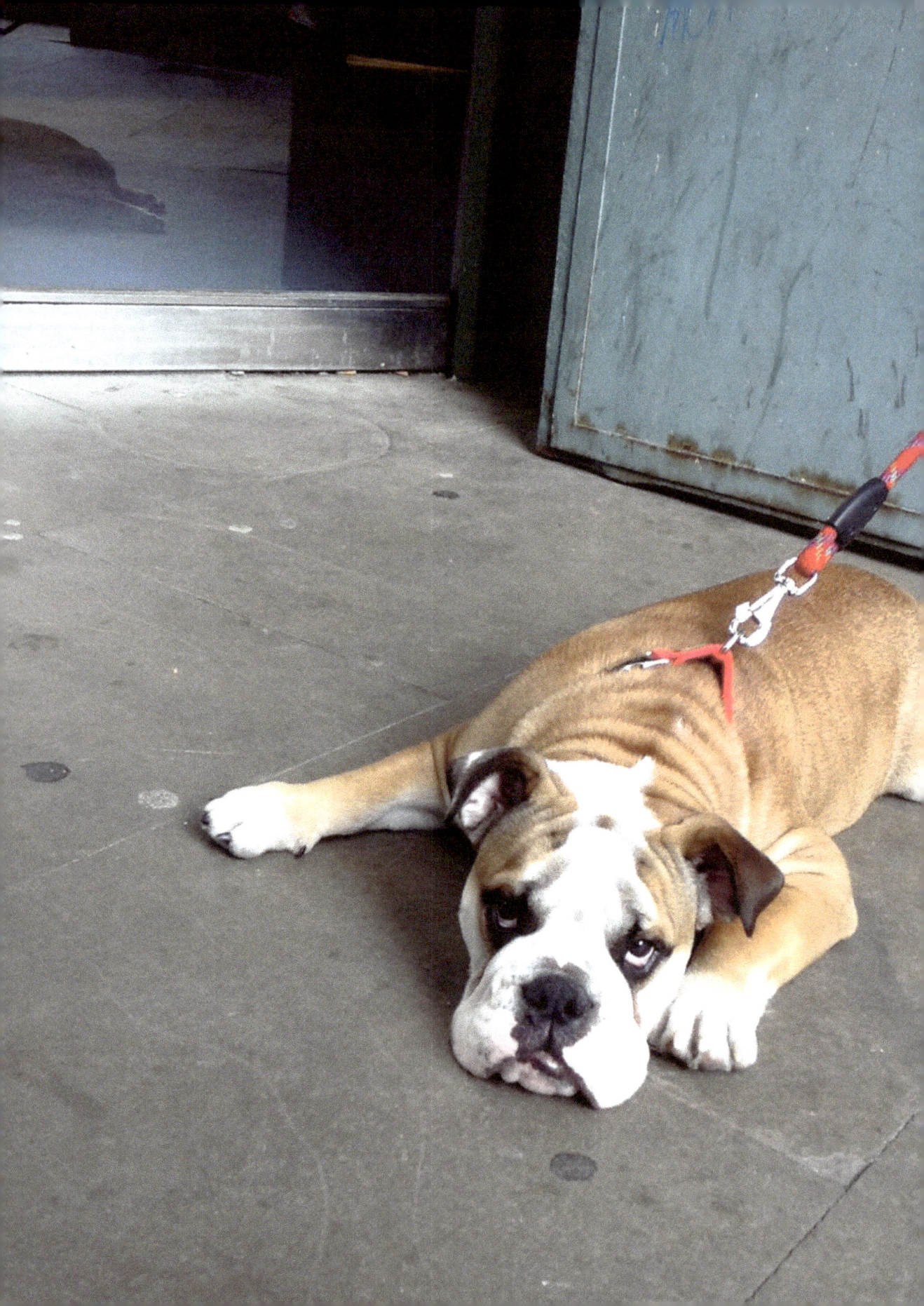

I have walked every day for excercise (and happiness!) for most of my life. Walking the Camino de Santiago was a MIRACLE! To walk every day, all day, well, that is just pure heaven! I haven't ever had the opportunity to walk every day, all day for 31 straight days, so I did wonder what it would be like. I also wondered if I would be able to do it!!! I have a job Monday through Friday, so I was not able to "practice" the actual Camino before I arrived. Instead, I did as best as I could and walked every minute I could fit in during the work week and then at least one seven-hour walk day on the weekend and almost always a five-hour walk day on the other day of the weekend. I did this for about 5-6 weeks before starting the Camino. I also added climbing stairs and steep hills as much as possible during the week (2-5 times each week). I climbed stairs for about 30-45 minutes.

I still did not know what to expect repeating long days of walking in a new environment for 31 days in a row. I did have a few extra days to "play with" at the end of the trip before my scheduled plane flight home but was hoping to spend those days exploring and relaxing on the coast. I also knew that I could take a bus at any point along the route, but I was determined to "hike across Spain" and in my mind that meant from the eastern border to the western coast (EVERY STEP and NO CHEATING!). While I was hiking, I was so true to this "calling" that in one town, the reserved albergue gave away my bed because I did not call ahead 3 days to confirm and then insisted on driving me to another albergue. After arriving at the albergue, I walked back to the first albergue and walked the steps I missed. I can now genuinely say that I hiked every step across Spain! M I R A C L E !

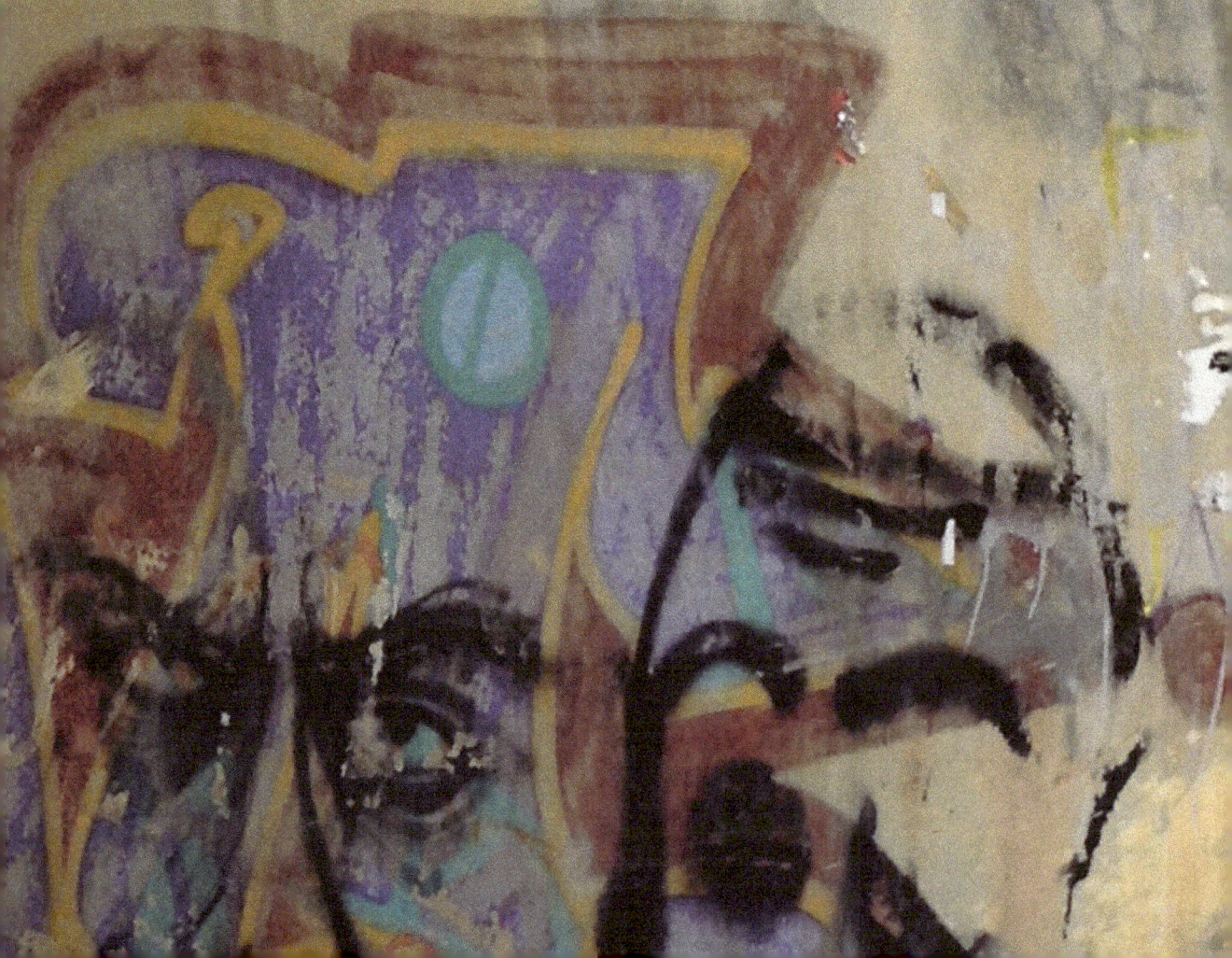

AN
08/08/02.

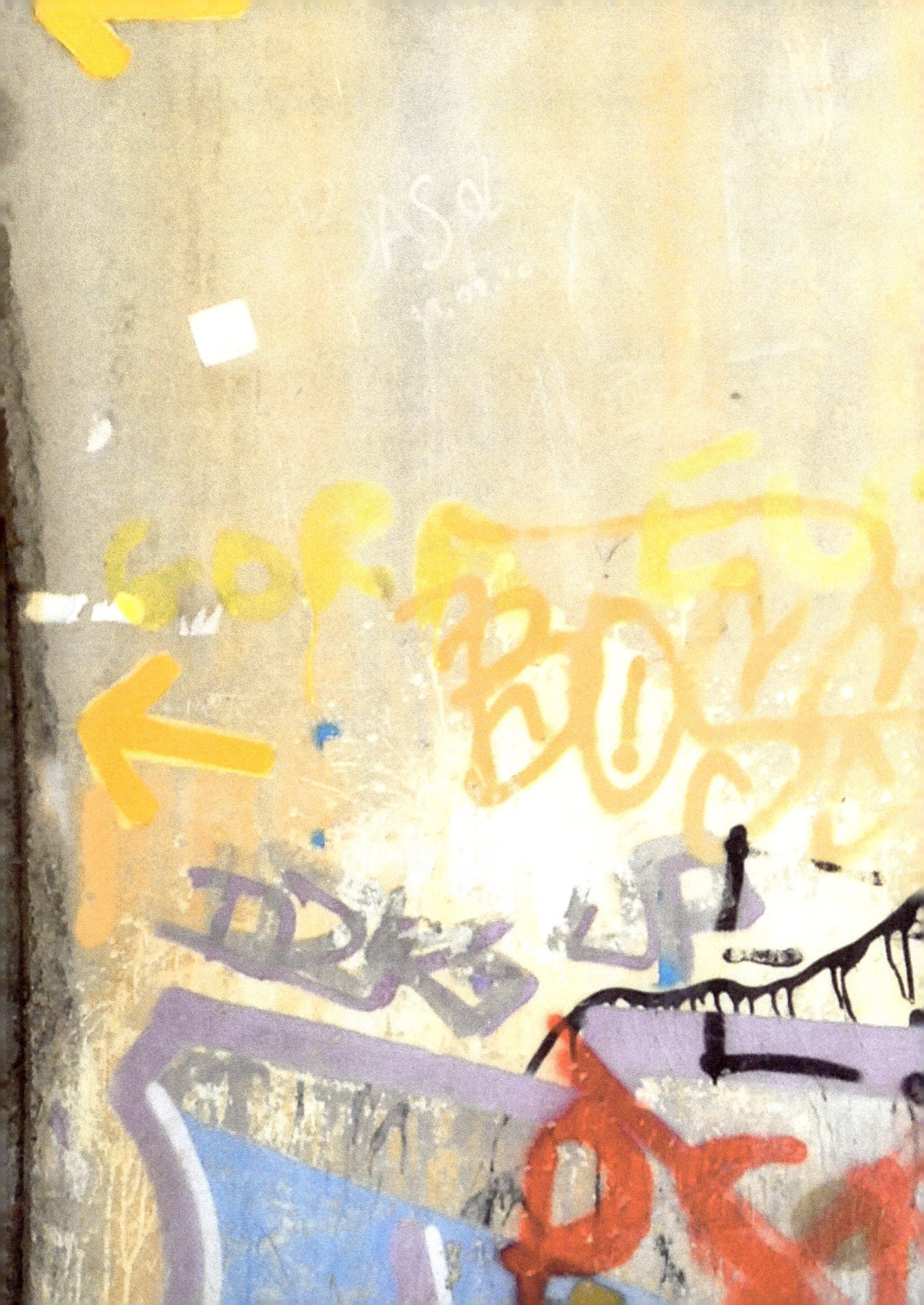

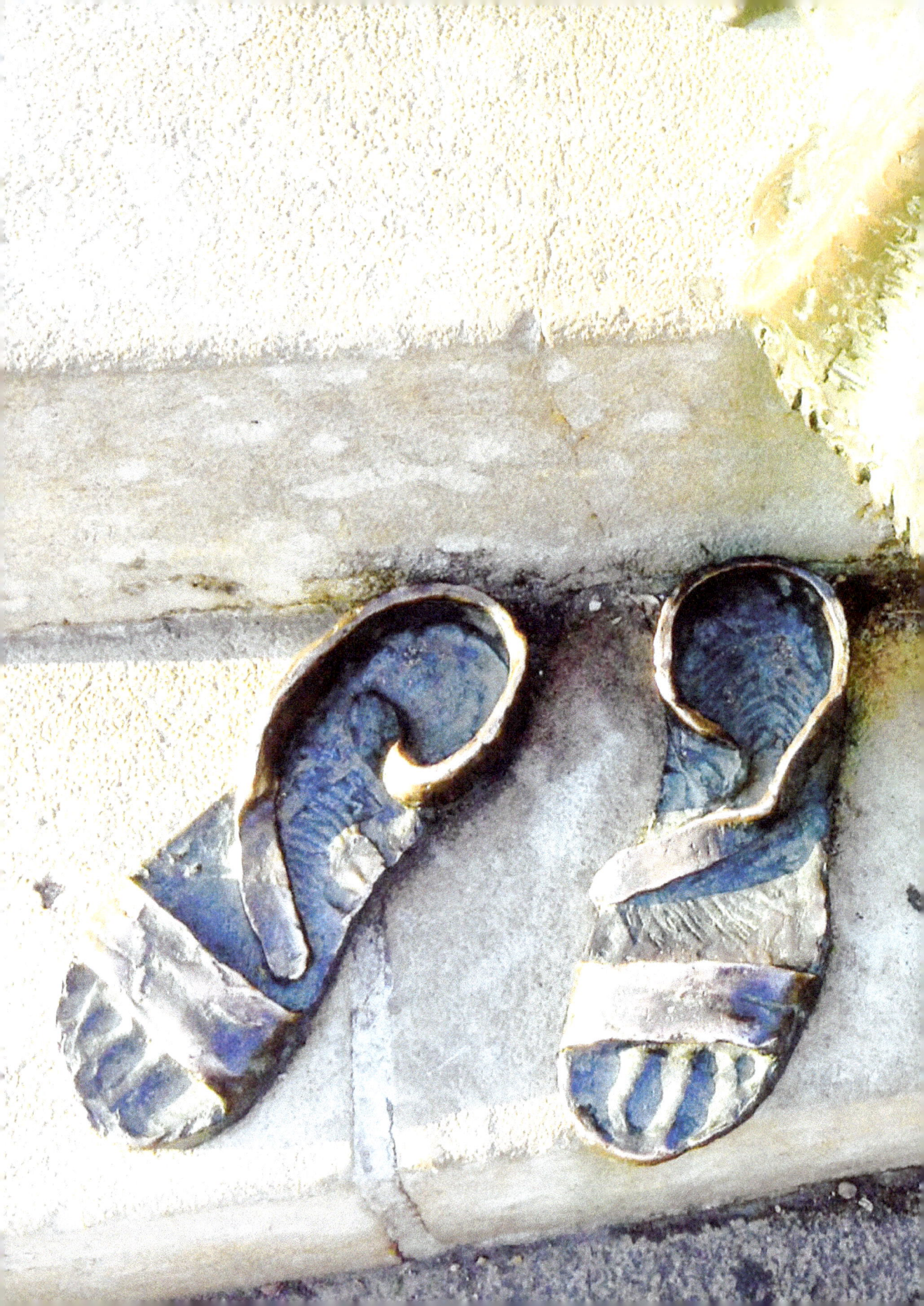

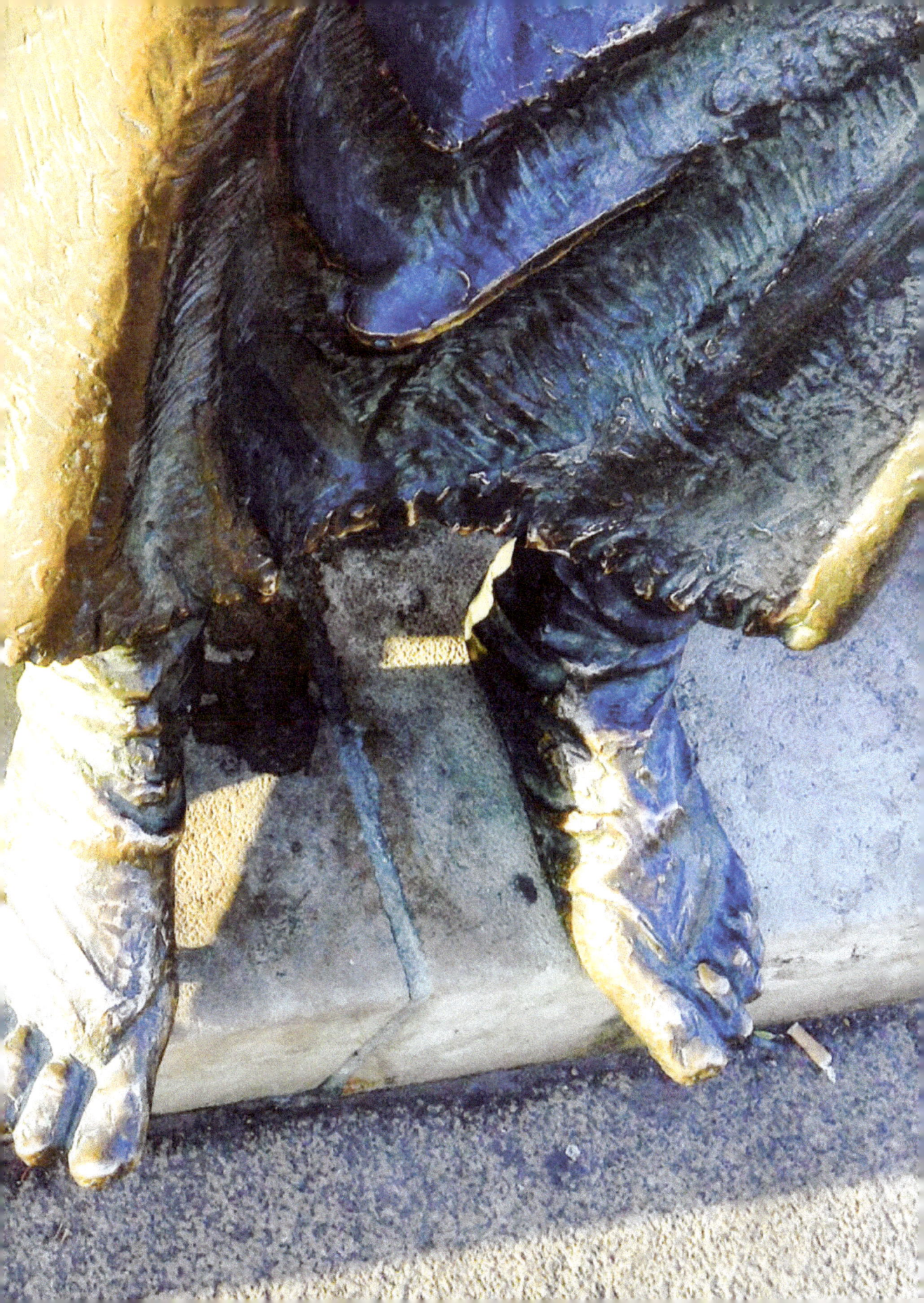

Even though it may appear as though wearing flip-flops on the Camino is reckless, it was actually a thoughtfully considered decision. They are perfect in the rain because I did not have to worry about them getting wet. They are so light and easy, and they combat high heat discomfort. They look cute with outfits, and they are my most beloved shoes for walking. I have worn flip-flops exclusively during the past 3 or 4 summers after reading about the health benefits of being barefoot or wearing shoes with little or no soles. I tried it and loved it! I also read that the soles of feet absorb the most chemicals/toxins of any part of our body, so that lead me to wear natural rubber flip-flops. The natural rubber flip-flops are surprisingly durable, mold to my feet and are extremely comfortable. It was a dream come true walking the Camino in flip-flops! So grateful! M I R A C L E ! ! !

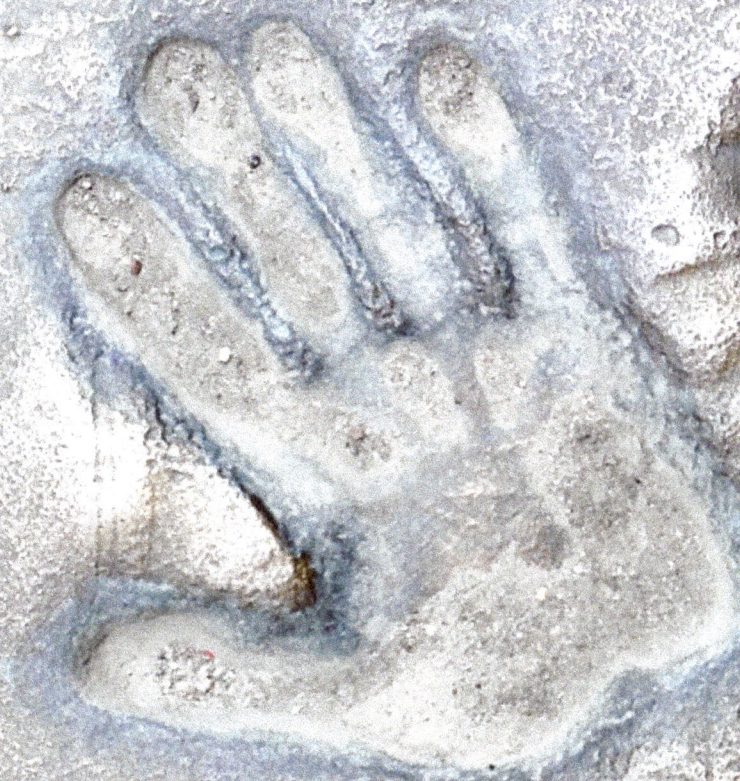

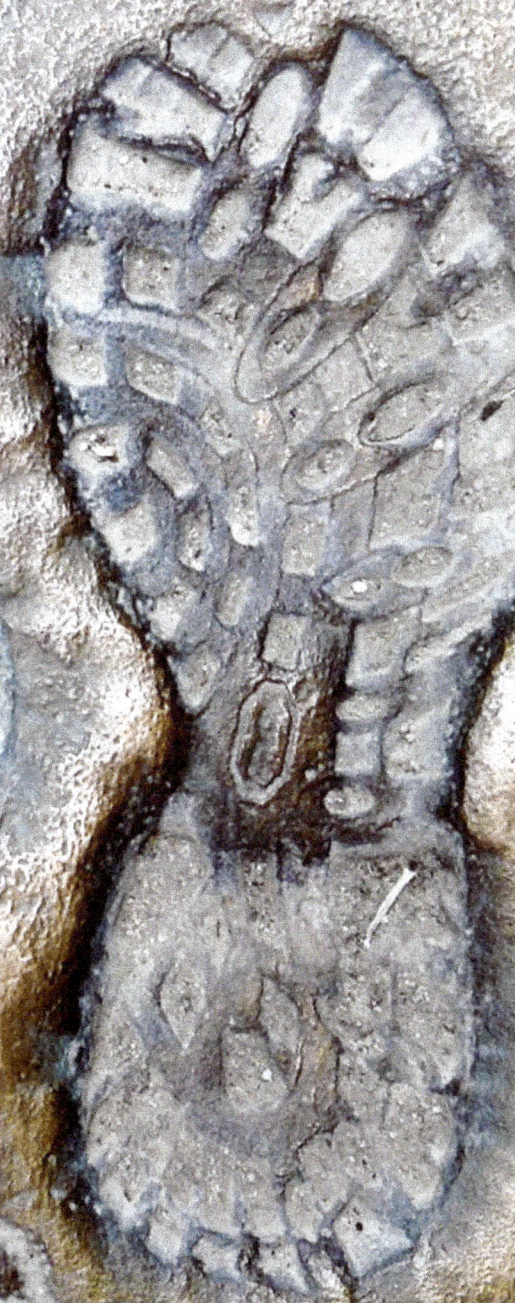

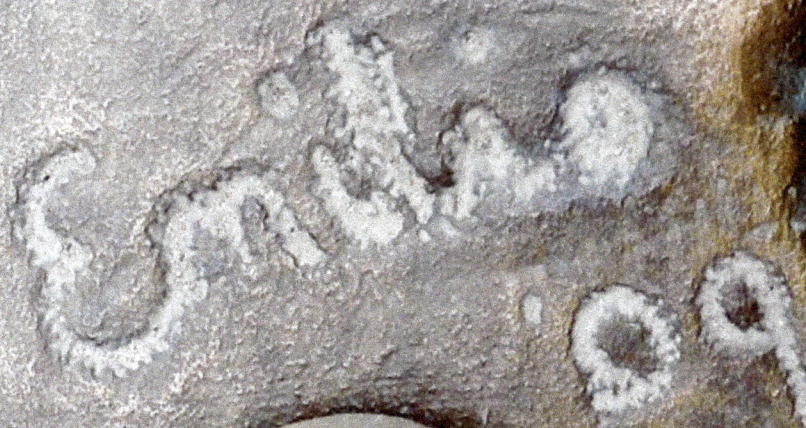

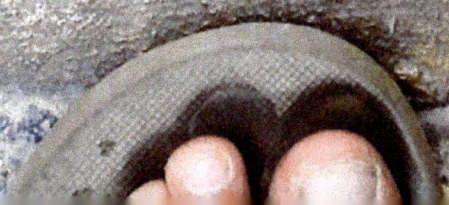

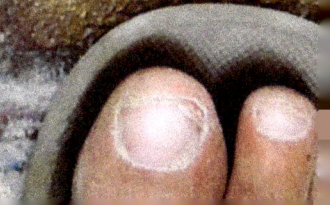

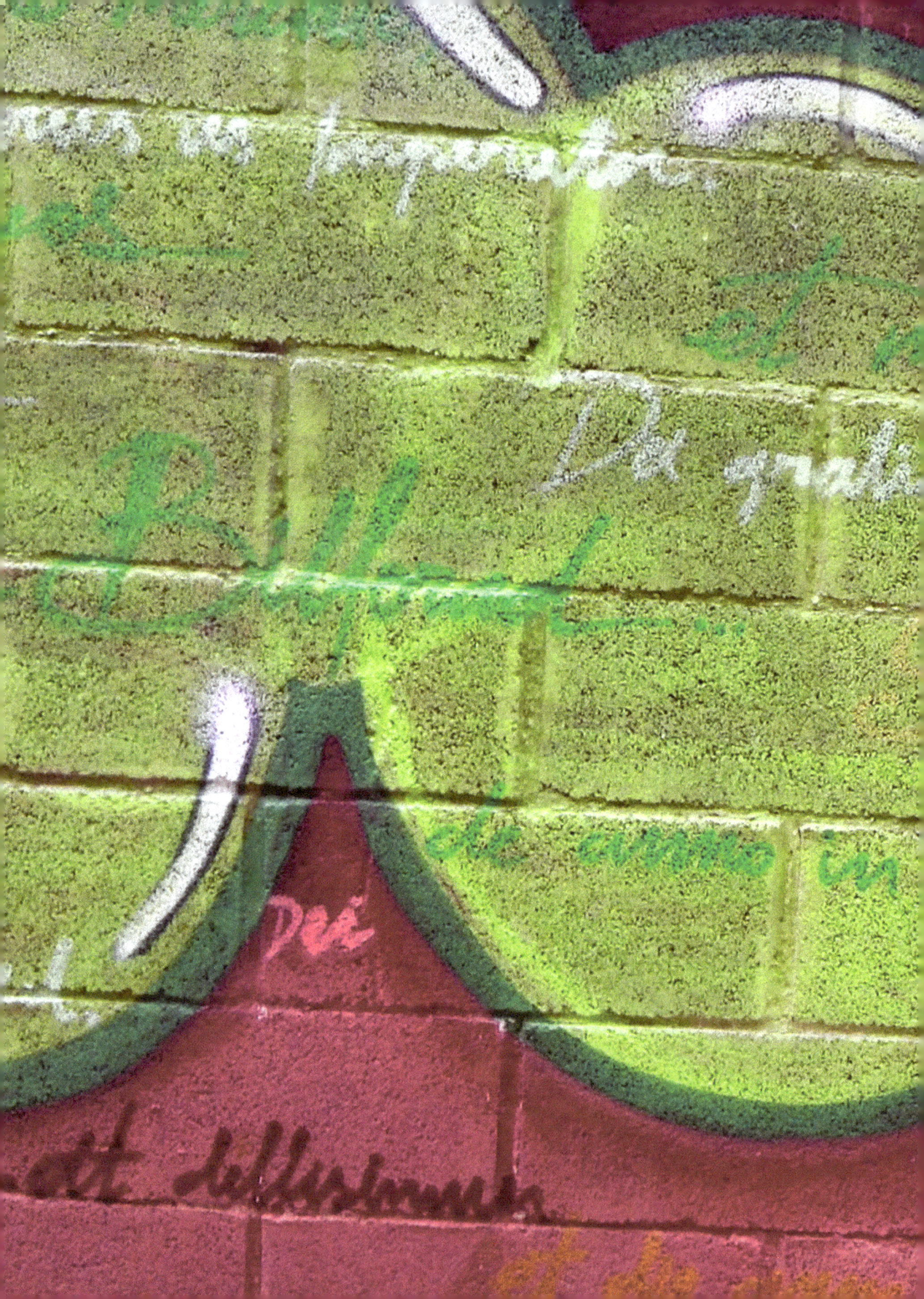

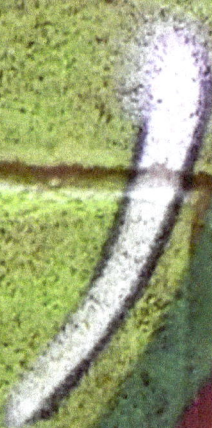

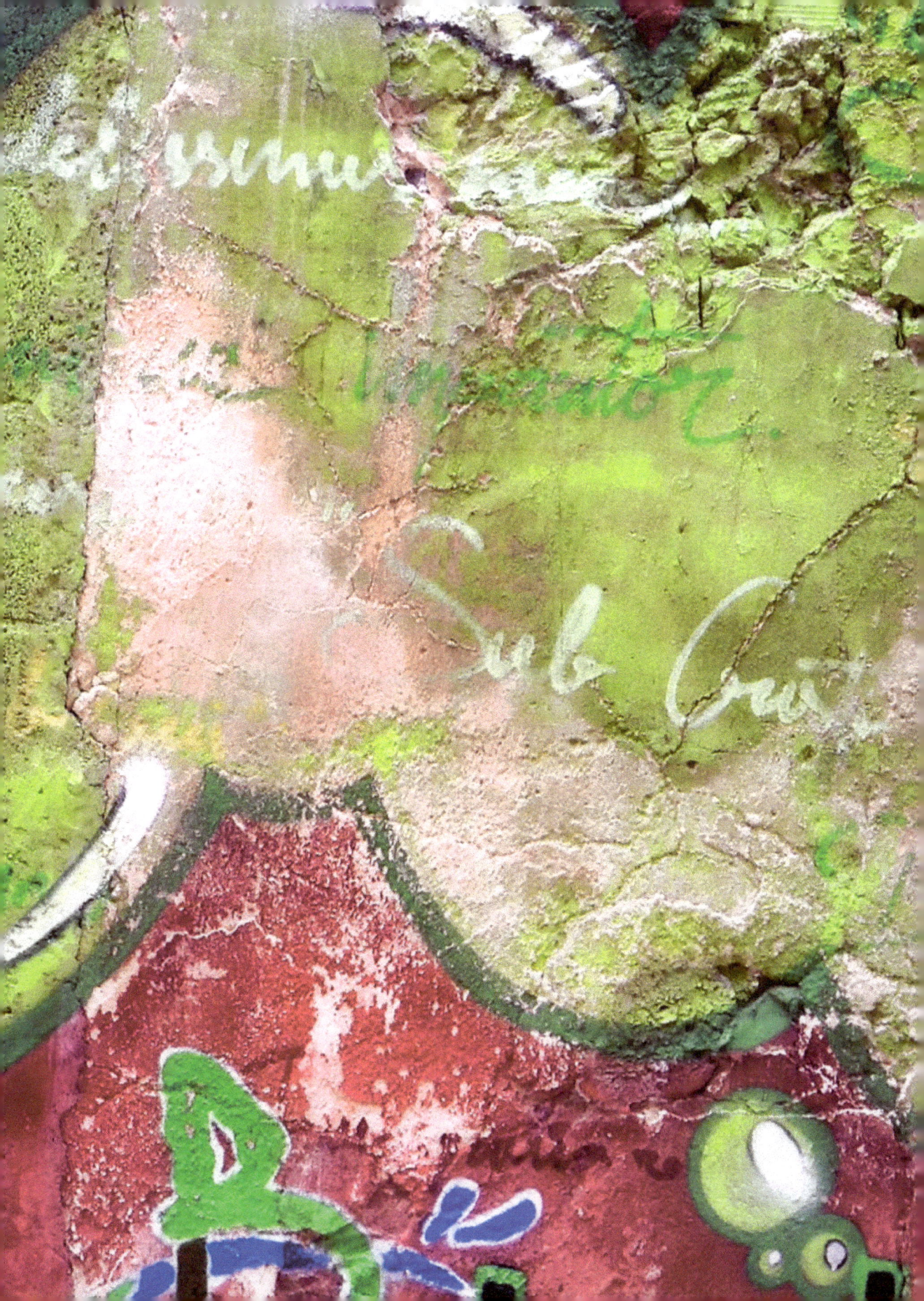

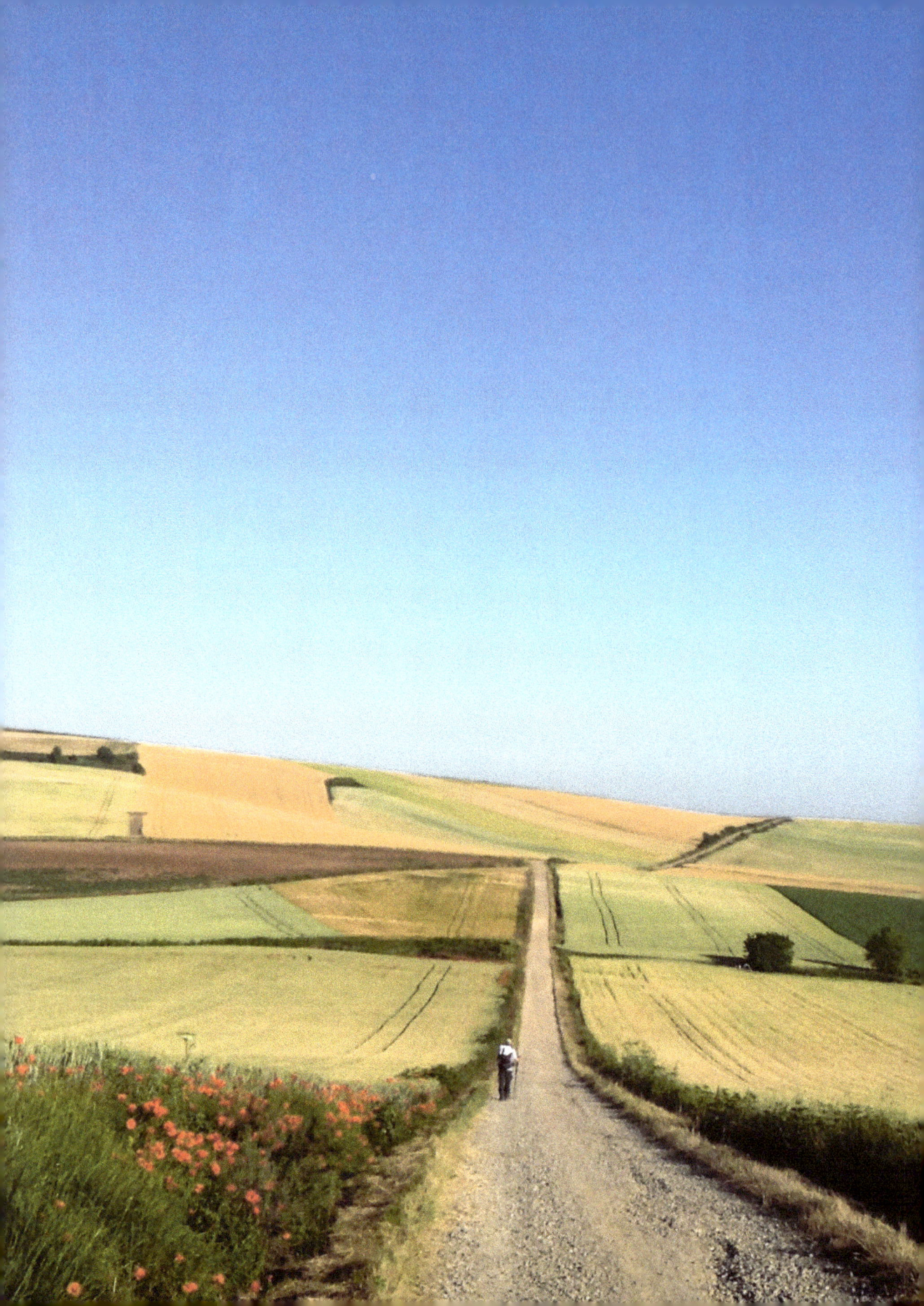

Schedule

MARCH
25 sit-ups/25 pushups every day
2 hours of walking every day
climbing stairs 2 times every week

APRIL
25 sit-ups/25 pushups every day
4-6 hours of walking every day
climbing stairs 3-4 times every week

MAY
25 sit-ups/25 pushups every day
5-8 hours of walking every day
climbing stairs 4 times every week

JUNE 14-JULY 14
25 sit-ups/25 pushups every day
8-10/14 hours of walking every day
climbing hills & mountains

551 MILES, 31 DAYS, FLIP-FLOPS!
M I R A C L E !!!

If I were to train for walking the Camino another time,
I would do everything the same except I would add climbing stairs
and/or steep hills almost every day.

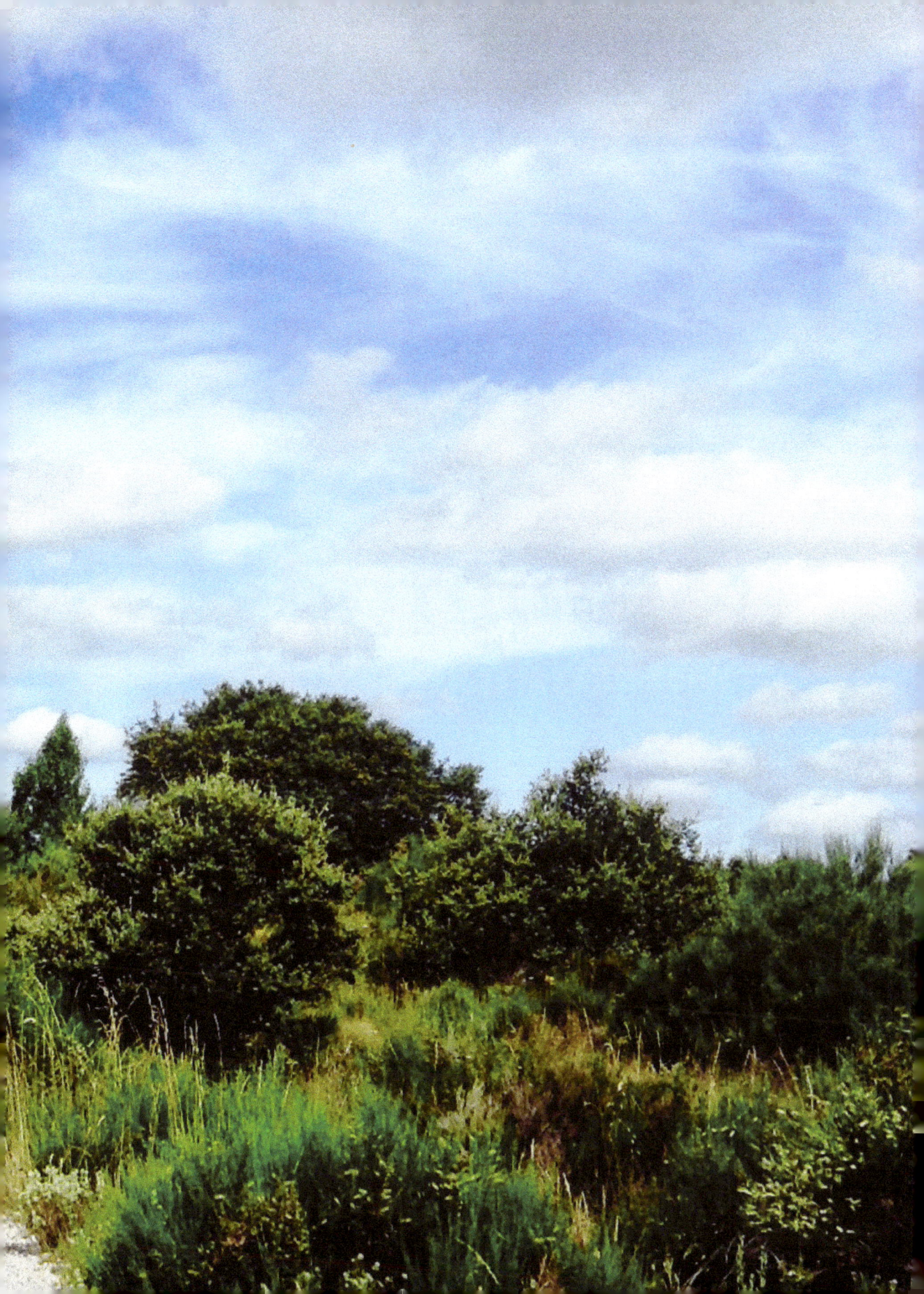

Plaza Mayor

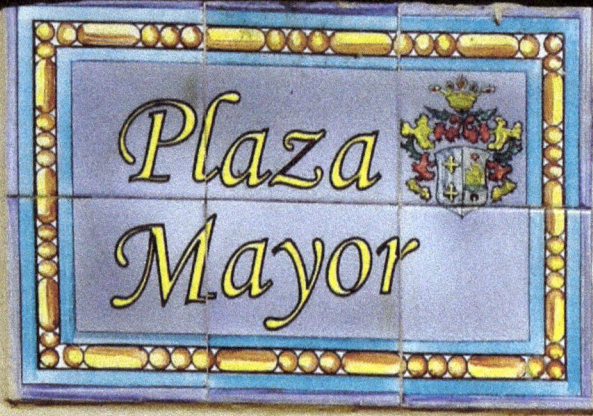

belongings
FOOD CLOTHING SHELTER

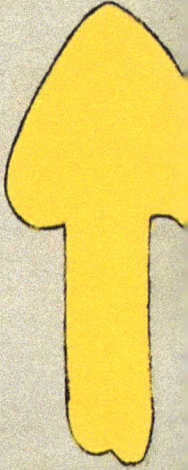

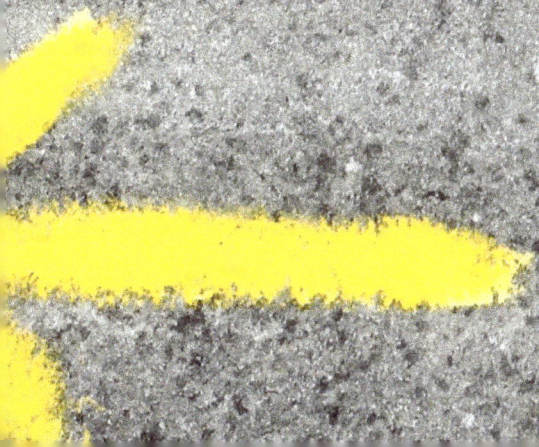
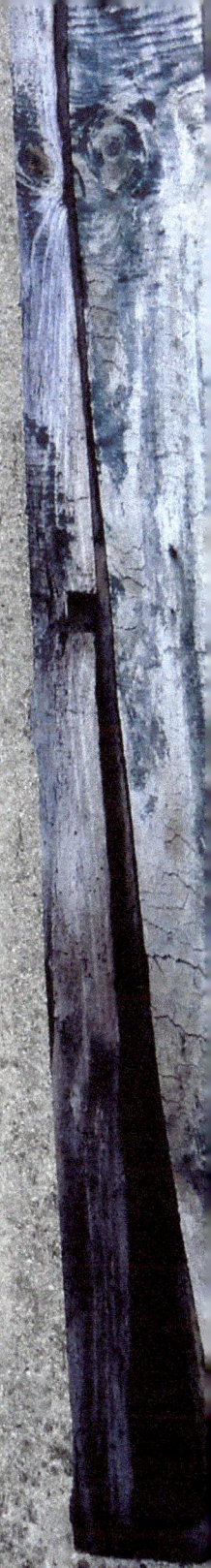

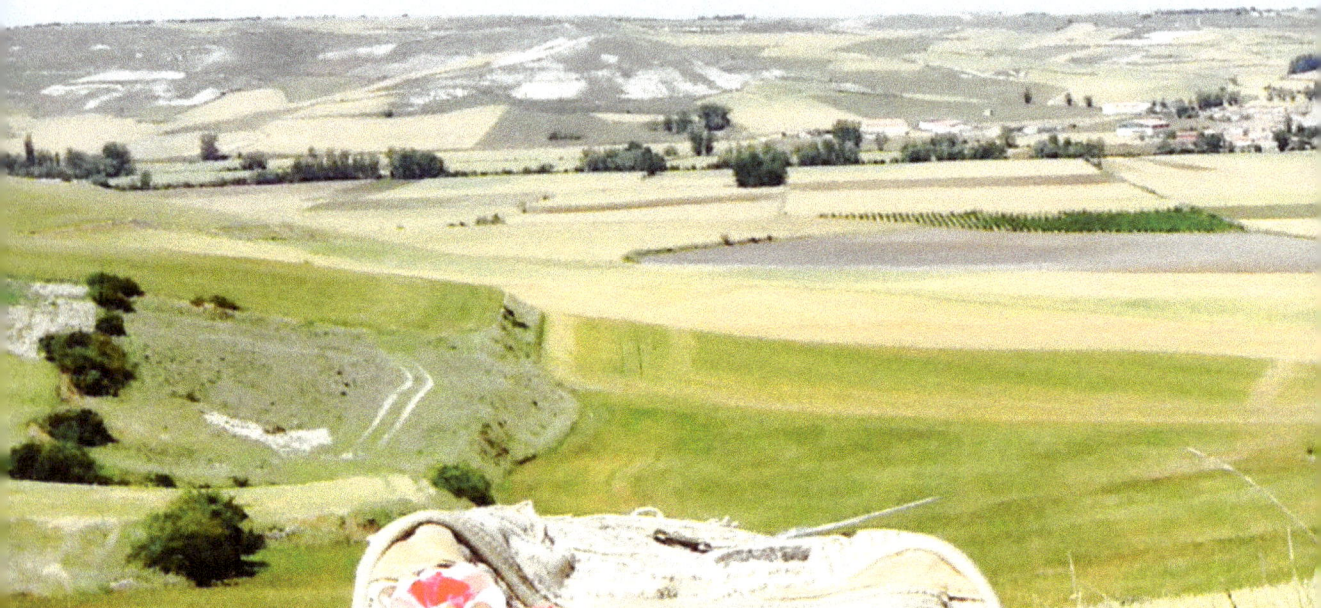

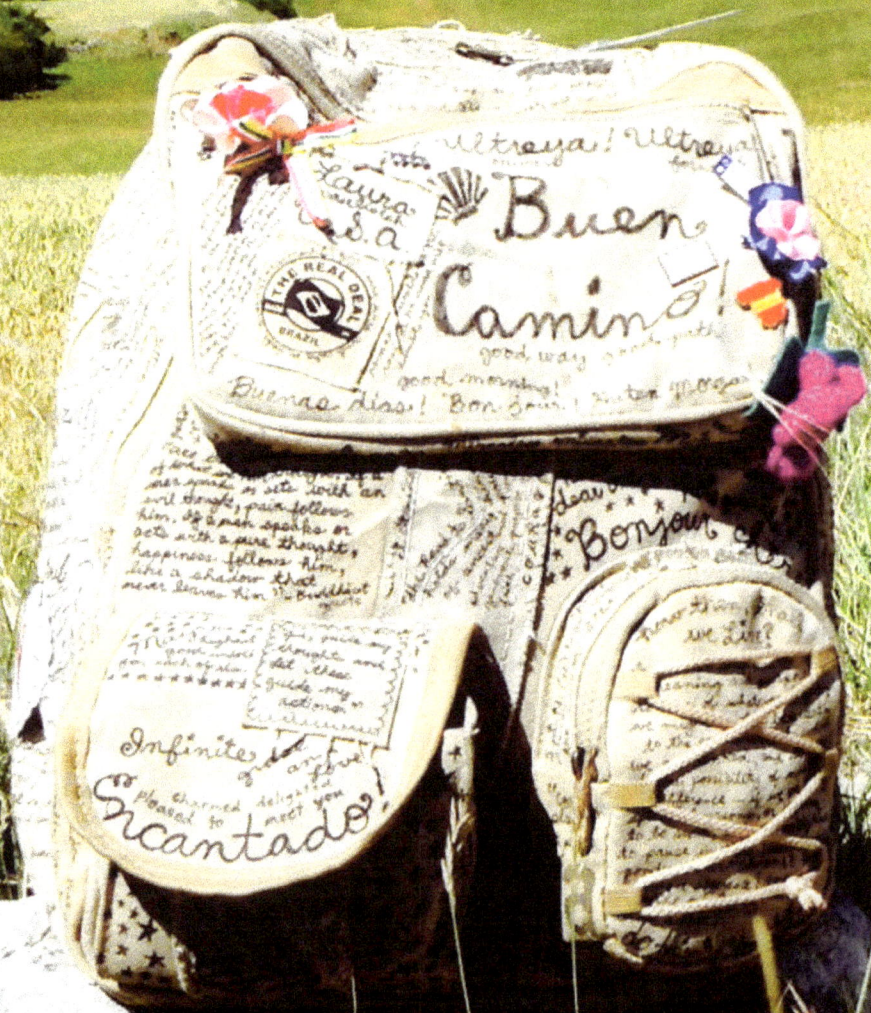

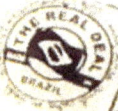

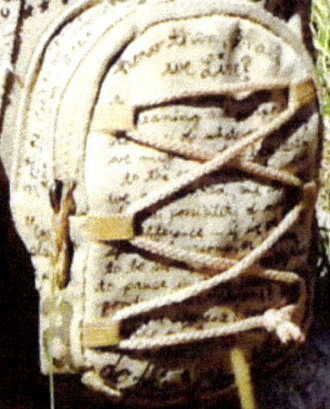

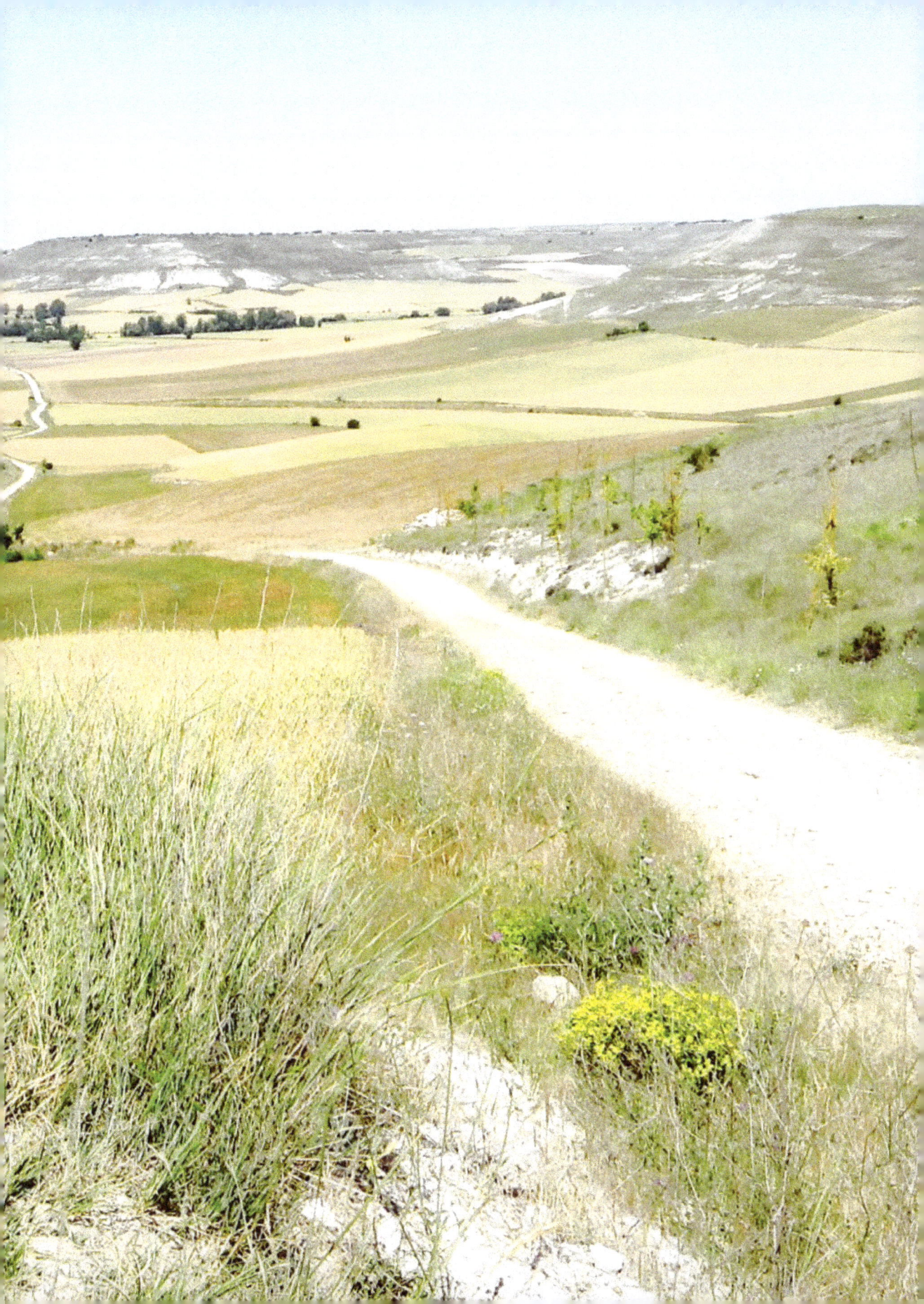

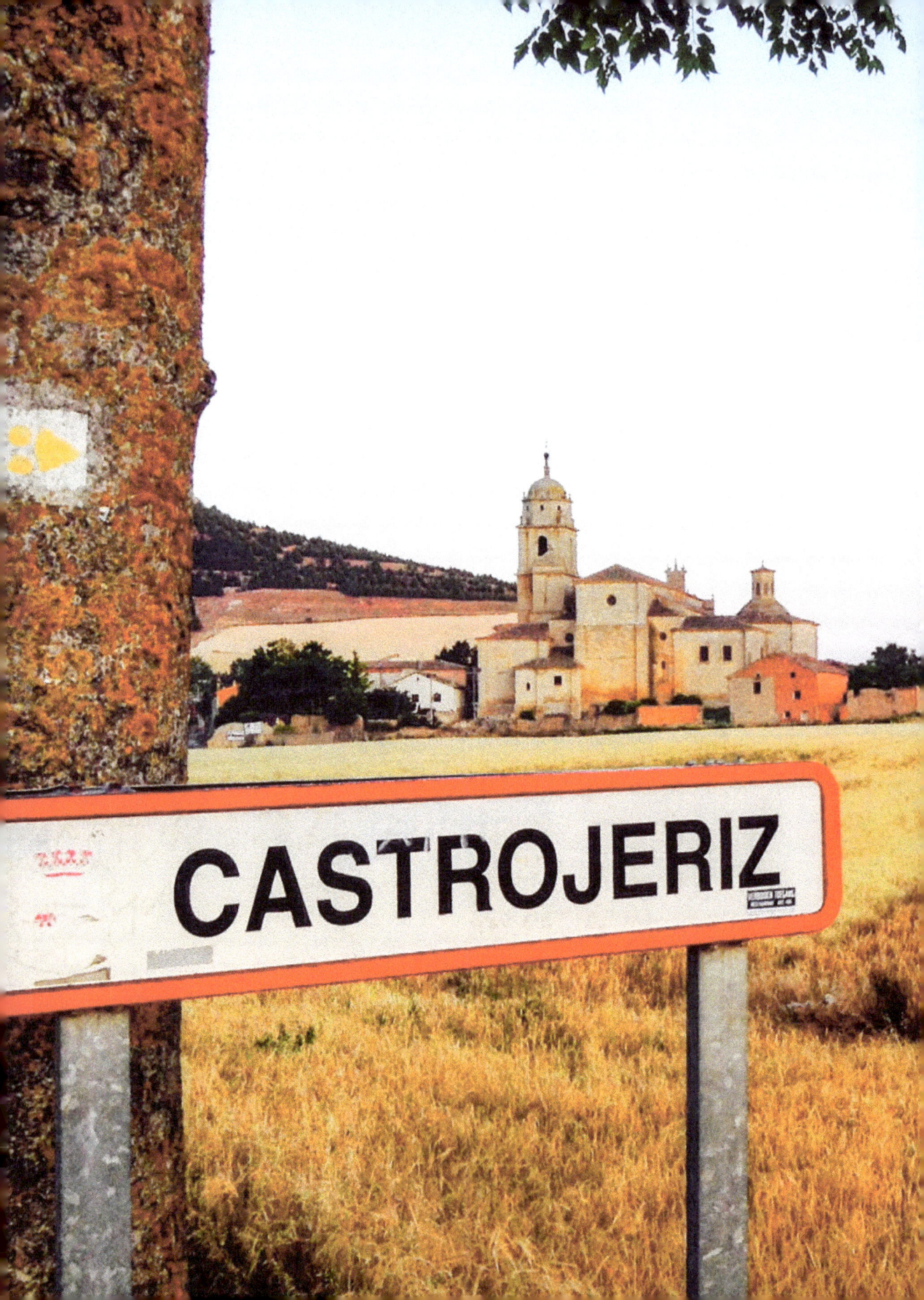

I love to walk, but I have no experience walking with a backpack. In addition to not knowing what it would be like to walk 20+ miles 31 days in a row, I also had no idea what it would be like carrying all of my belongings. For many months, all I knew was that I WANTED A LIGHT BACKPACK!!!!! I spent extensive energy thinking of and scheming ways to make my pack as light as possible. Now I consider my experience a miracle! I invested a lot of money in purchasing quality, key belongings and then benefited extremely from the rewards. Just like life at home, walking the Camino with only the most necessary and well-planned belongings, I walked all of my steps with ease! M I R A C L E !

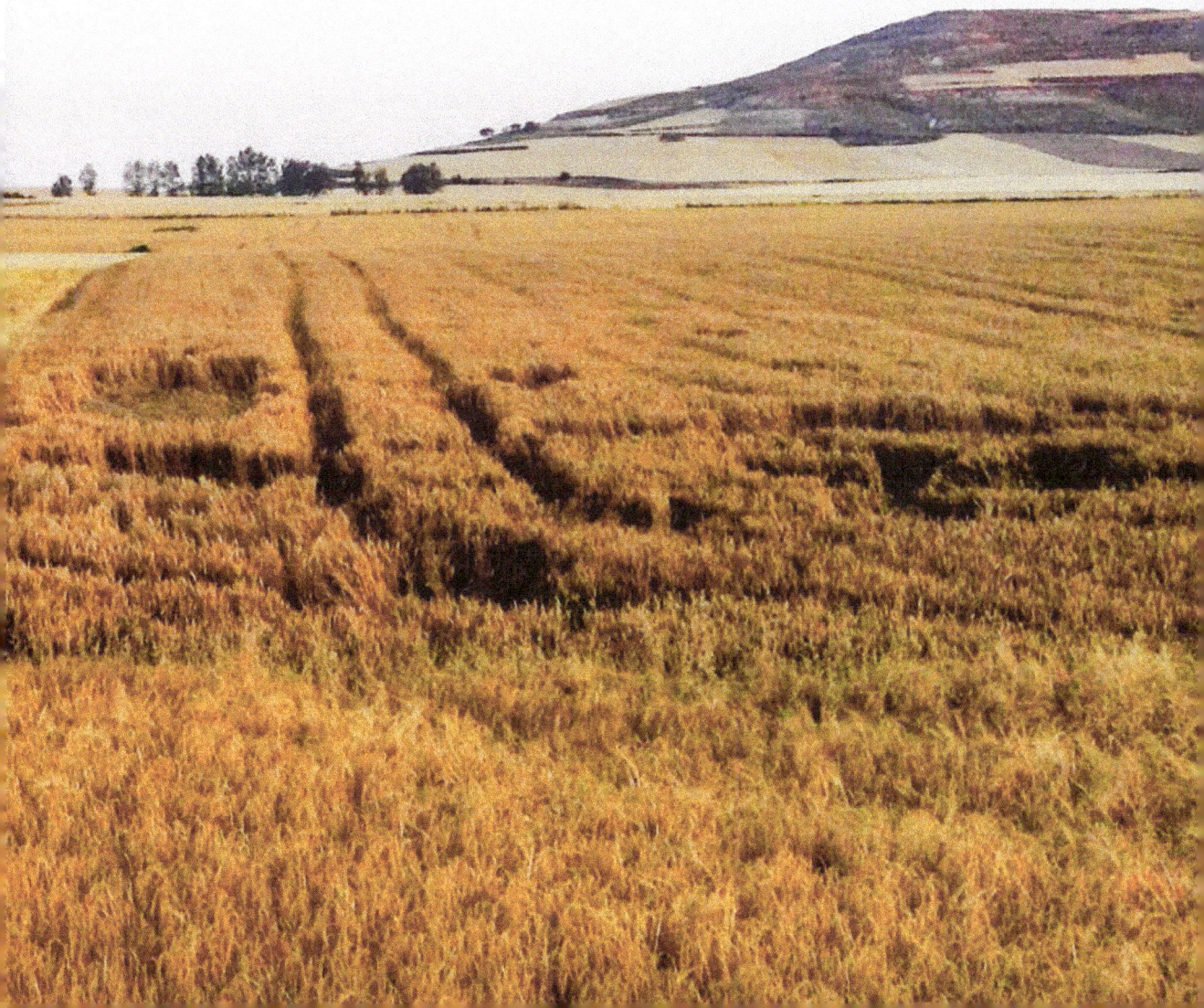

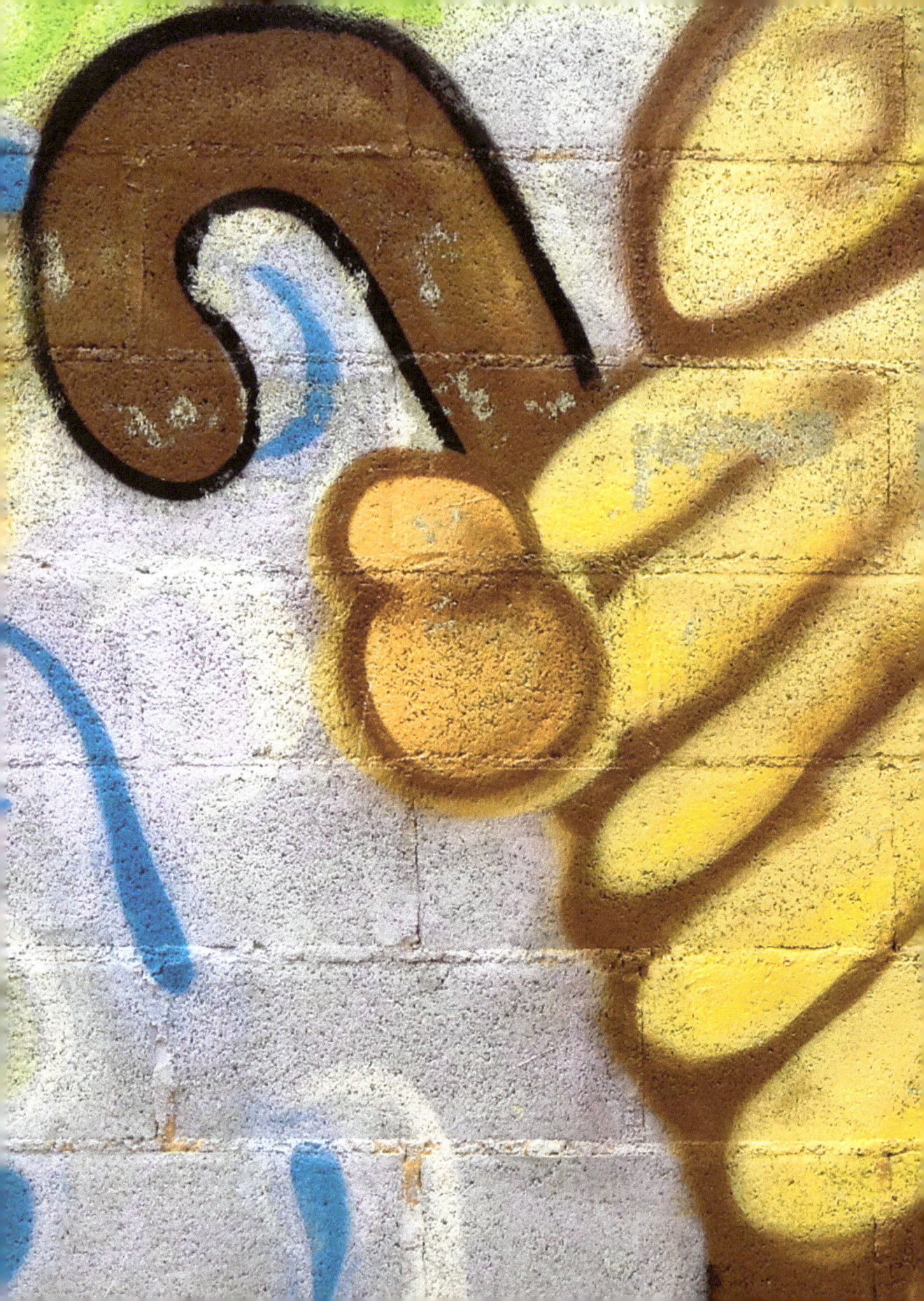

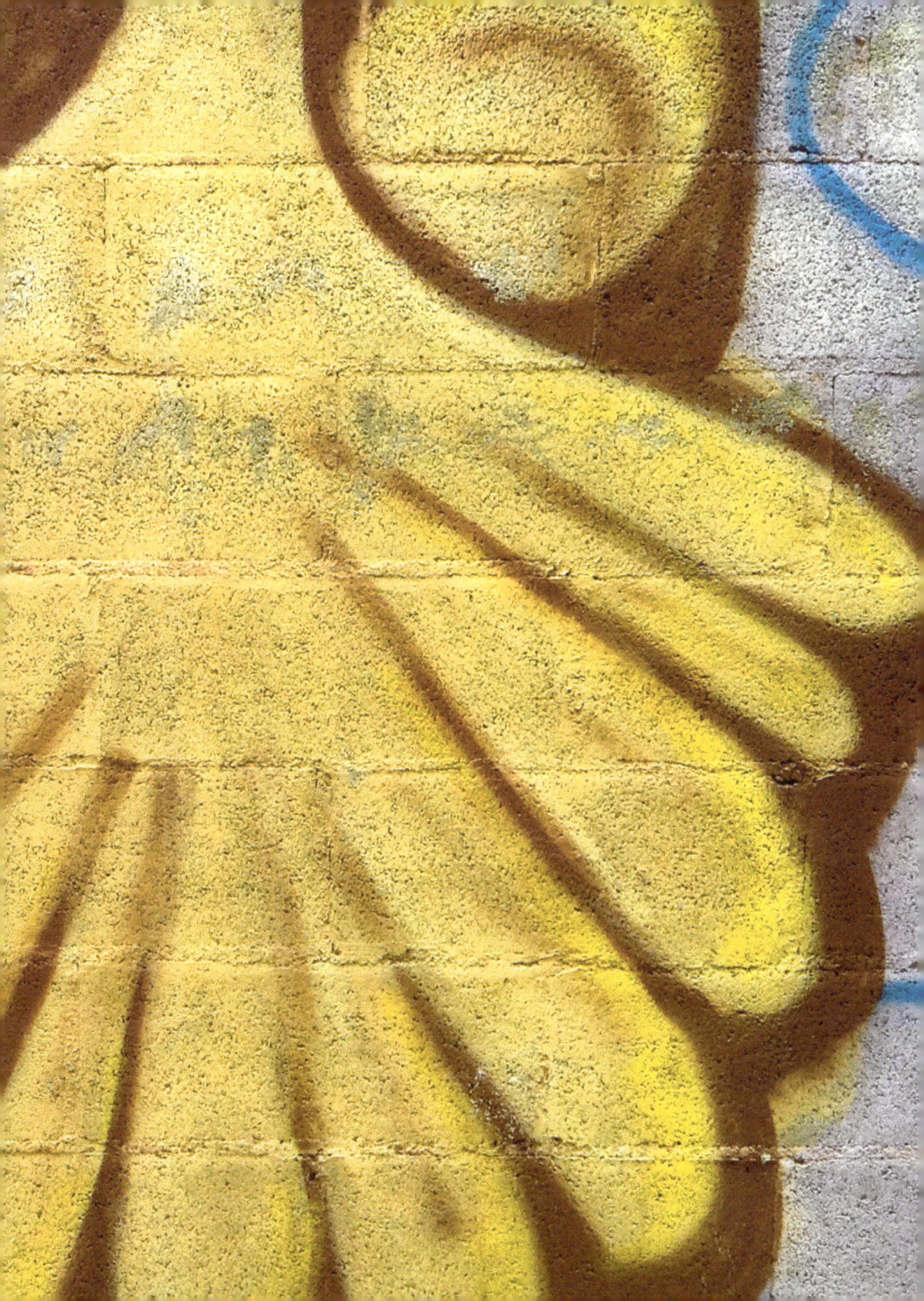

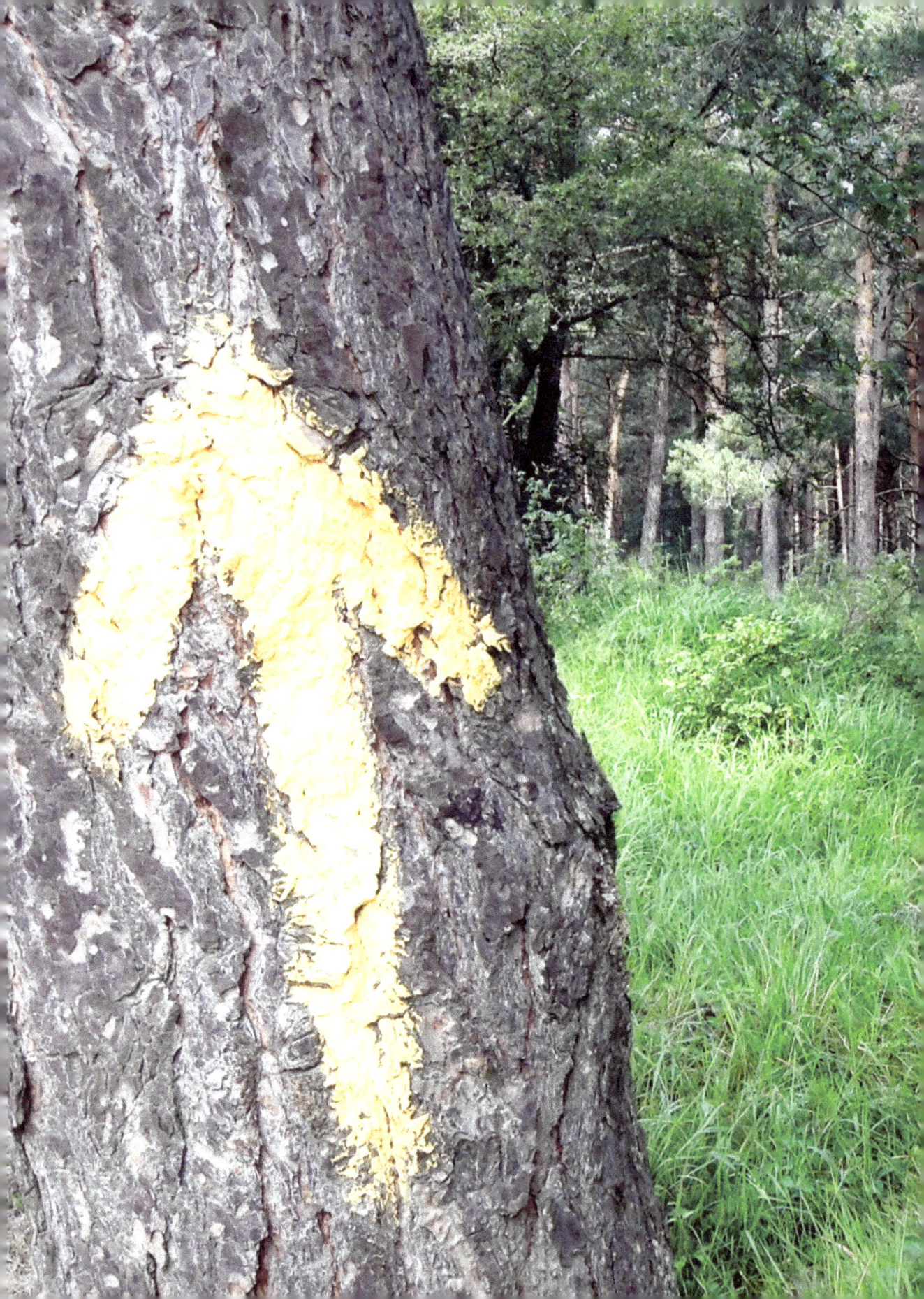

Belongings

Clothing
2 skirts, 2 tube tops
2 tube dresses, 1 tank shirt
2 undergarments

Shoes
Flip-flops
Cloth slipper shoes
(mailed extra flip-flops)

Supplies
Silk towel/scarf/shawl
Silk sleeping liner
Soapnuts (for laundering)

Toiletries
Toothbrush
Toothpowder
Coconut oil soap
(1/2" x 1/2" square)

Outdoor Gear
Sunglasses
Parasol
2 large plastic garbage bags
(for waterproofing)

Food
Cheese
Olive oil
Chorizo

Water
Steel water bottle with
filter (carried empty & then
filled with any water along the way)

Spirit
iPod
Weightless rice paper notes
(each page had 2 days of
information & then biodegradable disposal!)

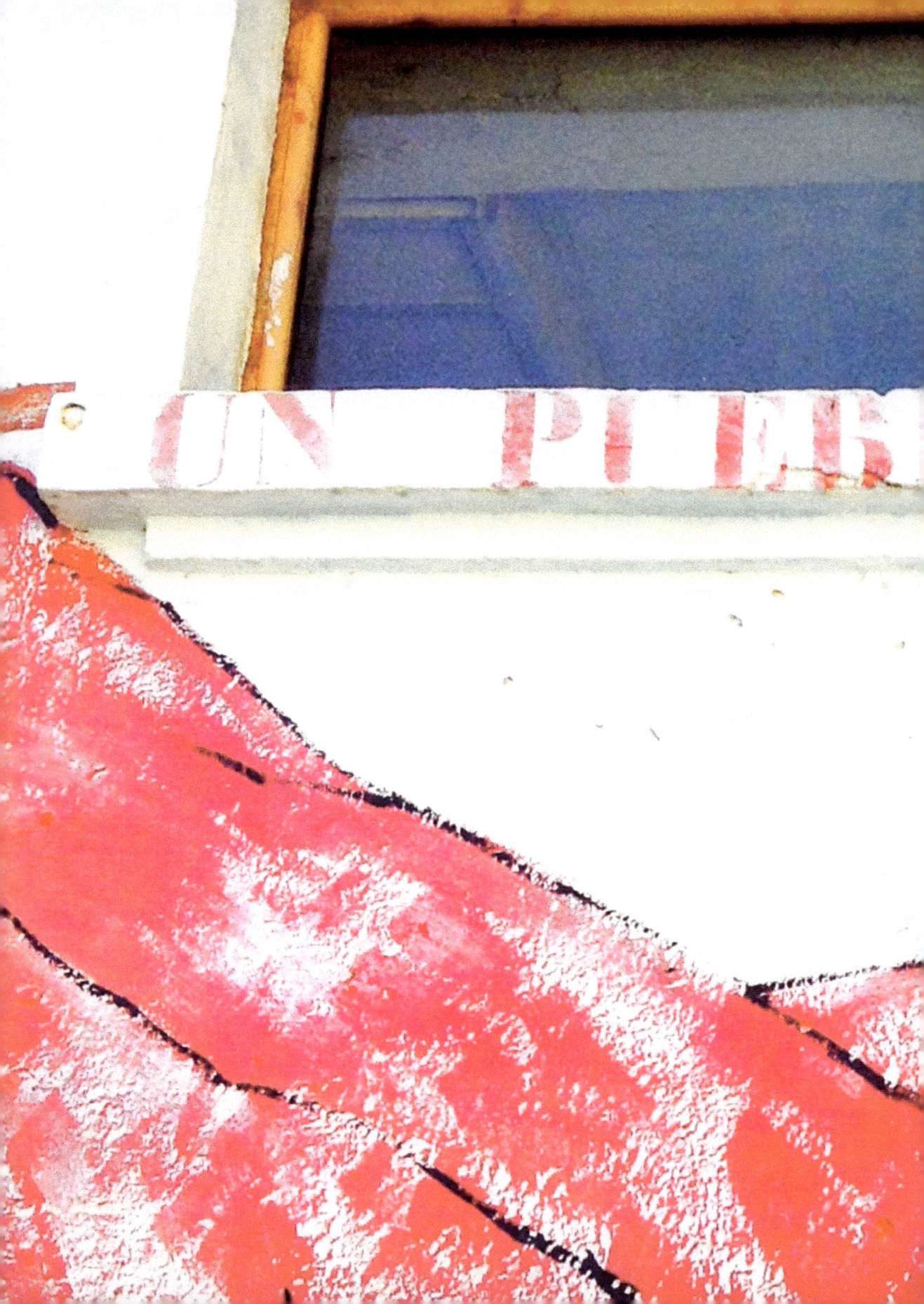

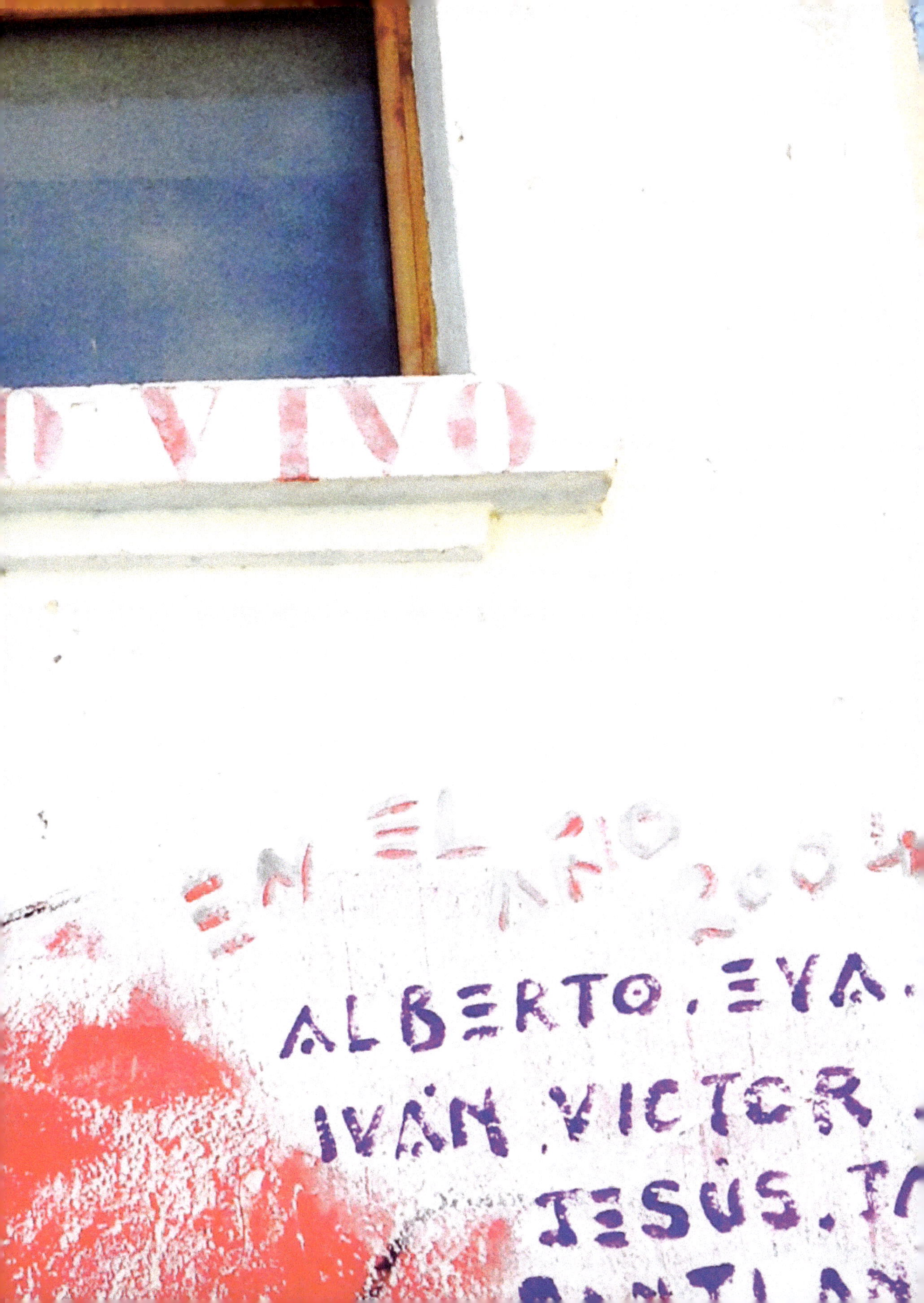

O VIVO

EN EL AÑO 2004

ALBERTO. EVA.

IVÁN. VICTOR.

JESÚS. T

I have mostly lived simply my whole life. At first it was by accident. My mother loved throwing unnecessary items away to keep the house tidy (sometimes even necessary items like homework). A few years before walking the Camino, I also became extremely minimalist. Circumstances required many, many moves in a short amount of time. By the 8th move in a brief time period, I didn't want to own any more belongings! I also was learning more and more about nutrition and chemicals in food/clothing/homes. Gradually, my life's belongings became only necessary items made with pure, real ingredients and materials.

I spend a lot of money investing in a few items that make life blissful. With this evolution has come unsurpassed freedom and joy. A few tricks that proved to be key on the Camino were investing in real silk bedding and other high quality items. Using a silk sheet set, a dear friend helped me make a sleeping bag liner (required by albergues to place on top of every communal mattress). It kept me warm, cool, comforted and protected from bed bugs.Silk has a tightly woven weave which is difficult for bed bugs to enter. With the remaining silk, we made a towel that I also used as a shawl/scarf. This was also one of my most valuable possessions. It was extremely light to carry, kept me warm and cool, and also dried immediately. The silk system was monumental in my Camino happiness and success. MIRACLE!

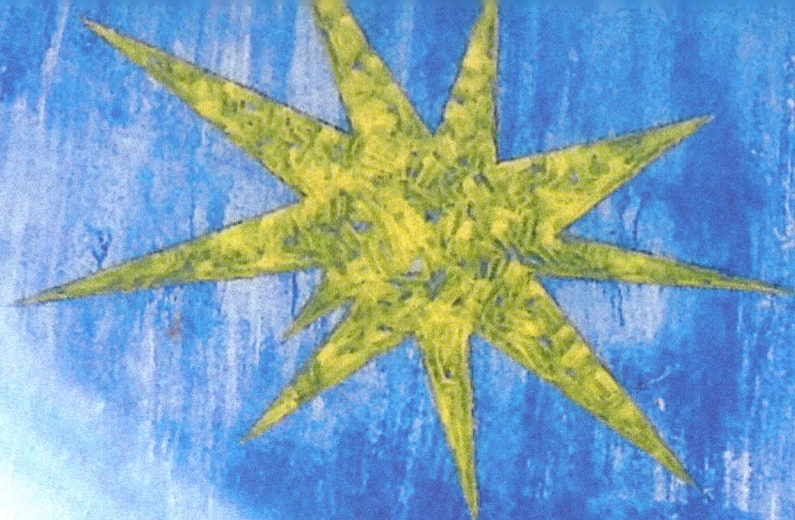

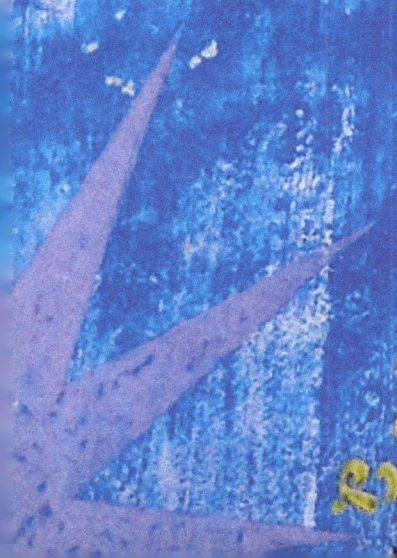

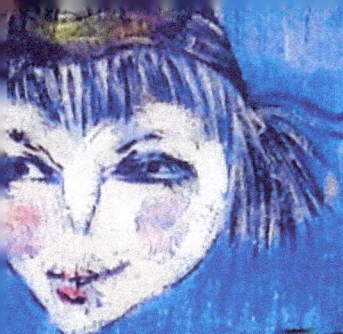

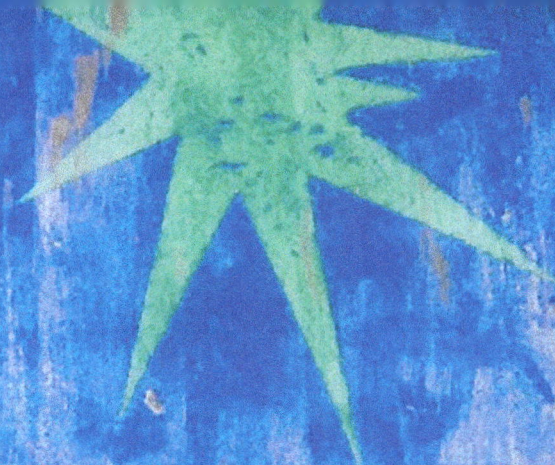

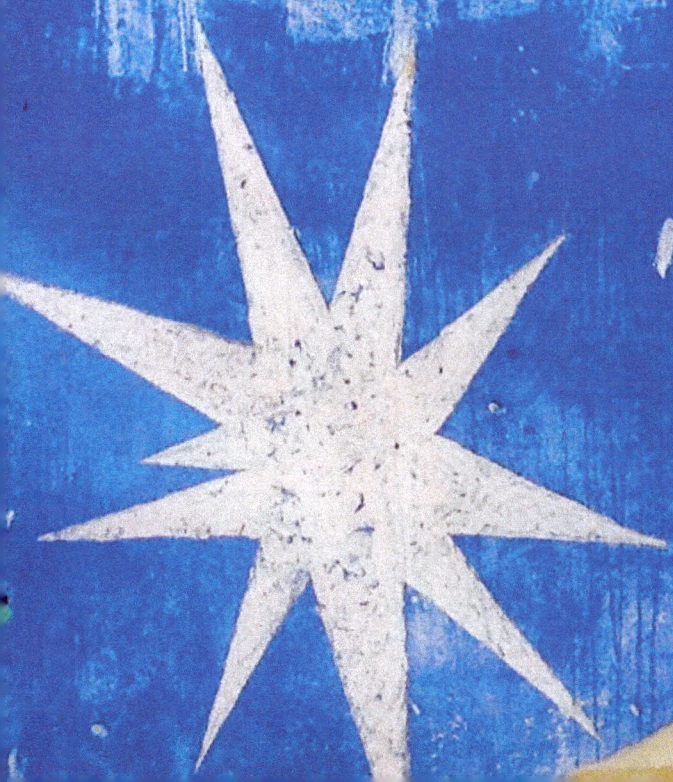

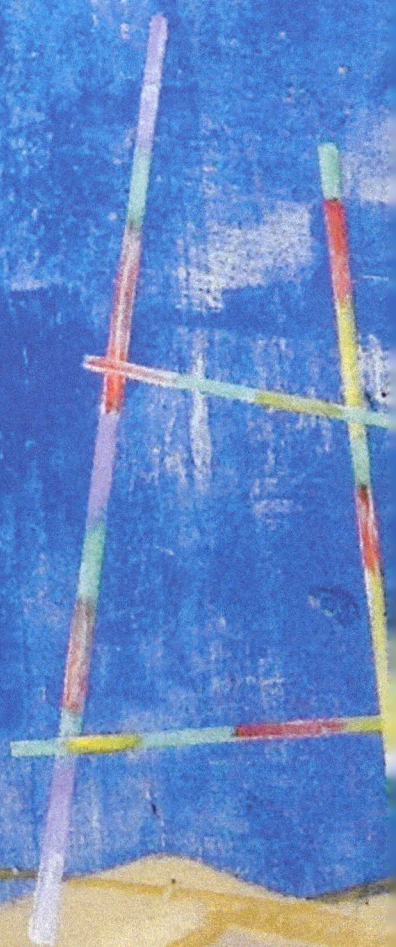

Guidance

"I cannot live without books!"-Thomas Jefferson

I love to read! At home I read every day and am always reading several books at a time. I am most grateful for the public library. I was completely willing to relinquish reading for the chance to walk the Camino, but at the last minute, I bought some books for my iPod. It wasn't necessary, but it was fun.

I also regularly turn to books for wisdom, guidance and comfort. I knew that I would not be able to carry the weight of my most guiding authors, so during the months before leaving, I wrote their words onto my backpack. It was valuable to have with me and added no extra weight.

I wrote travel tips to remember like translated phrases of greetings or other translated words to know. I wrote addresses of friends and family to send postcards. I wrote emergency information and phone numbers. I wrote the inspiring words of Byron Katie, Deepak Chopra and many more. All of the words offered guidance, comfort and joy. M I R A C L E !!!

*Byron Katie *Martha Beck *Deepak Chopra *The Toltecs *Wayne Dyer
*Damian McElrath *Thich Naht Hahn

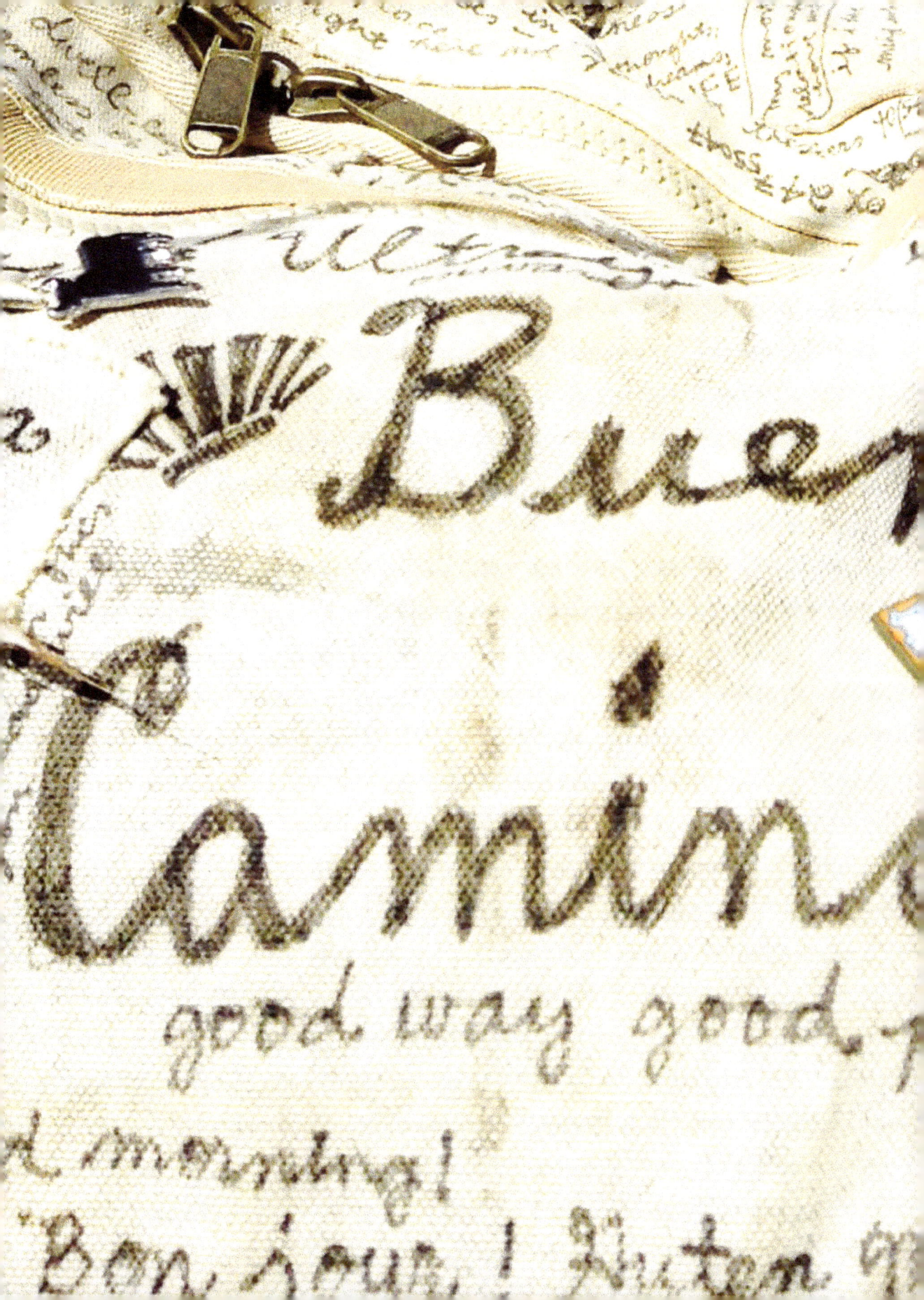

Buen
Camino
good way good
morning!
Bon jour! Guten

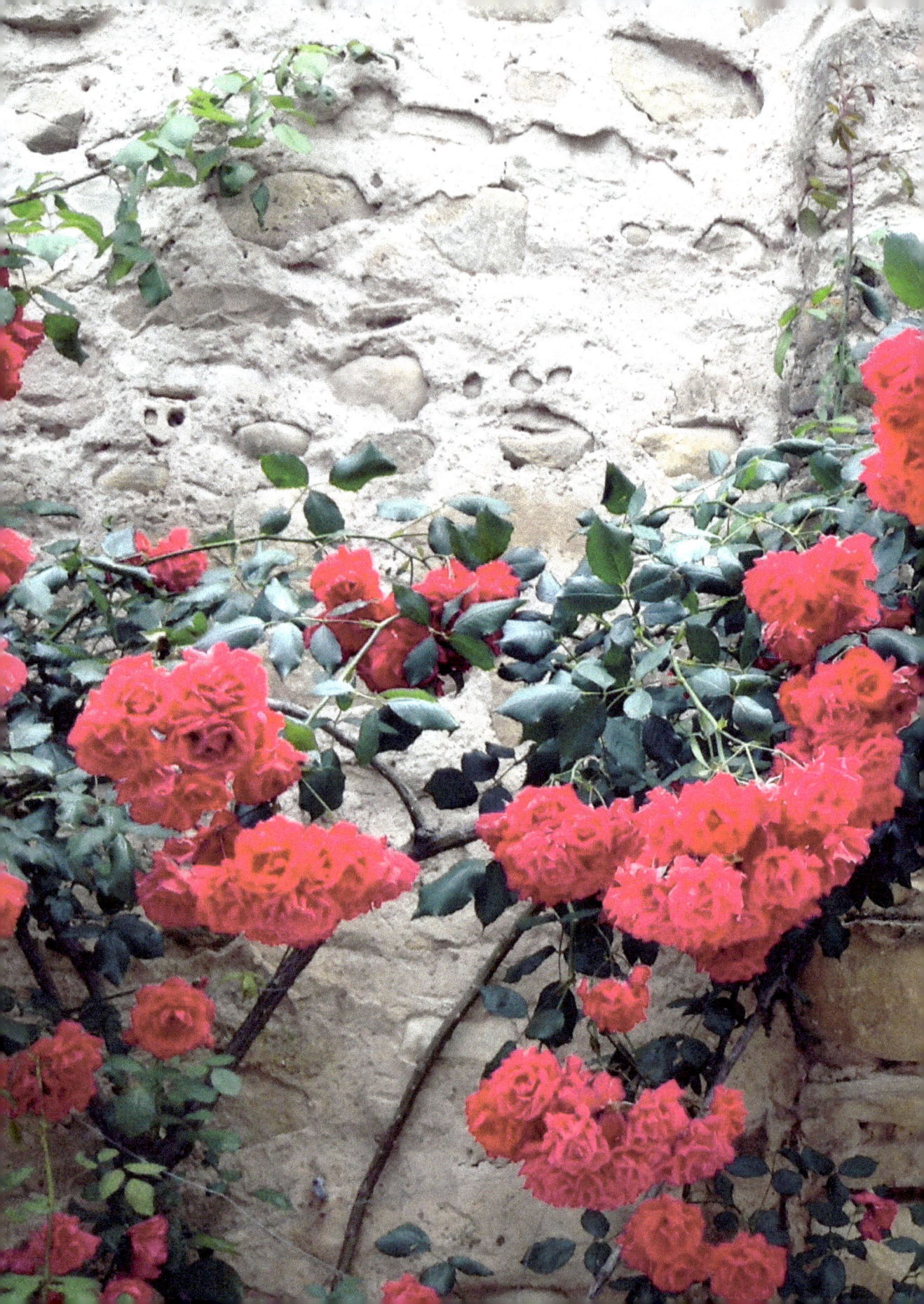

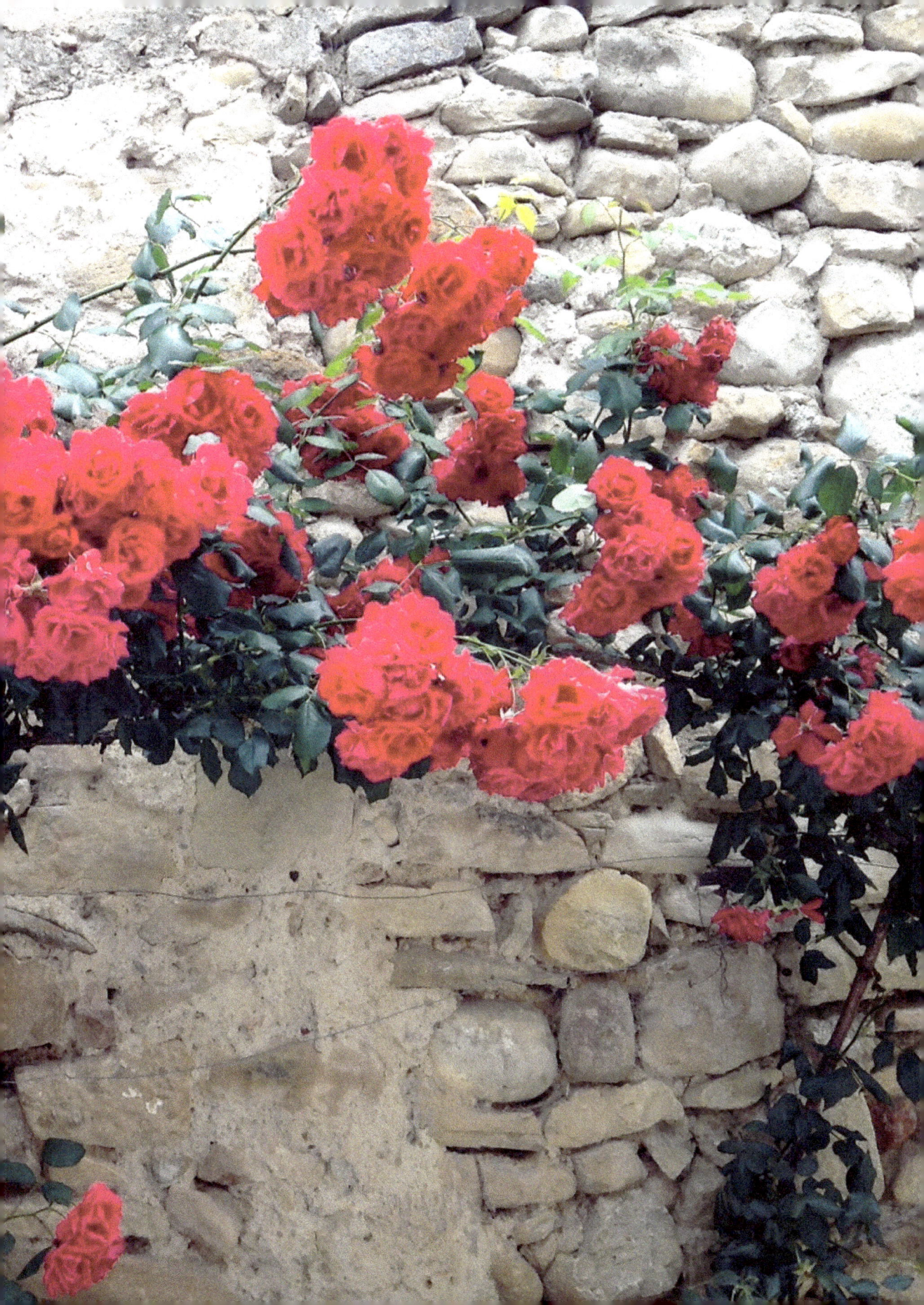

S
RVICIO

 CORRe

Kindness of Others

"No act of kindness, no matter how small, is ever wasted" -Aesop

I love Spain's postal system! One mistake I made during my Camino experience is not trusting my ability to communicate in Spanish and to navigate the postal system. Before leaving for the Camino, I spent several weeks preparing boxes of supplies to send to myself in Spain along the Camino. I knew the post office would keep a package for a pilgrim for 15 days. I did not know how long it would take for the packages to arrive in Spain, so I sent them about 3 weeks before my arrival. The packages contained new flip-flops, grass-fed beef jerky, dried salmon, dried anchovies, beef fat, dried liver powder, dried gelatin powder, toothpowder, a small 1/2" X 1/2" soap square, 7-10 soapnuts, a week's worth of small maps and notes and torn out daily reading pages. I sent 5 boxes, one each to Pamplona, León, Astorga, Sarria, Santiago. None of the packages arrived in time!

When I realized my mistake in Pamplona, I quickly redid my strategy. I had researched shops that I knew would have the highest quality pure foods, so I bought large quantities of these foods and sent the packages ahead to myself. In every postal office employees treated me with the utmost kindness, patience and generosity. I was awed by their munificence! I also was so grateful to receive all of the missed packages once I had returned home to the United States. Spanish postal system: M I R A C L E !

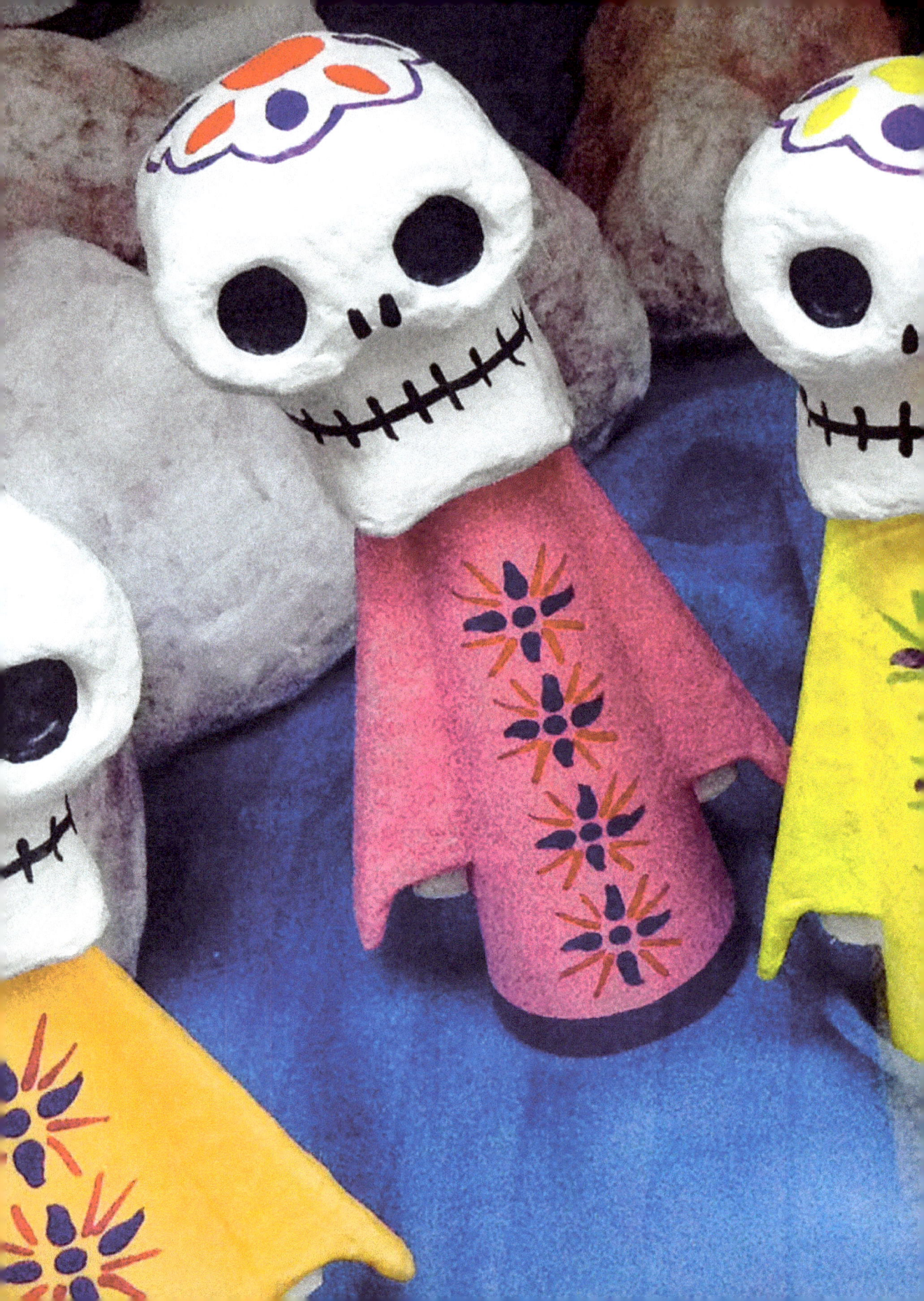

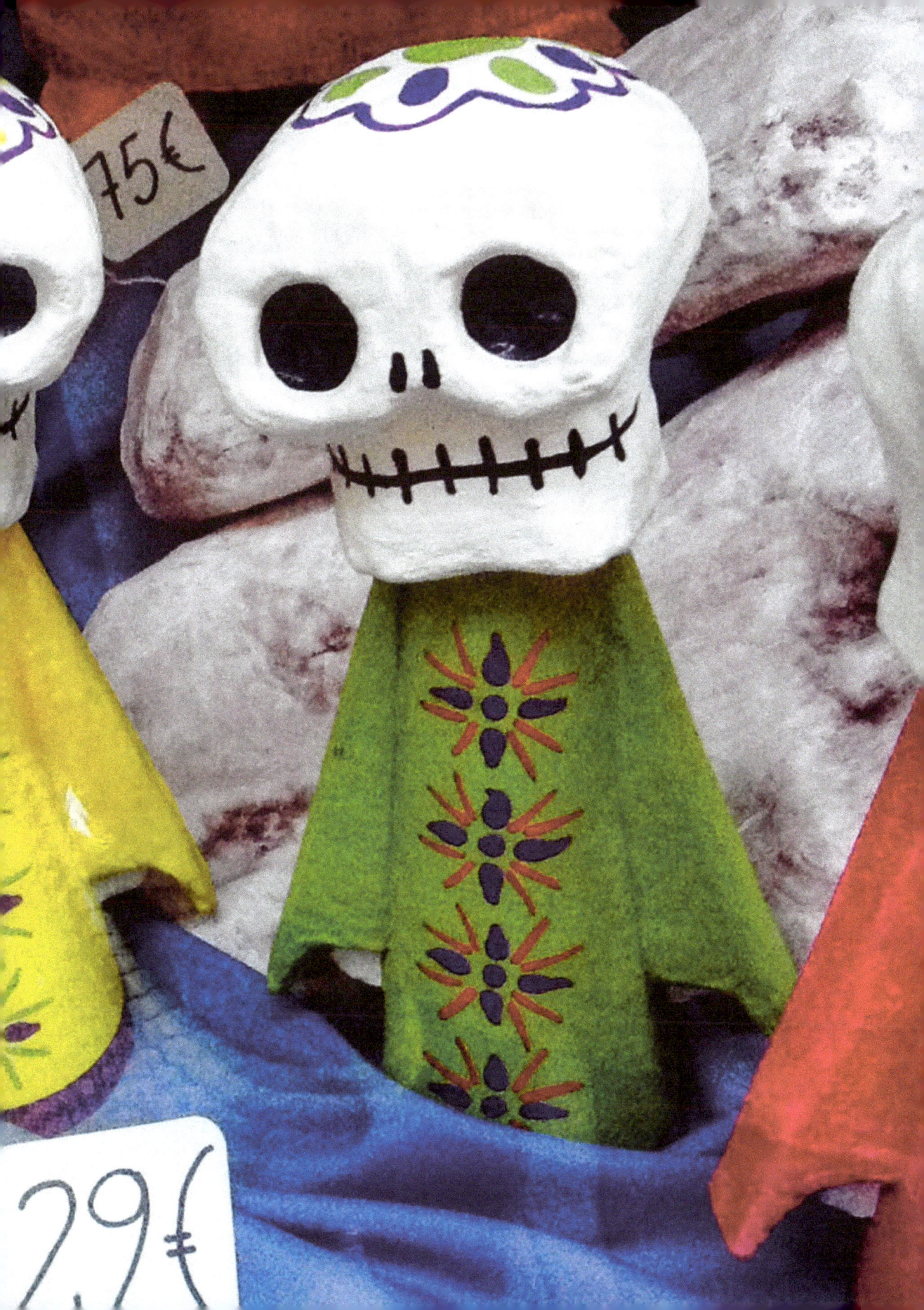

POSTAL SYSTEM INFORMATION
(CORREO INFORMACION)

*Paseo Sarasate 9
31080 Pamplona (Navarre)

Perez Caldo 44
26080 Logrono (La Rioja)

*Plaza Conde de Castro 1
09080 Burgos

Jardines de San Francisco s/n
24080 León

*Alférez Provisional 3
24700 Astorga (León)

Calle General Vives 1
24400 Ponferrada (León)

*Calle Calvo Sotelo 183
27600 Sarria (Lugo)

*Orfas 17
15703 Santiago de Compostela (A Coruña)

example: PAULISICH. LAURA (PEREGRINO)
LISTA de CORREOS
ORFAS 17
15703 SANTIAGO de COMPOSTELA (A Coruña)

translations
post office: correo
general delivery: lista de correos
"Post Restante to Santiago" (will keep 30 days)

*the offices I used while hiking the Camino Francés

FITNESS
BRAZIL

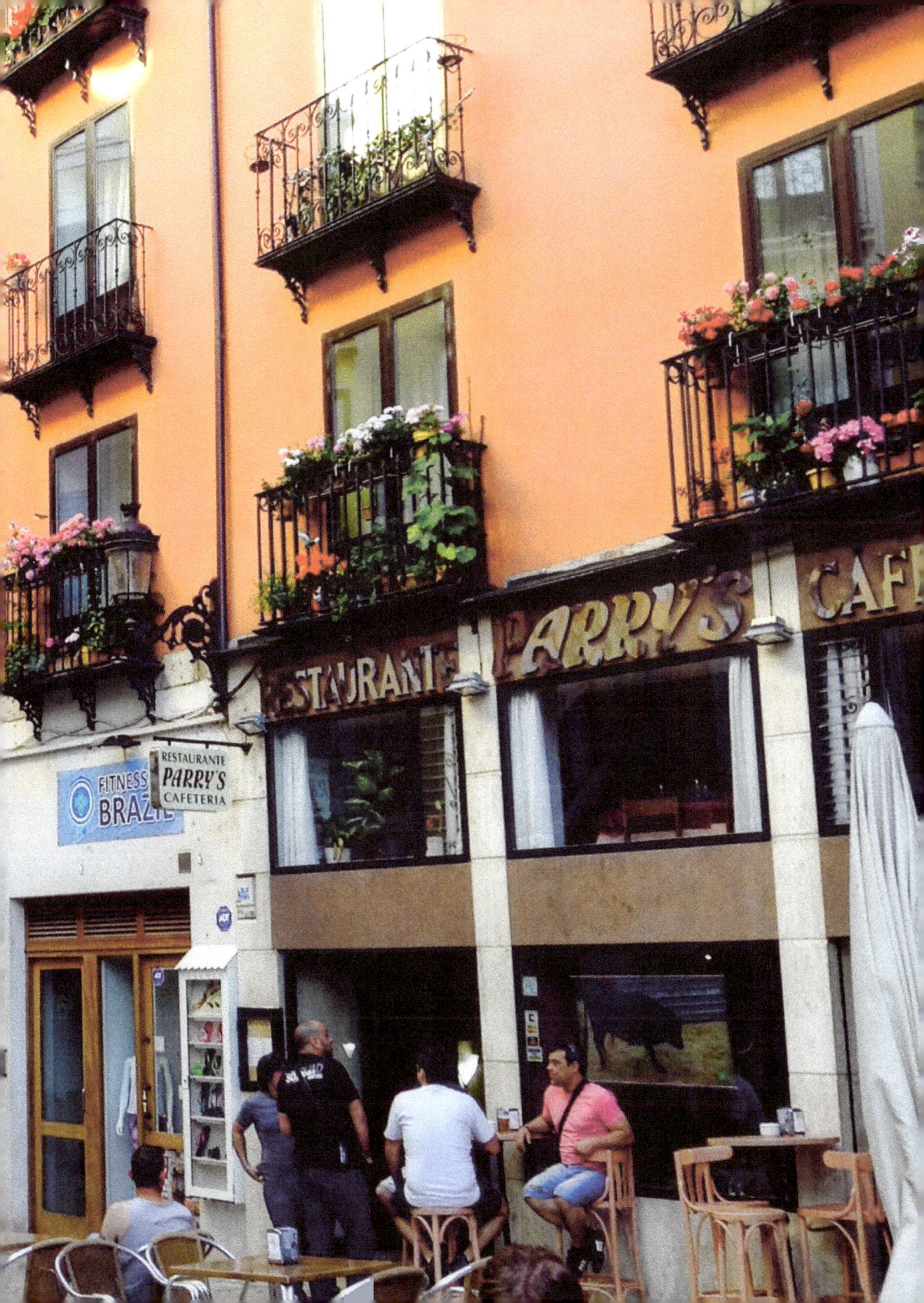

RESTAURANTE
PARRY'S
CAFETERIA

RESTAURANTE PARRY'S CAF

BUYING GUIDE

Clothing
www.gaiaconceptions.com
Stash Simplicity Mini Skirt $75
Tube Dress $85
Eos Shirt $60
all in sandalwood natural dye

Silk
www.sleepnbeauty.com
100% Mulberry Silk Sheet Set (Twin) $440

Filtering Water Bottle
www.clearlyfiltered.com
Stainless Steel Filter Bottle $46.95

Backpack
www.rawganique.com
Reincarnation Recycled Tarp Road Warrior Backpack $95

Undergarments
www.cottonique.com
Women's Low-Rise Contoured Brief (2-pack) $27.75

Flip-flops
www.feelgoodz.com
Classicz Sand $24.99
Lizzielooms Felicity $29.99

Parasol
www.jedicreations.com
Cotton Waterproof Hand Parasols in Solid Color with Bonnet $50

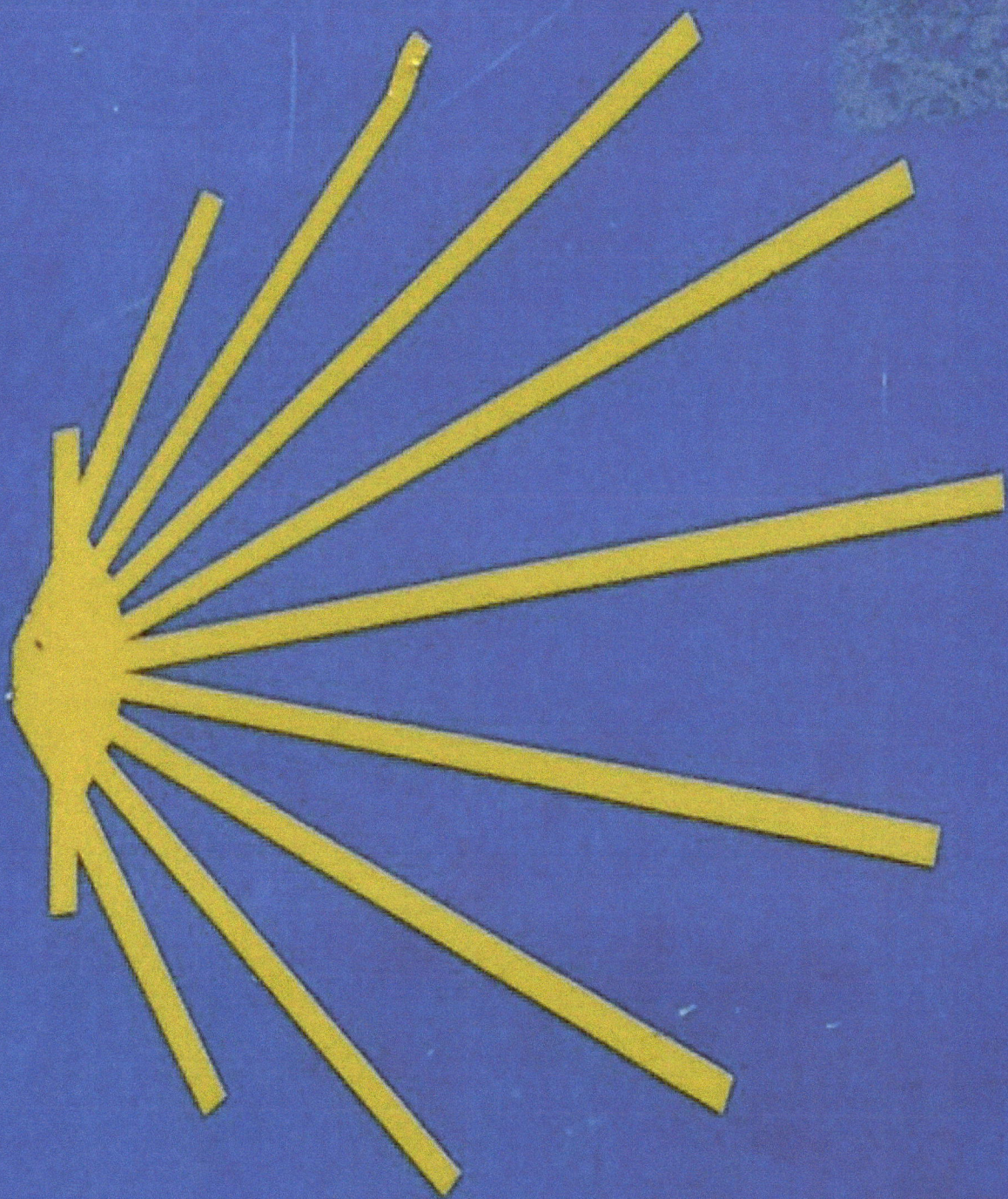

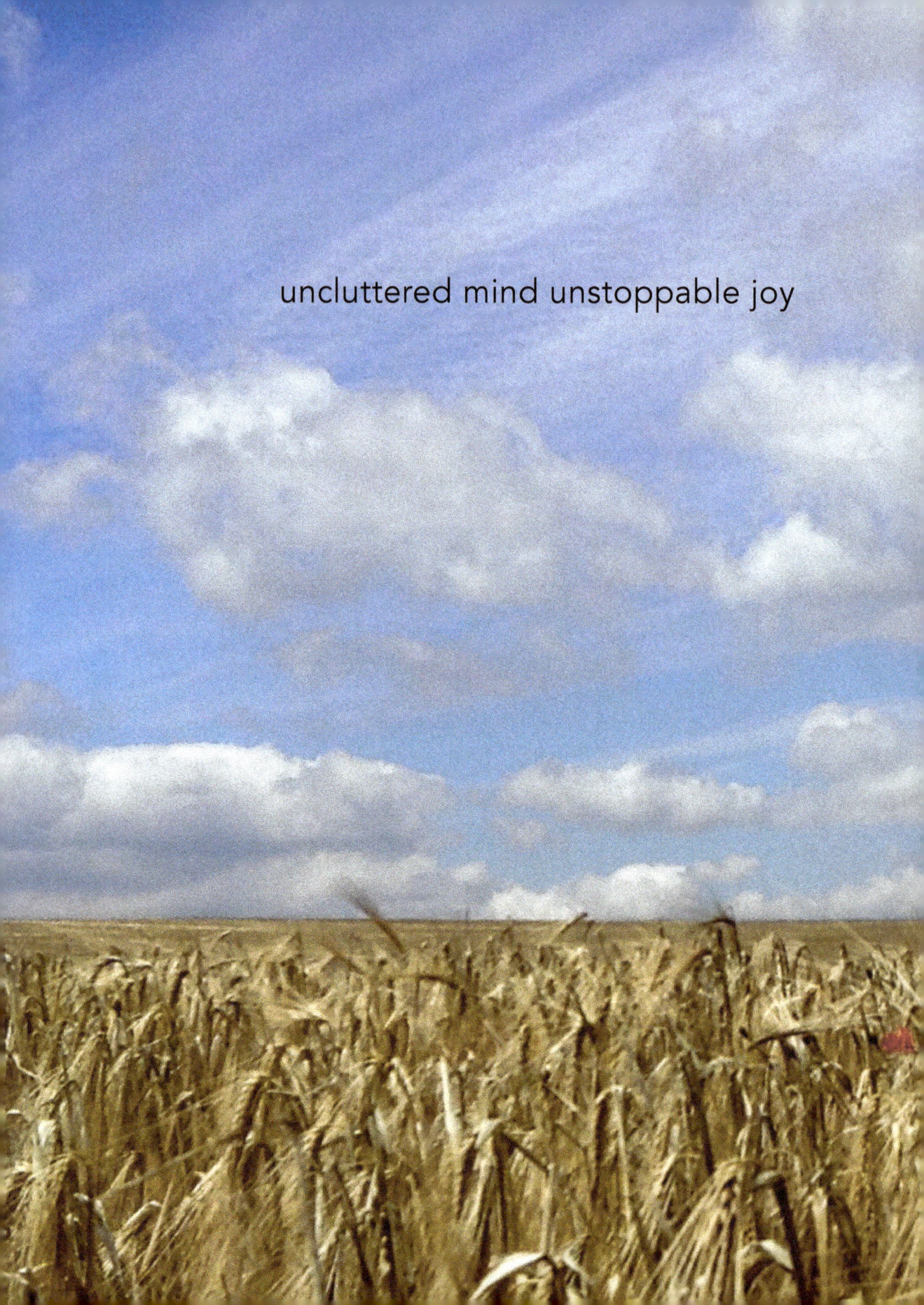

uncluttered mind unstoppable joy

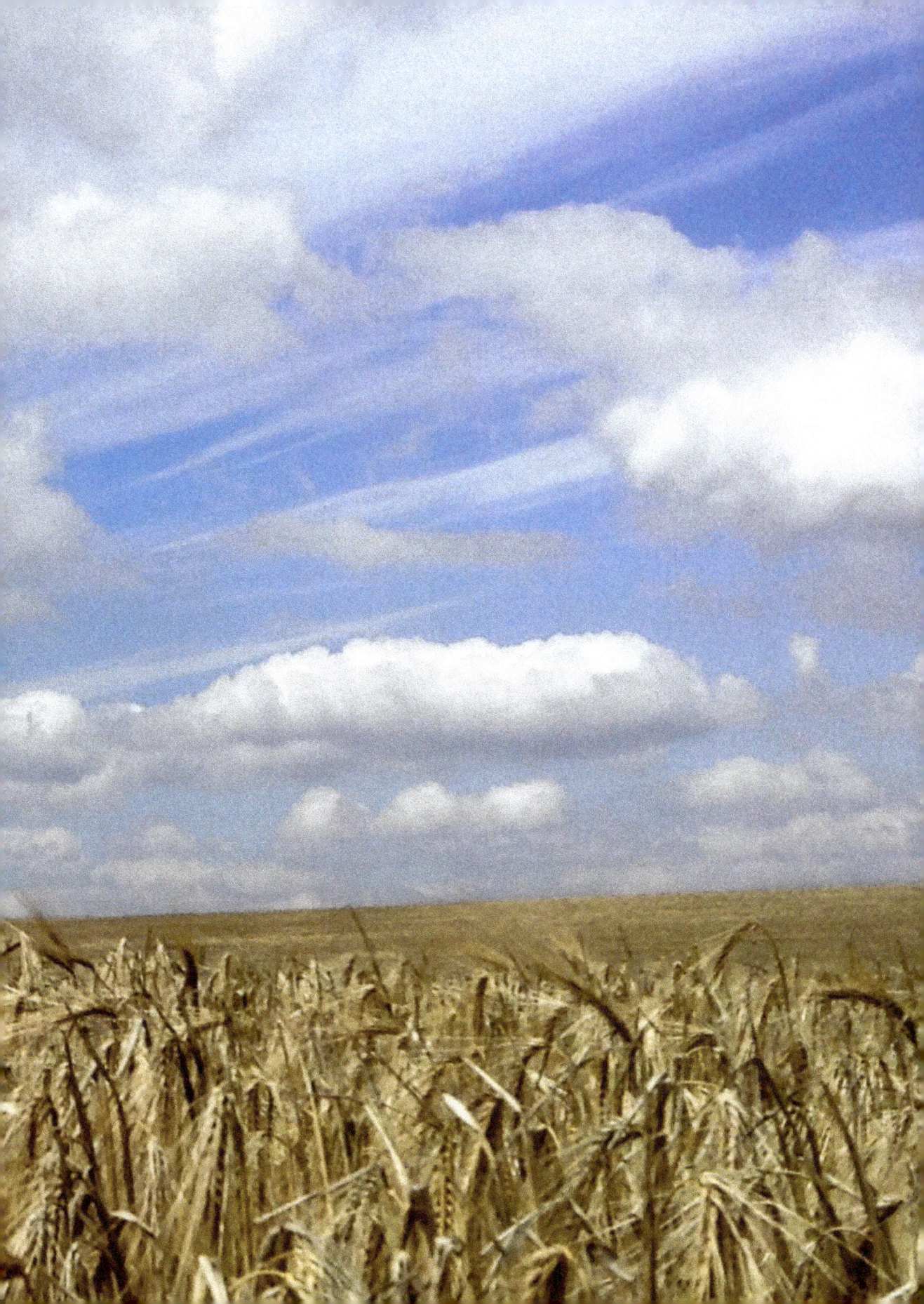

food

CHEESE CHORIZO OLIVE OIL

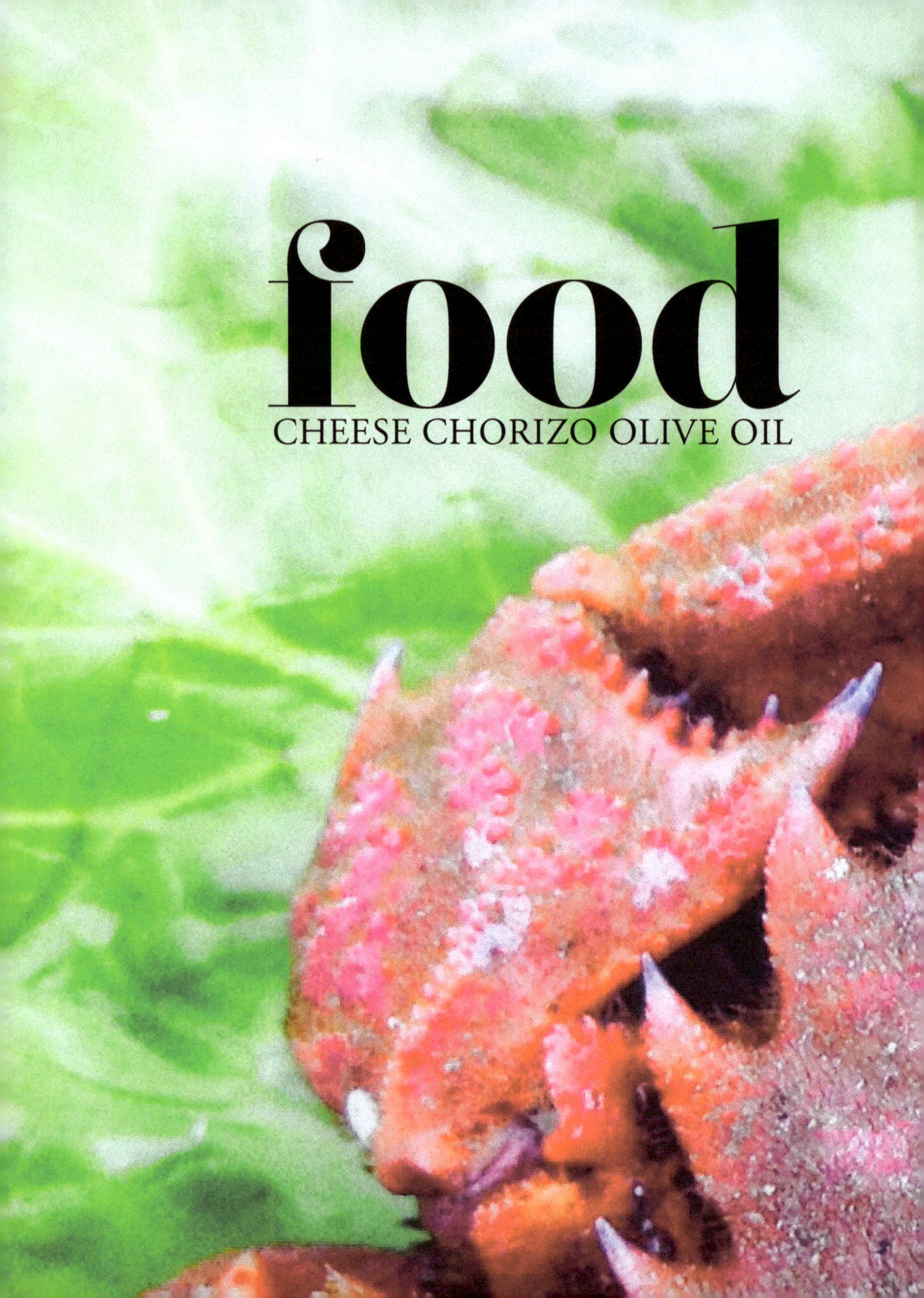

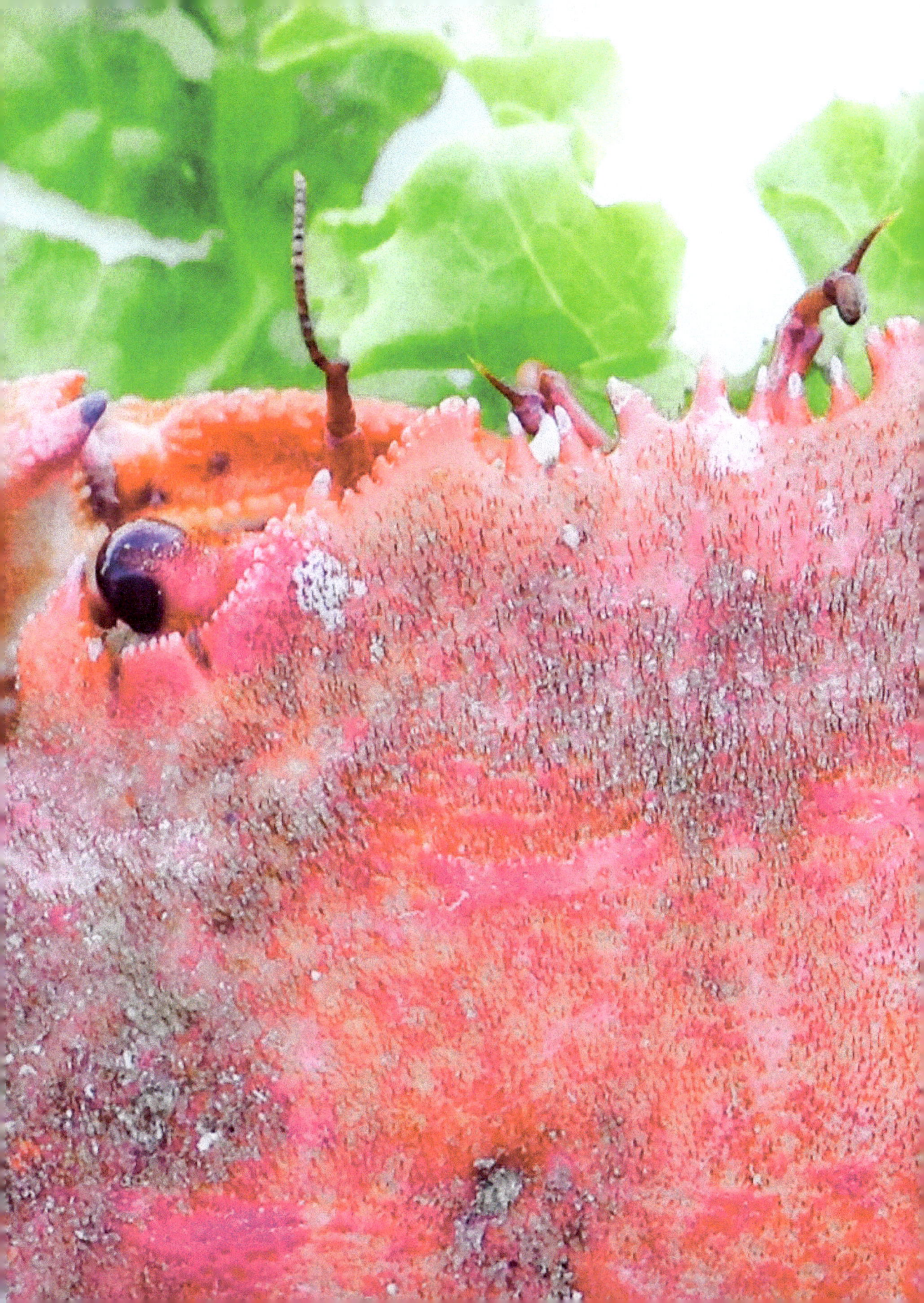

"There is a nutritional basis for modern physical, mental and moral degeneration."
-Dr. Weston Price

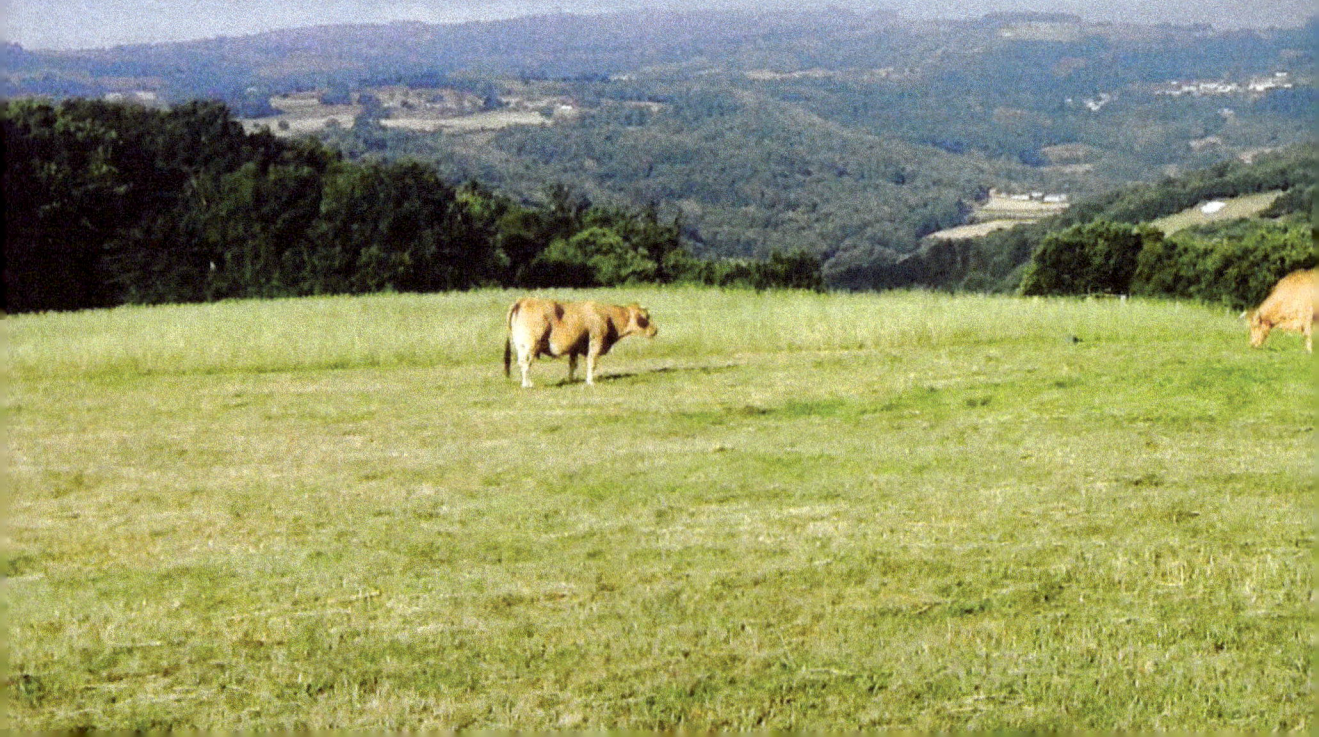

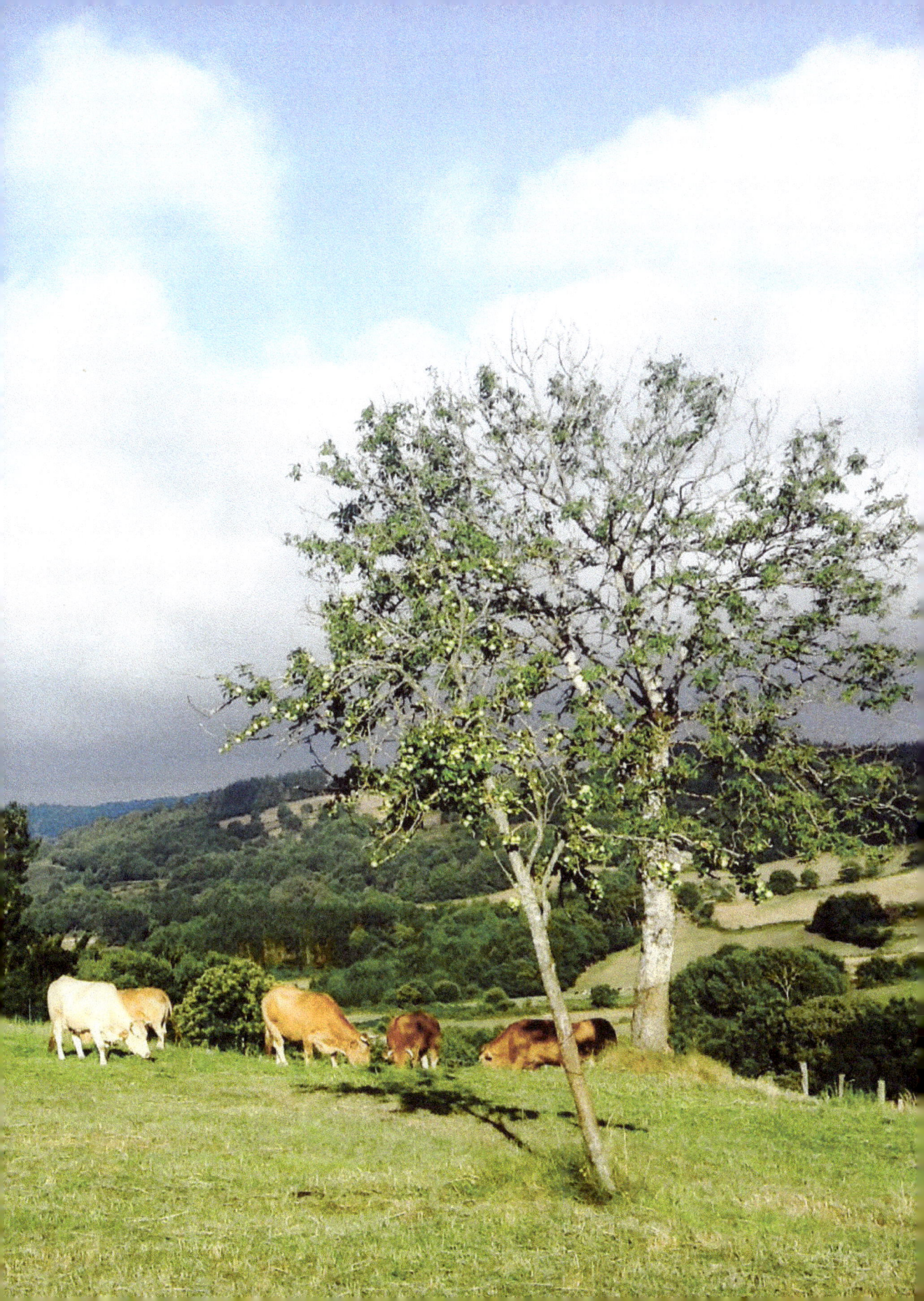

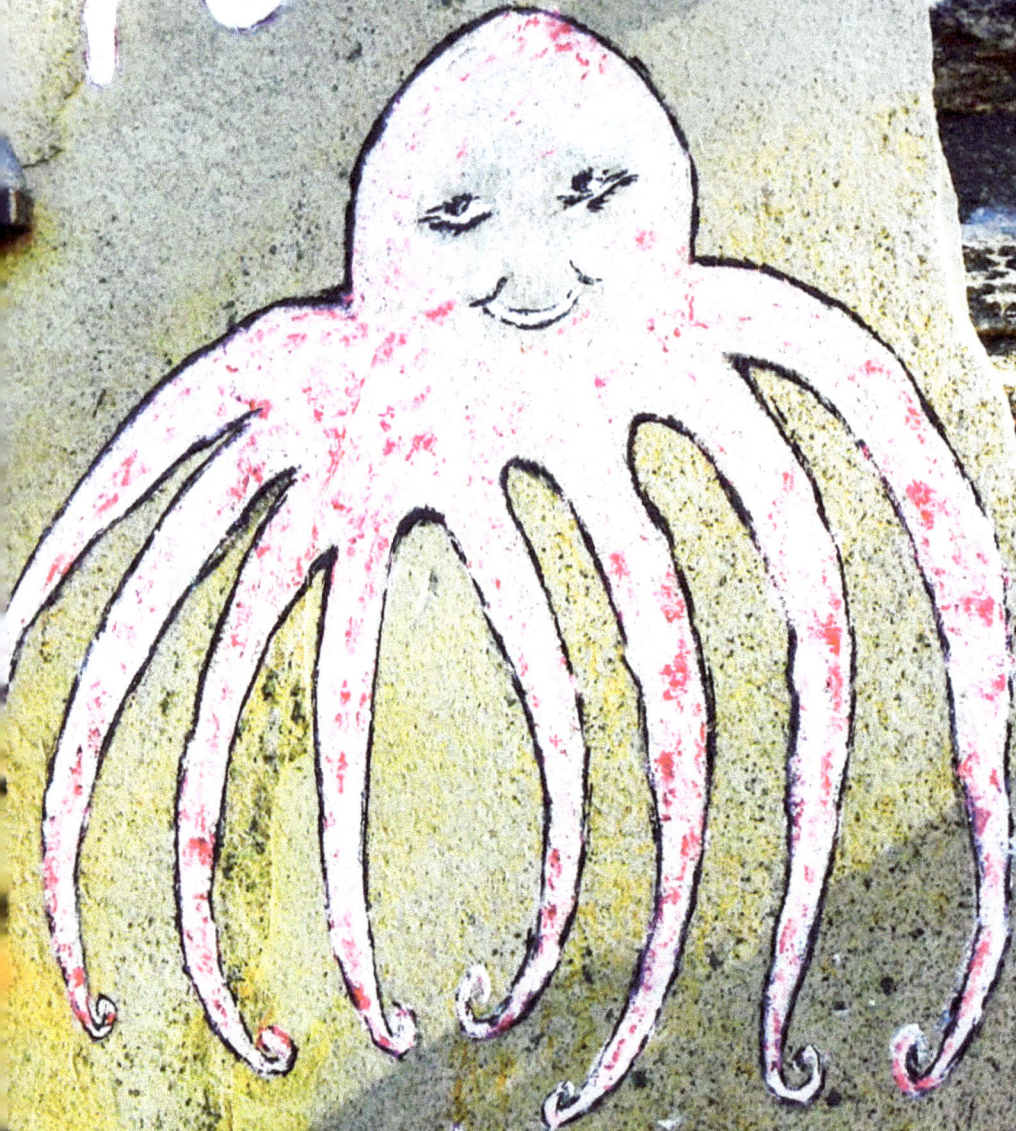

During the months of preparation, I revisited many nutrition books to remind myself of foods that I could find while hiking that would meet my nutritional requirements. It was great fun because I had forgotten some of the information. For instance, chorizo meets several vitamin and 4 mineral requirements. I knew that if I could find chorizo made from animals with natural diets I would be able to eat it without compromising my meticulous dietary habits. I also found out that paprika meets all mineral and almost all vitamin requirements. Spain produces world-renowned paprika!

Chorizo was looking like the ideal food because it is made with pork fat and paprika, it is fermented, and I could carry it without refrigeration. Aged cheeses would also be portable but had to be unpasteurized and from grass-fed animals to be the most nutritionally beneficial. I started researching sources for food. I started with the Weston Price Foundation Spain chapters but had no luck. I then searched endlessly online for chorizo, cheese, and olive oil sources. With months of research and the beautiful foods of Spain, I was able to remain in ketosis while meeting all of my nutritional needs. M I R A C L E !

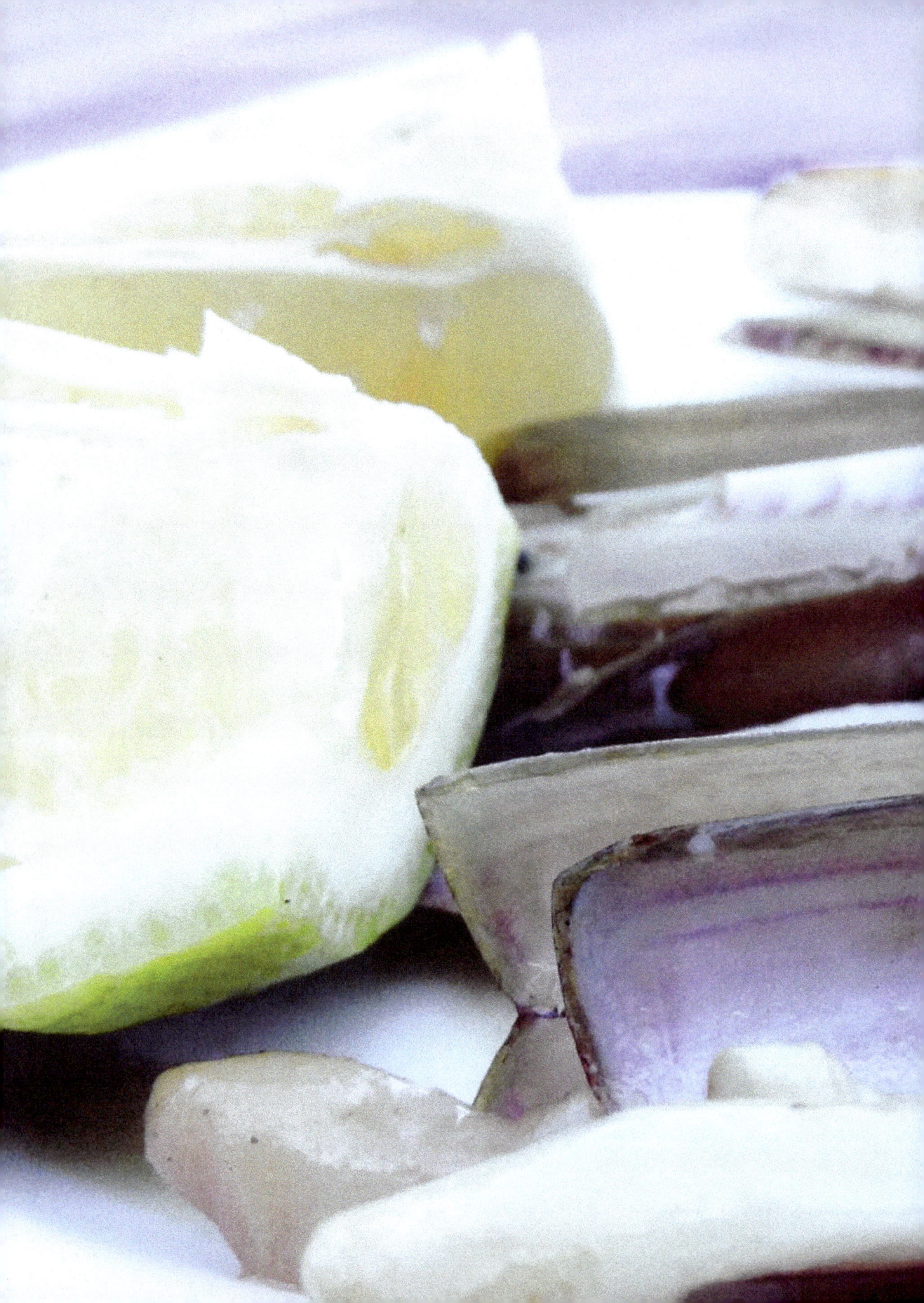

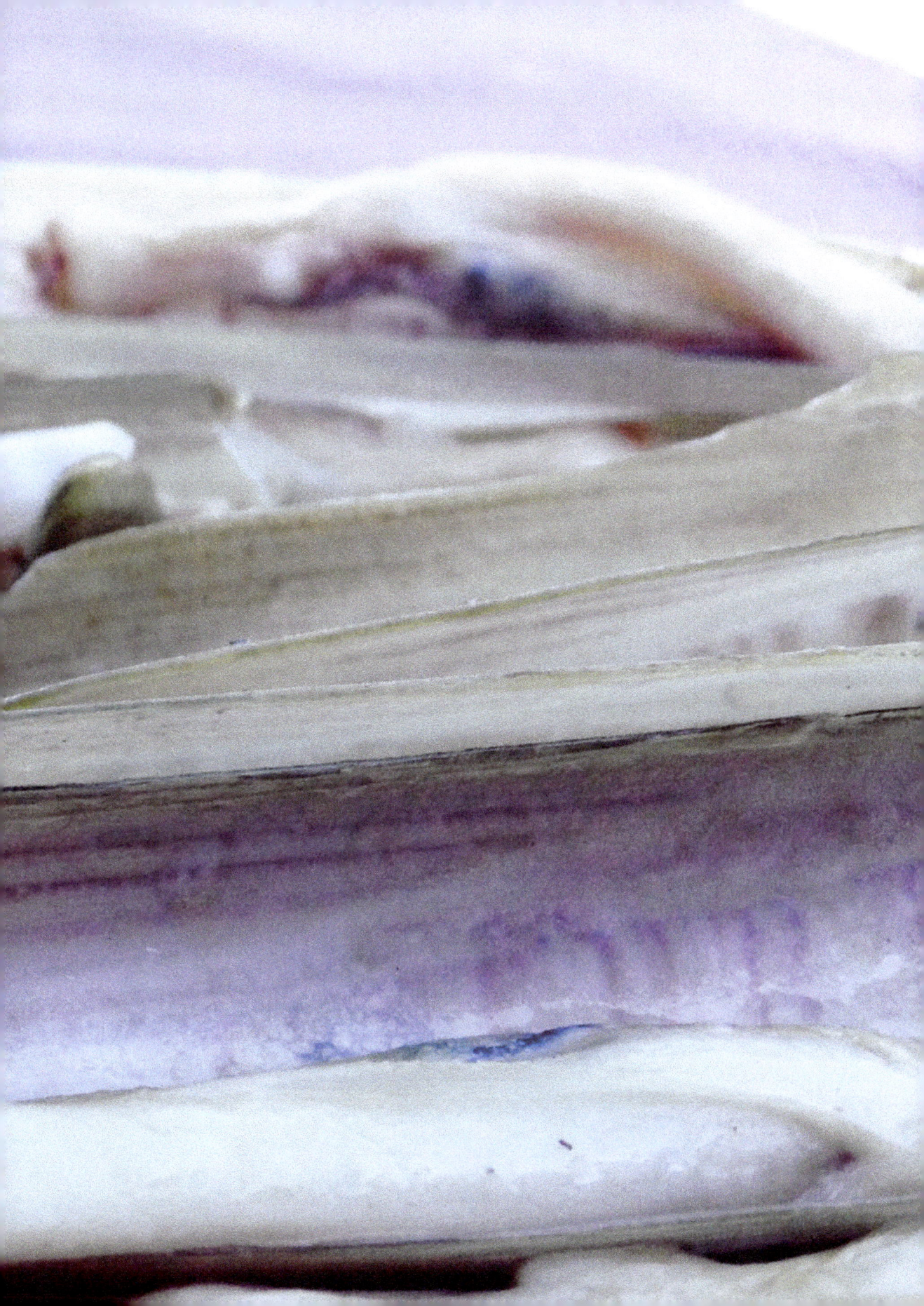

STAYING IN KETOSIS

I have an impeccable diet at home, and I knew this would be one of my biggest challenges while walking the Camino. At home, it has taken me a few years to find the best sources of food the U.S.A. has to offer. I knew that while walking, it would be impossible to locate farmers and talk to them about their animals, the diets of their animals and their soil conditions. I had heard that in all of Europe it is much easier to find foods grown, raised and prepared using traditional methods. I also assumed that the use of chemicals to grow animals, fields, and other foods would not exist as much as in the United States.

My first ideas of "safe" foods to eat were olive oil and seafood. I remembered reading in a book about nutrition that the island of Crete has some of the most healthy humans, and the author wrote that many of the farmers would drink olive oil for breakfast. I had never thought of this idea before, and it really made an impact on me. Because the majority of my calories come from fat, I knew that I would be okay because I would be traveling to some of the most famous olive oil territories in the world! M I R A C L E !

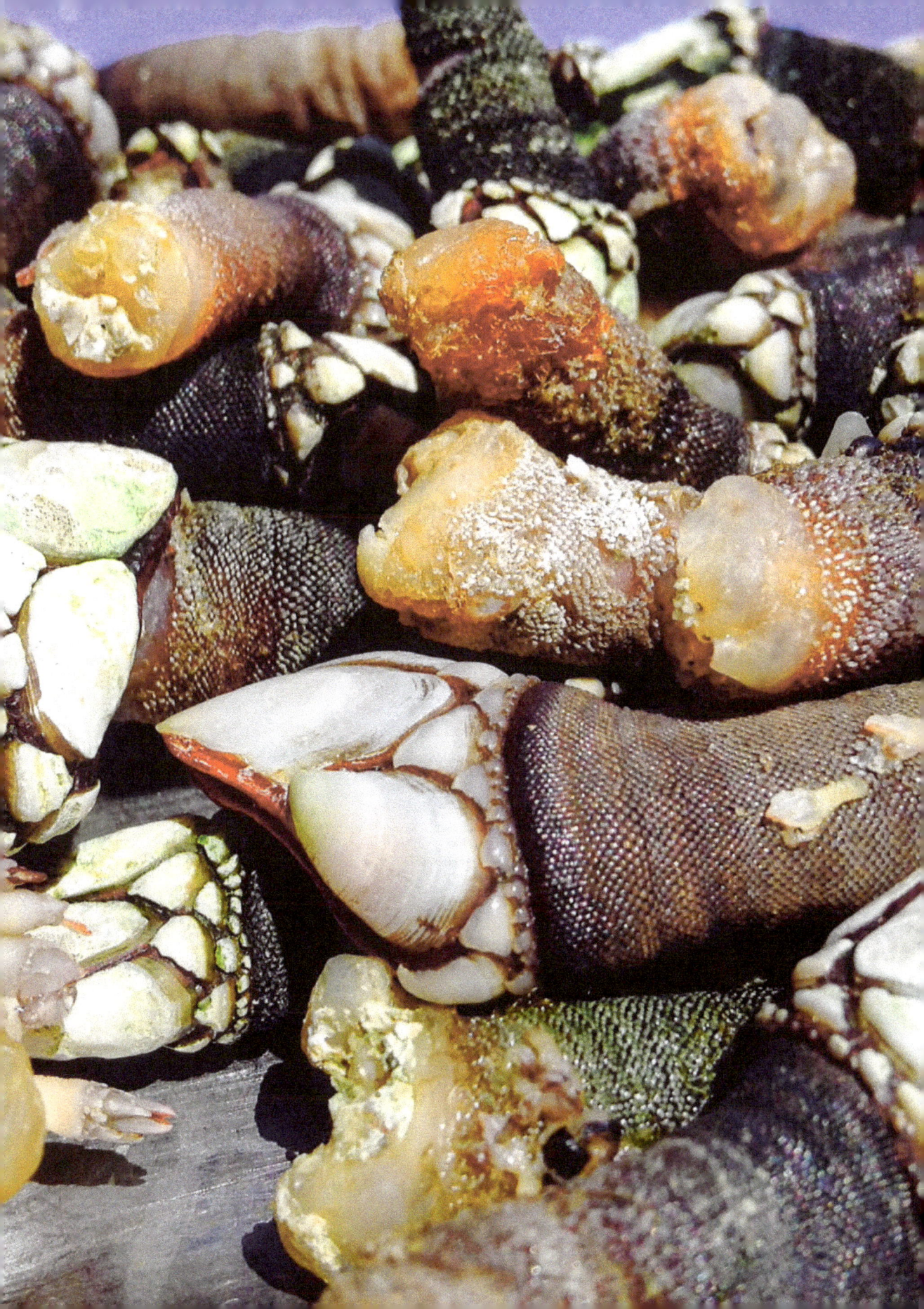

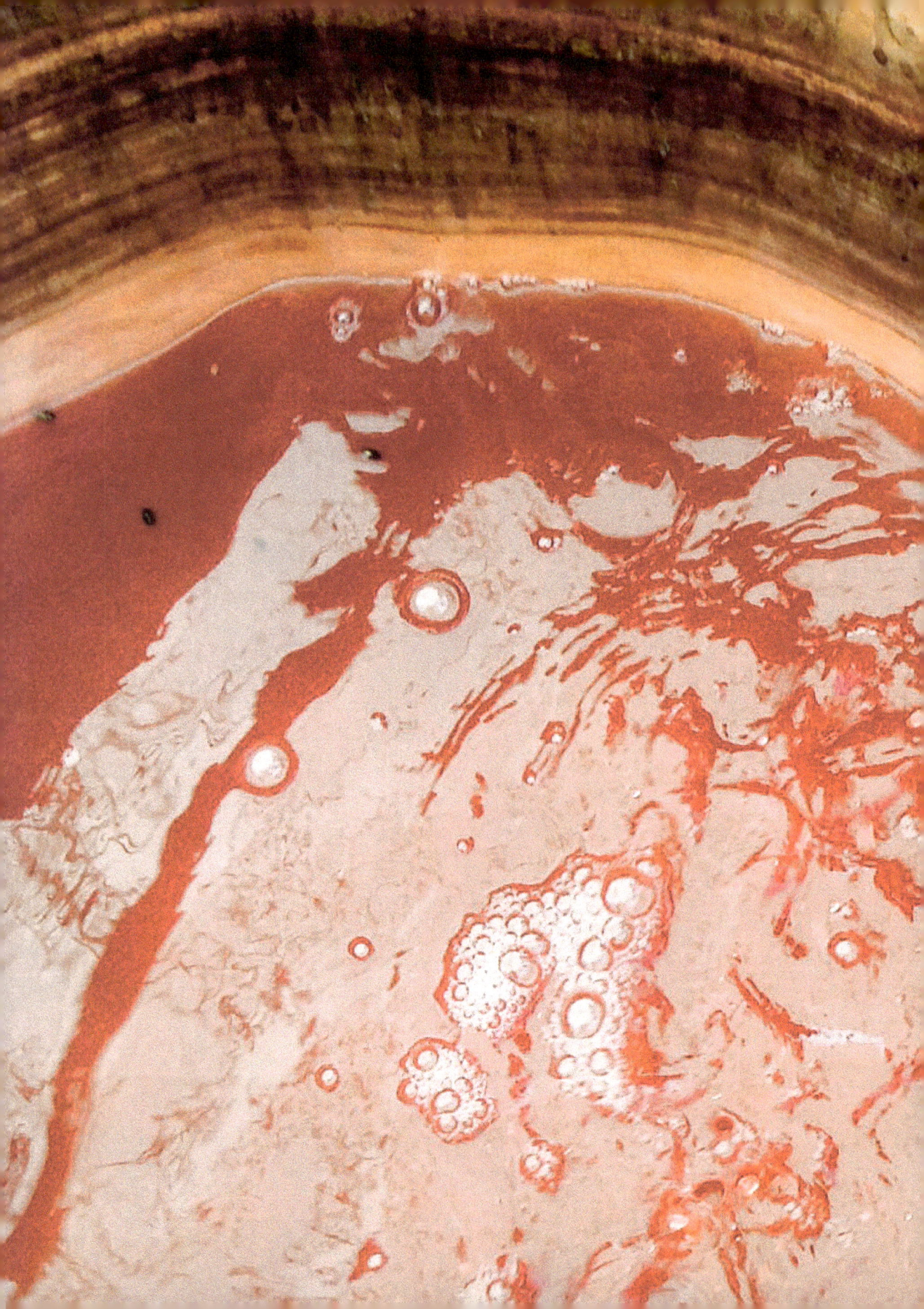

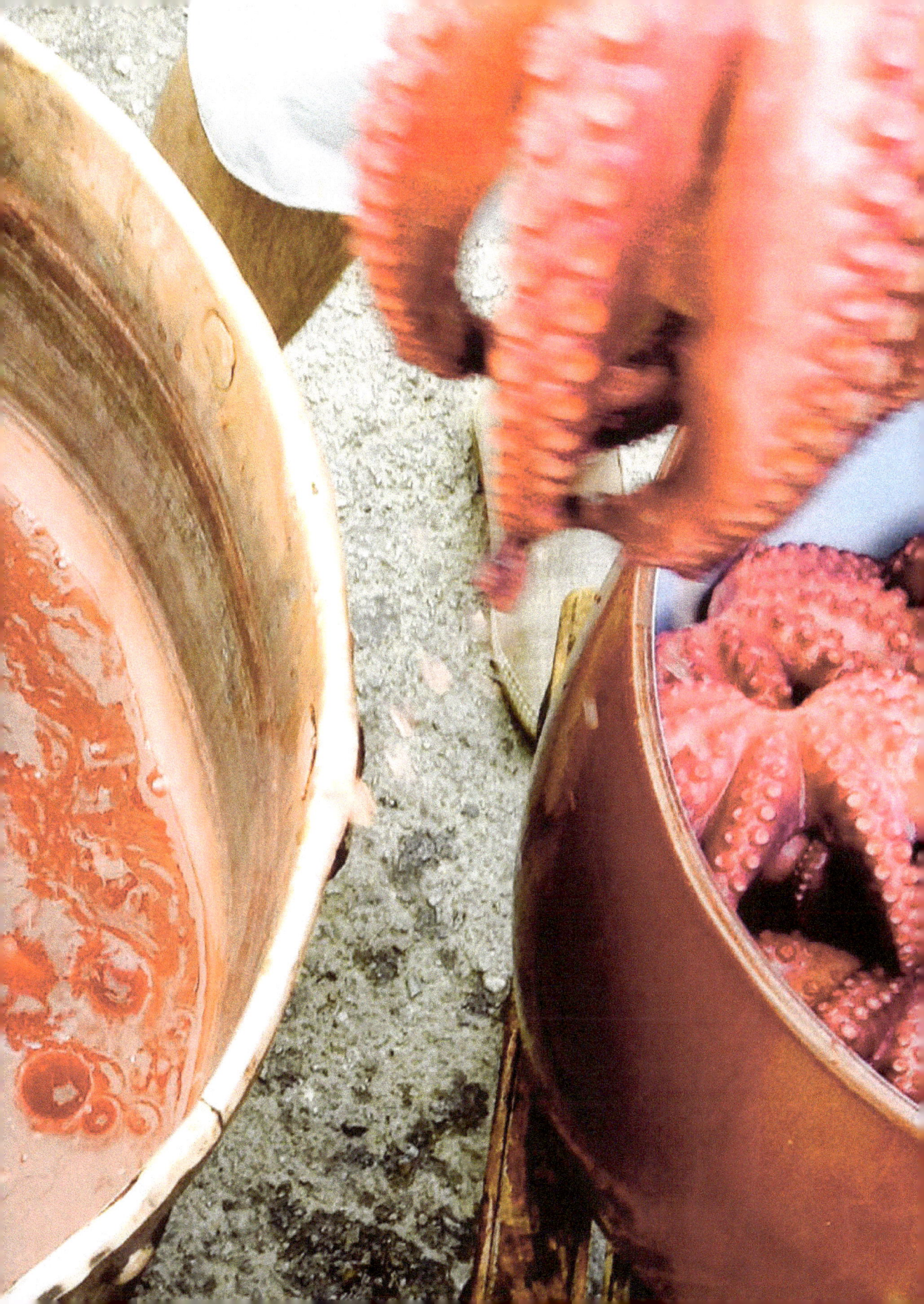

"Dr Steve Phinney and Dr Jeff Volek
have noted that a sugar-burner has only about 2,000 calories' worth of
energy stored in [his/her] body while a fat-burner has over 40,000 calories'
worth of fuel-more than twenty-times as much!"
-Jimmy Moore & Maria Emmerich *The Ketogenic Cookbook*

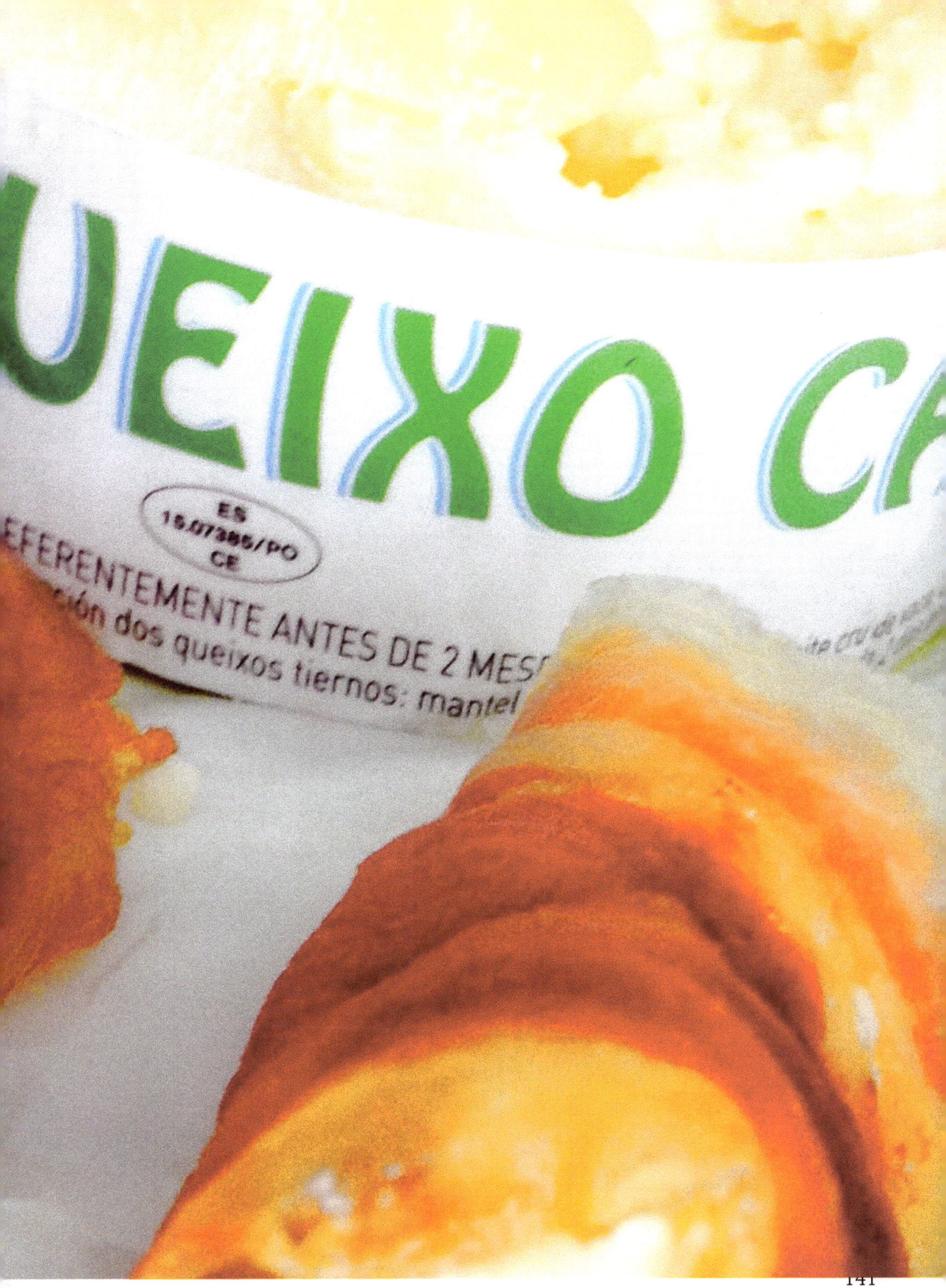

UEIXO CA

ES
18.07386/PO
CE

EFERENTEMENTE ANTES DE 2 MES
ón dos queixos tiernos: mantel

NUTRIENT-DENSE FOODS

by Mathieu Lalonde, PhD, Harvard University
Nutrient Density Score Ranking

1. Organ meats and oils

2. Herbs and spices

3. Nuts and seeds

4. Cacao

5. Fish and seafood

6. Pork

7. Beef

8. Eggs and dairy

9. Vegetables (raw and unprepared)

10. Lamb, veal, and wild game

11. Poultry

12. Legumes (raw or cooked edible)

13. Processed meat

14. Vegetables (cooked, blanched, canned, pickled)

15. Plant fats and oils

16. Fruit

17. Animal skin and feet

18. Grains and pseudocereals (cooked)

19. Refined and processed fats and oils

20. Animal fats and oils

21. Grains (canned)

22. Processed fruit

- Jimmy Moore & Maria Emmerich

amespea

Arzúa co

zúa Chee

zúa Kase

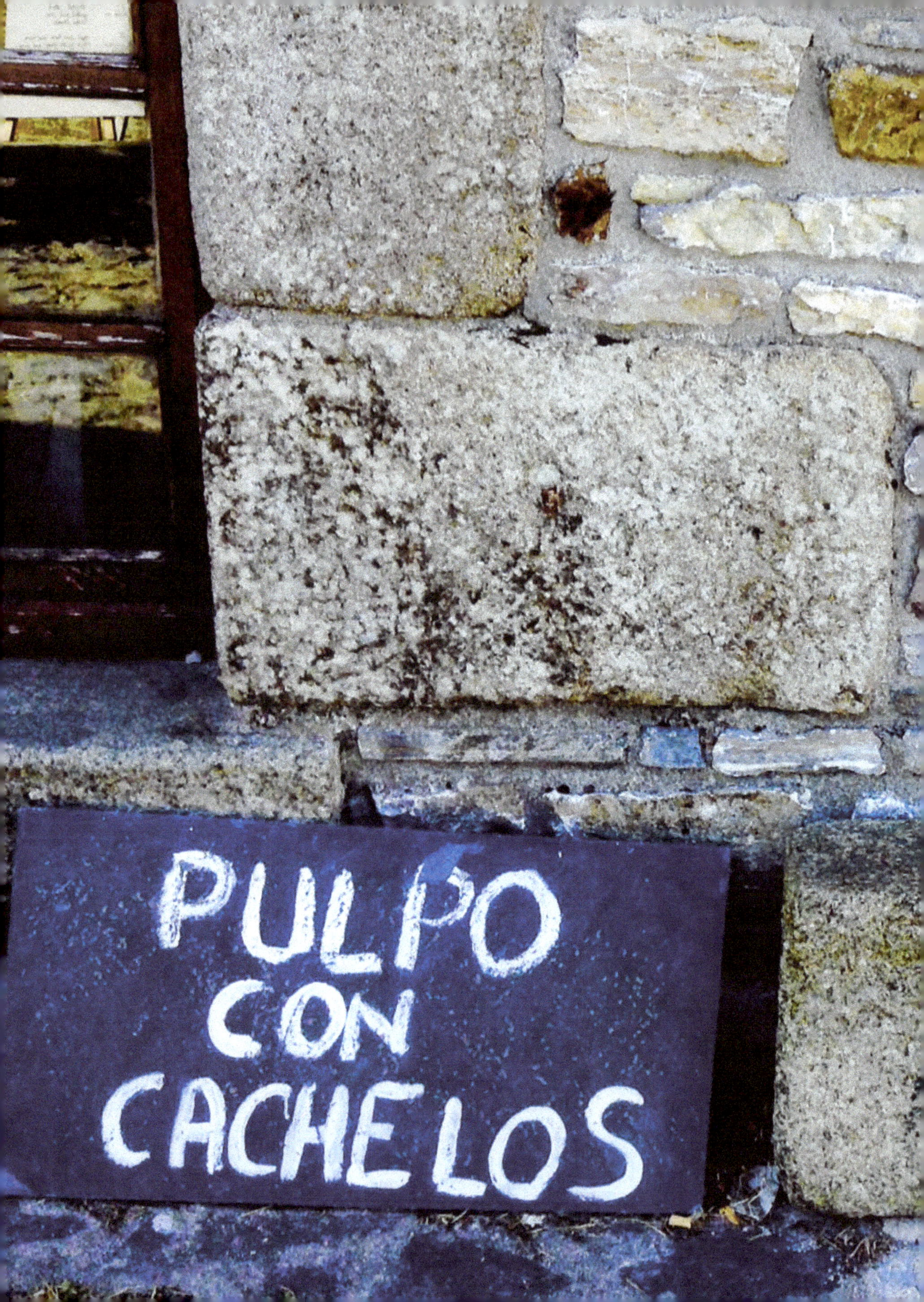

PULPO
CON
CACHELOS

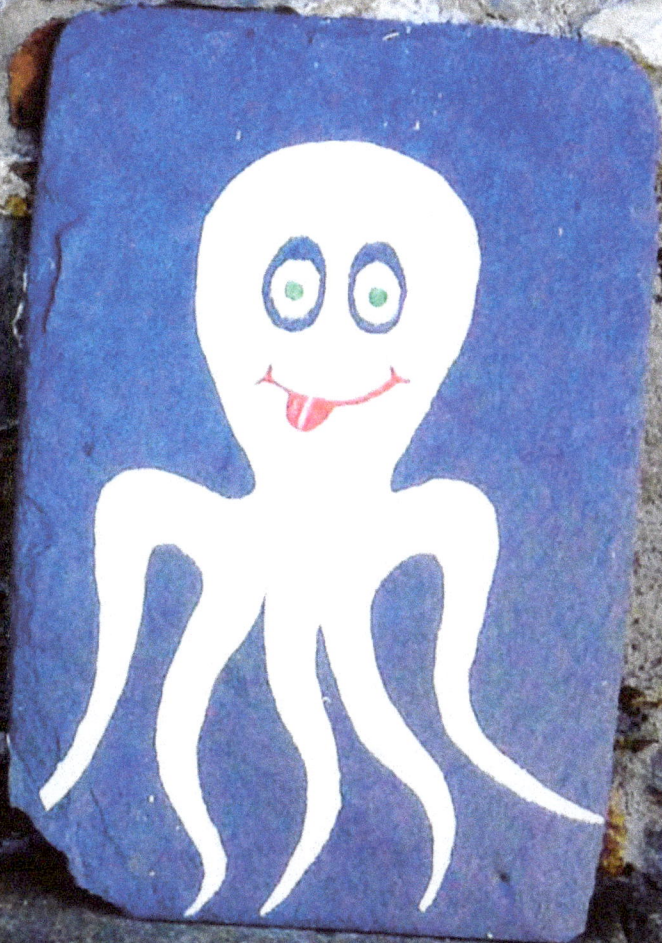

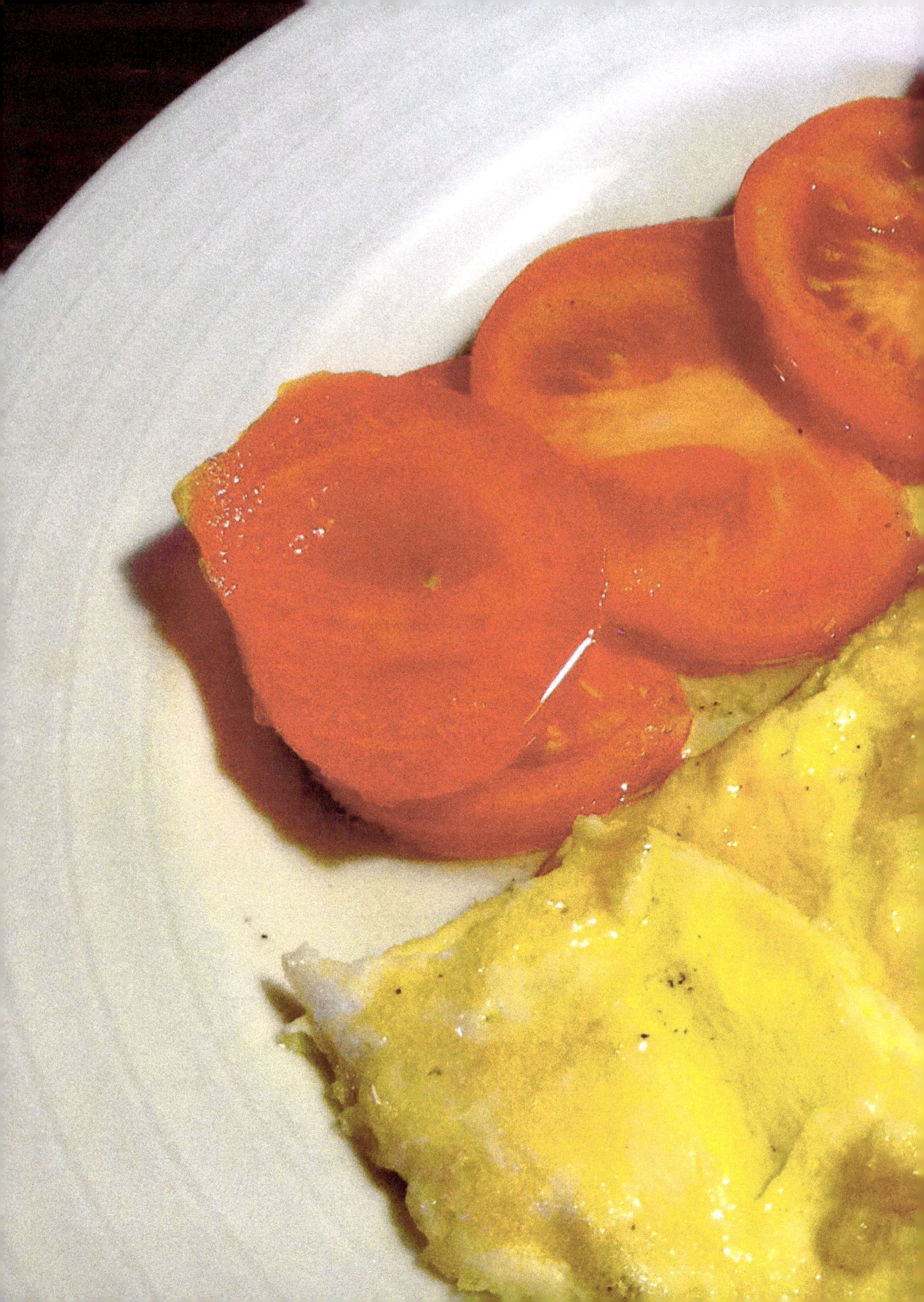

FOODS I ATE ON THE CAMINO

1. aged raw-milk cheese from pastured animals
2. Ibérico de bellota (semi-wild pig eating 100% Holm Oak acorn diet)
3. traditionally-made chorizo from pastured animals
4. traditionally-made and chemically-free/organic olive oil
5. canned sardines in olive oil & sea salt
6. canned octopus in water
7. local organic bottled & canned asparagus in water & sea salt
8. canned cod liver in oil
9. avocado
10. local eggs from small village homes
11. tomatoes, red lettuce, basil, cucumbers
12. 100% cacao
13. paprika
14. bacon made with only salt from pastured animals
15. fresh octopus, barnacles, crab, clam, squid

FOODS I EAT AT HOME

*eggs *bison/beef/lamb/chicken/goose/elk meat/organs *many fresh organic herbs & homemade spices *wild Alaskan salmon *salmon roe *oysters *clams *pork belly *bison/beef/chicken bone broth *pork/chicken/lamb/beef/bison/duck fat *cave-aged, raw-milk cheese *butter/ghee/clarified butter *créme fraîch *heavy cream *olive/coconut/cod liver oil *homemade pickles *lemon/lime *avocado *homemade mustard *homemade sauces & mayonaise *arugula/watercress *Himalayan salt

HIGH-FAT FOODS
(& percentage of calories that come from dietary fat)
by Jimmy Moore

1. AVOCADOS - 82.5% fat

2. BUTTER - 100% fat

3. WHOLE EGGS - 61% fat

4. COCONUT OIL - 100% fat

5. BACON - 69.5% fat

6. SOUR CREAM - 88.5% fat

7. 70% GROUND BEEF - 59.5% fat

8. FULL-FAT CHEDDAR CHEESE - 74% fat

9. COCONUT - 88% fat

10. DARK CHOCOLATE - 65% fat

11. CREAM CHEESE - 88.5% fat

12. LIQUID FISH OIL - 100% fat

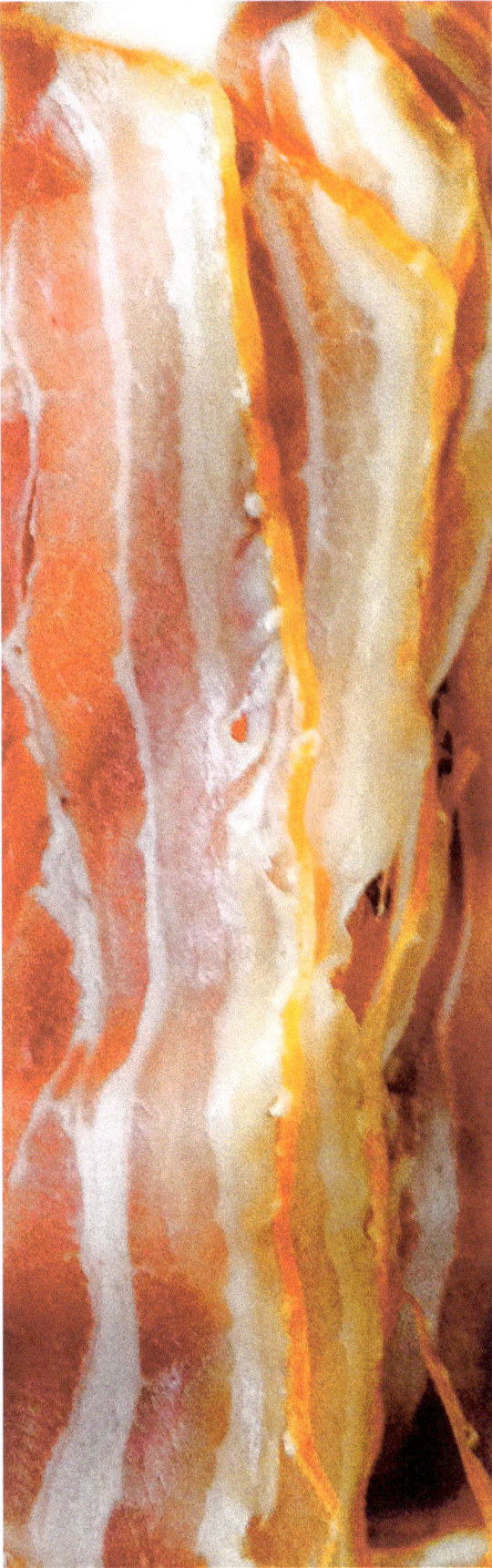
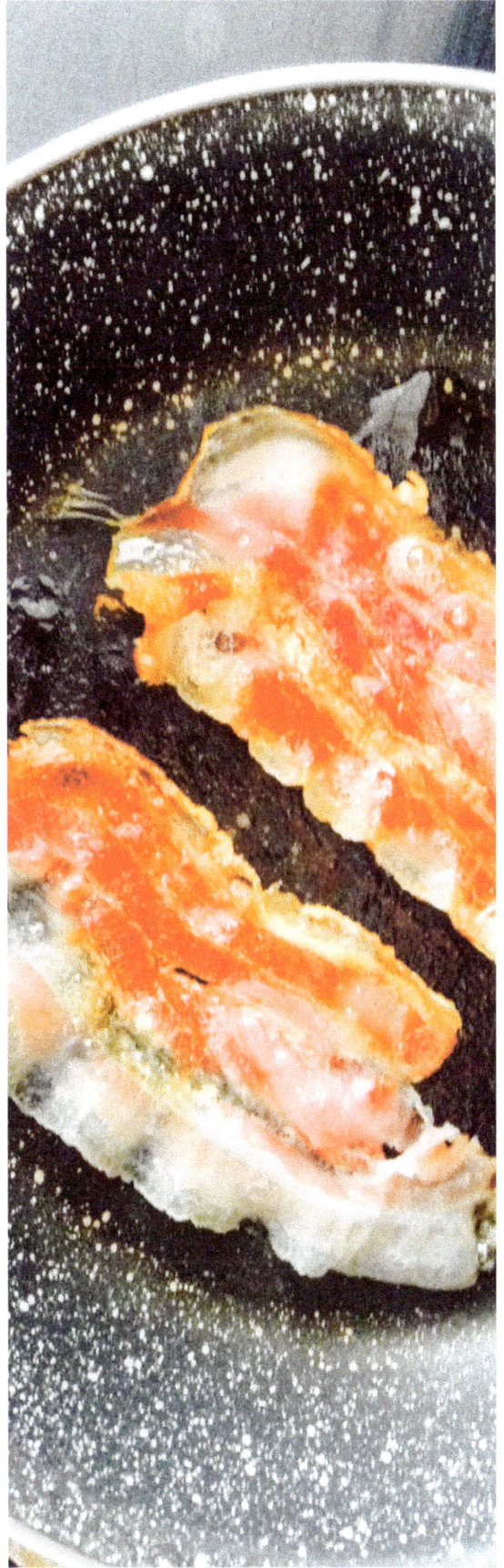

HELPFUL FOOD-FINDING RESOURCES

Paris
OLIVIERS & CO., 60 rue Vieille du Temple (Marais) www.oliviers-co.com/en, olive oil (harvest date month & year generally Oct-Jan. extra virgin cold-pressed) FROMAGERIE DUBOIS Saler's cheese (97-99 rue Saint Antoine)

St-Jean-Pied-de-Port
MEAT SHOP (rue de la Citadelle) Ibérico de bellota, raw grass-fed cheese

Pamplona
CASA TORRENS, San Miguel, 12 (+34 948 224 286) wild mushrooms, farm products, Ibérico de bellota, raw grass-fed cheese, most gracious customer service

Logrono
DE TORRE GOURMET, Garcia Morato, 25 (+34 941 241 018) www.detorregourmet.com Raw grass-fed cheese, Ibérico de bellota, Navarre white asparagus, 100% cacao, organic olive oil ***I purchased many foods here and then sent them ahead in weekly boxes to the future cities I would be visiting. I was able to carry a week's worth of food in my backpack and stay true to my impeccable diet while remaining in ketosis! The staff was miraculously helpful slicing the Ibérico de bellota and cheese and packaging them in individual daily serving sizes then air-sealing!

Burgos
DELICATESSEN OJEDA, Vitoria, 5 Plaza del Cordón (+34 947 20 4832) Raw grass-fed cheese, Ibérico de bellota, glass-bottled gourmet mushrooms, organic olive oil, cod liver tin***I purchased many foods here too and then sent them ahead in weekly boxes to the future cities I would be visiting. The post office is close to this store, so I made more than one trip!

Astorga
MEAT SHOP (located in the historic centre not far from the post office) I loved this beautiful area for exploring & discovered a butcher shop offering traditionally-made meats, dairy, & delicious bacon made only with salt. MUSEO DEL CHOCOLATE 100% cacoa, Avenida de la Estación, 6

Santiago
CHARCUTERIA LOLITA CARDEL (market in the plaza near the Cathedral)

U.S.A.
www.eatwild.com
Find Real Food WAPF phone app
www.localharvest.org

NUTRITION RESOURCES

The Ketogenic Cookbook by Jimmy Moore & Maria Emmerich

Keto-Adapted by Maria Emmerich

Secrets to a Healthy Metabolism by Maria Emmerich

Keto Clarity by Jimmy Moore

Cholesterol Clarity by Jimmy Moore

Eat Fat, Lose Weight by Mary Enig & Sally Fallon

Nourishing Traditions by Sally Fallon

Know your Fats by Mary Enig

Nutrition and Physical Degeneration by Weston A. Price

Good Calories, Bad Calories OR *Why We Get Fat* by Gary Taubes

Fat and Cholesterol are GOOD for You by Uffe Ravnskov

Primal Body, Primal Mind by Nora Gedgaudas

Deep Nutrition by Catherine Shanahan

Real Food by Nina Planck

Traditional Foods are the Best Medicine by Ronald Schmid

Primal Blueprint by Mark Sisson

The Paleo Diet by Loren Cordain

Paleo Solution by Robb Wolf

Twinkie Deconstructed by Steve Ettlinger

The Dorito Effect by Mark Schatzker

France
Échiré (famous butter 83.5% fat)

Saint-Jean-Pied-de-Port
Gâteau Basque sheep cheeses & local ham & fish

Pyrenean foothills
Queso de Roncal (unpasteurized sheep's milk cheese)

Pyrenees
meat cooked a la llosa civet stew with wild boar or goat

Northern provinces
game is abundant

Navarra & Rioja
veal from Navarra = well-known; chorizo from Pamplona = very good (these areas
eat a lot of meat)

La Rioja area
chorizo sausage cordero lechal (thick slices young lamb roasted over fire with
grapevine in fire for smoky flavor)

Salamanca, Granada & Burgos
chorizo & Morcilla sausage

Castile
cordero (lamb) cochinillo (suckling pig)(both meats roasted in wood or clay ovens)

Melide
pulpo (boiled octopus)

Arzúa
known for its delicious creamy cheese

Galicia
famous for oysters, lobsters and crabs

Santiago
barnacles

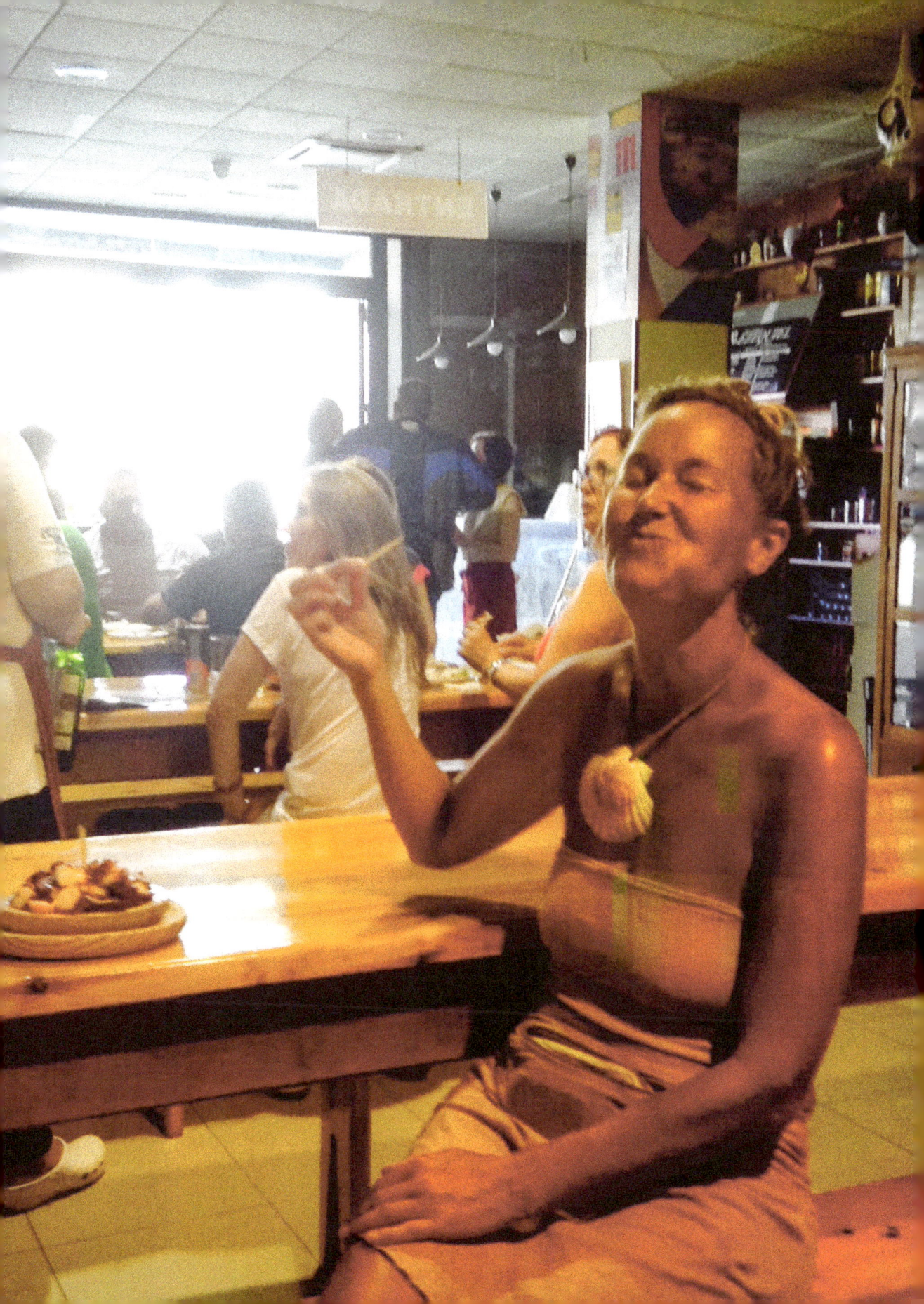

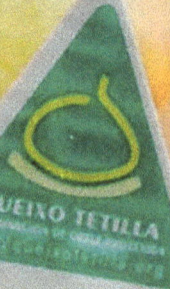

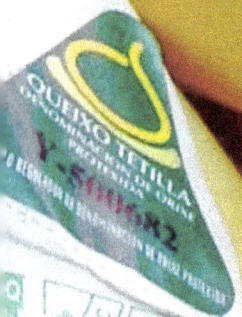

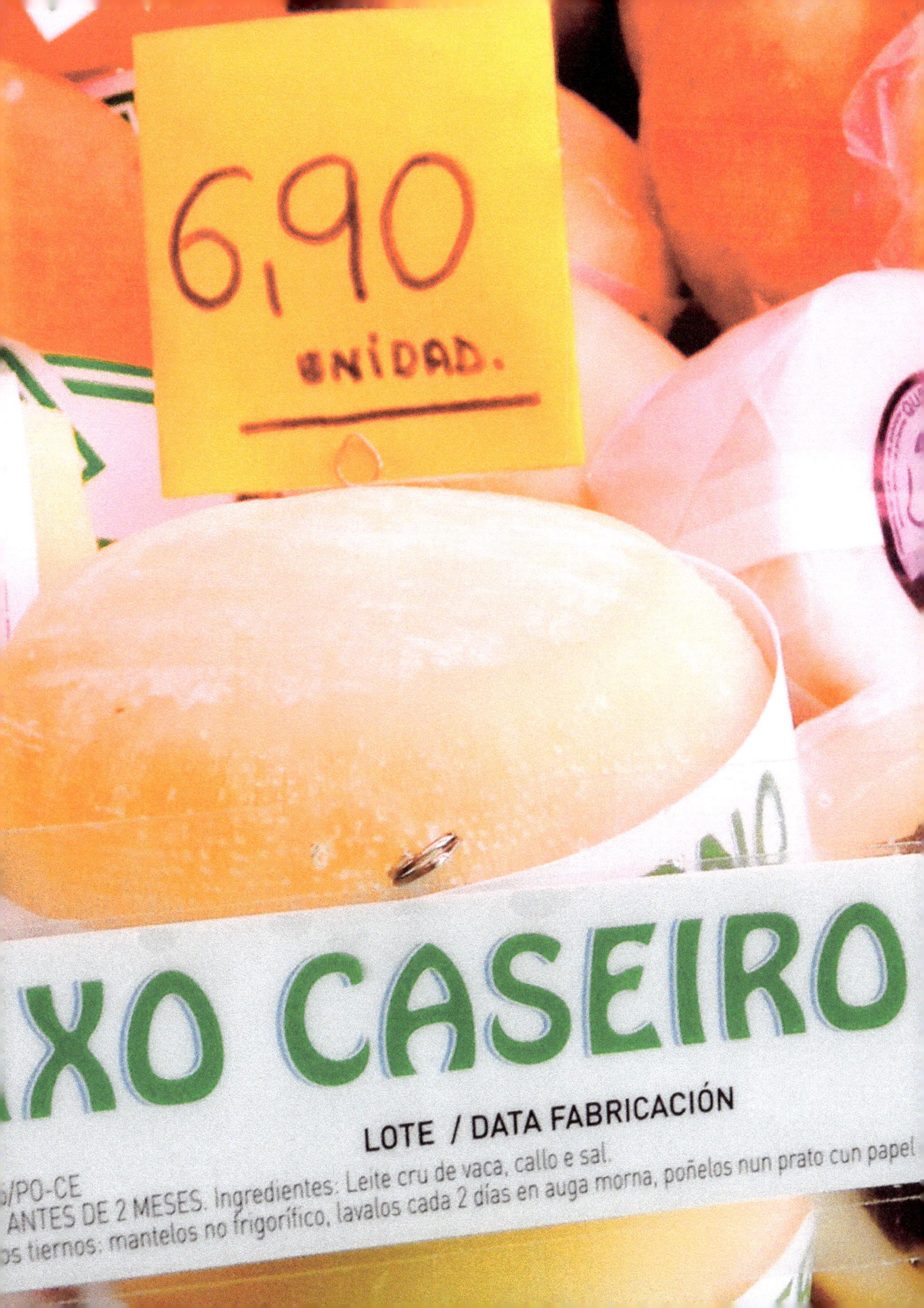

6,90
unidad.

XO CASEIRO

LOTE / DATA FABRICACIÓN

/PO-CE
ANTES DE 2 MESES. Ingredientes: Leite cru de vaca, callo e sal.
os tiernos: mantelos no frigorífico, lavalos cada 2 días en auga morna, poñelos nun prato cun papel

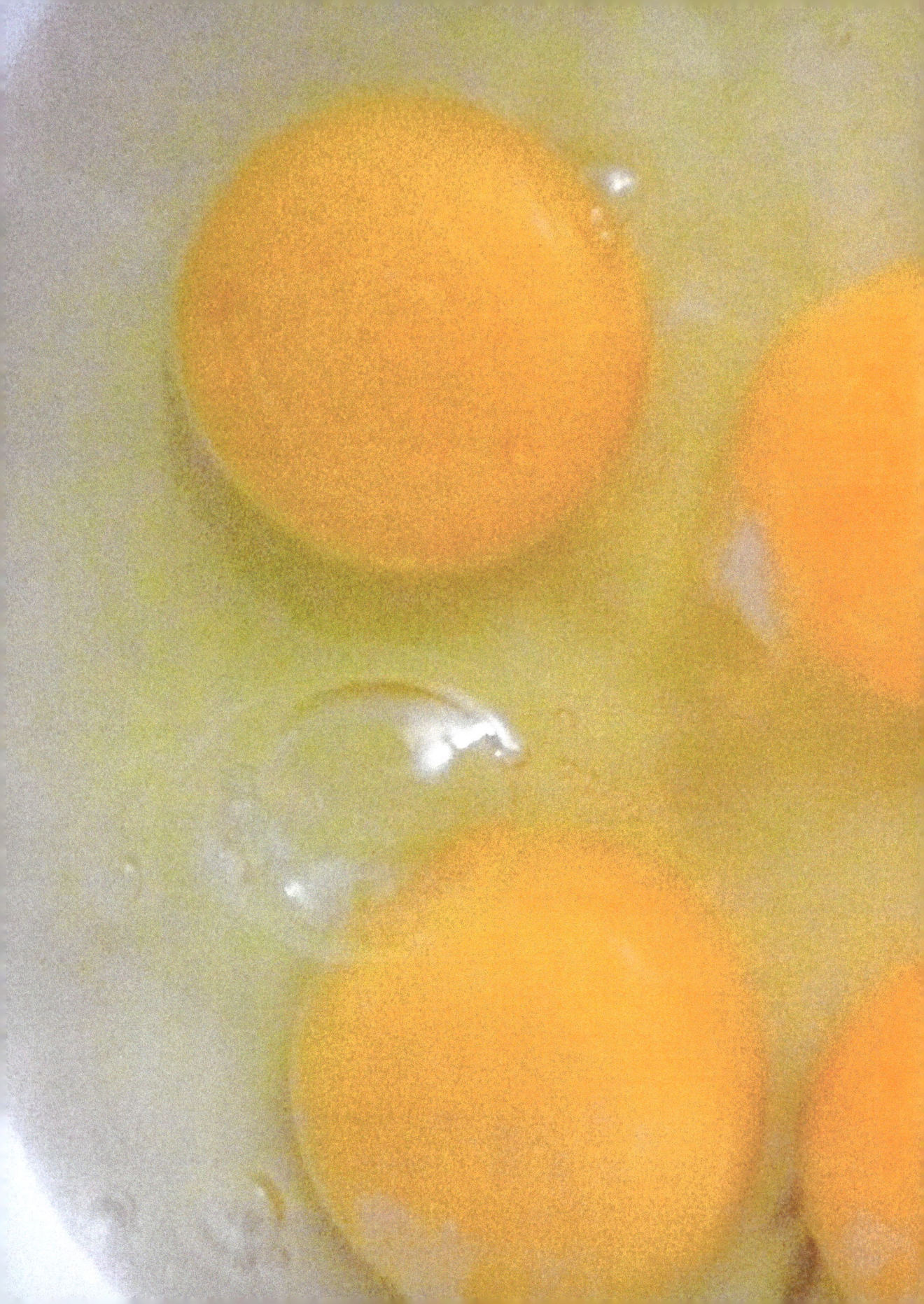

"Healthy eggs come from healthy chickens, sunlight, fresh air, exercise, healthy food (same as us!). Chickens raised on open pastures in the sun, eating bugs, worms and greens. The chickens raised in the sun have eggs with bright yellow yolks that look like the sun. The bright color of the yolk means the egg is rich in nutrients and came from a healthy chicken. Eating healthy starts by knowing where your food comes from"
-Suzanne Gross and Sally Fallon Morell
The Nourishing Traditions Cookbook for Children

*eggs pictured from family chickens Logoso, Spain

SPAIN FOOD GEMS

Ibérico de bellota: 100% acorn-fed, semi-wild foraging pig

Paprika: the valley of La Vera hand-harvested, dehydrated, smoked slowly by oak-wood fires over 10-15 days turning peppers by hand finely ground in traditional stone mills

mercados: covered food markets
cocina de mercado: market cooking; straightforward cooking techniques simple cafés serving fresh products surrounding them in the markets
*individually owned stalls offer cured sausages and diverse cheeses

saffron: the most expensive spice in the world

Conservas Ramón Peña in Cambados, Galicia: more workshop than factory; everything is natural as done at home; detailed, meticulous, no shortcuts; bay leaf, garlic, hand-packed mussels; traditional/artisinal methods, finest raw materials

Cordero: lamb/sheep roast suckling lamb slid from the wood-burning oven of centuries old, tile-walled mesón

le Chazo: suckling lamb

asadores: traditional restaurants that roast in wood ovens

Restaurante Asados Nazareno in the ancient market town of Roa: "the Cristóbal family preparing one dish to perfection lechazo, or roast cordero lechal (suckling lamb) master roaster, octogenarian Javier Cristóbal, places them on wide earthenware dishes and slides them into the restaurant's deep, wood-burning ovens no herbs, no garlic, just some manteca (lard) salt & a touch of water the quality of the animal must be perfection: 24 days old, 22-24 lbs, nearly wild, need to walk for food, the mothers eating the dry herb"

wood-roasted meats: "ancient city of Segovia stands out for its numerous centuries-old mesones serving cochinillo (suckling pig) a certified cochinillo de Segovia is no more than 21 days old and weighs 10-12 lbs, slow-roasted whole in oval earthenware dishes with minimal condiments- lard, salt and touch of water"

bacalao: dried salt fish

merluza a la gallega: steamed hake in a Galician paprika sauce

a la llosa: local trout cooked on a slate slab over hot coals

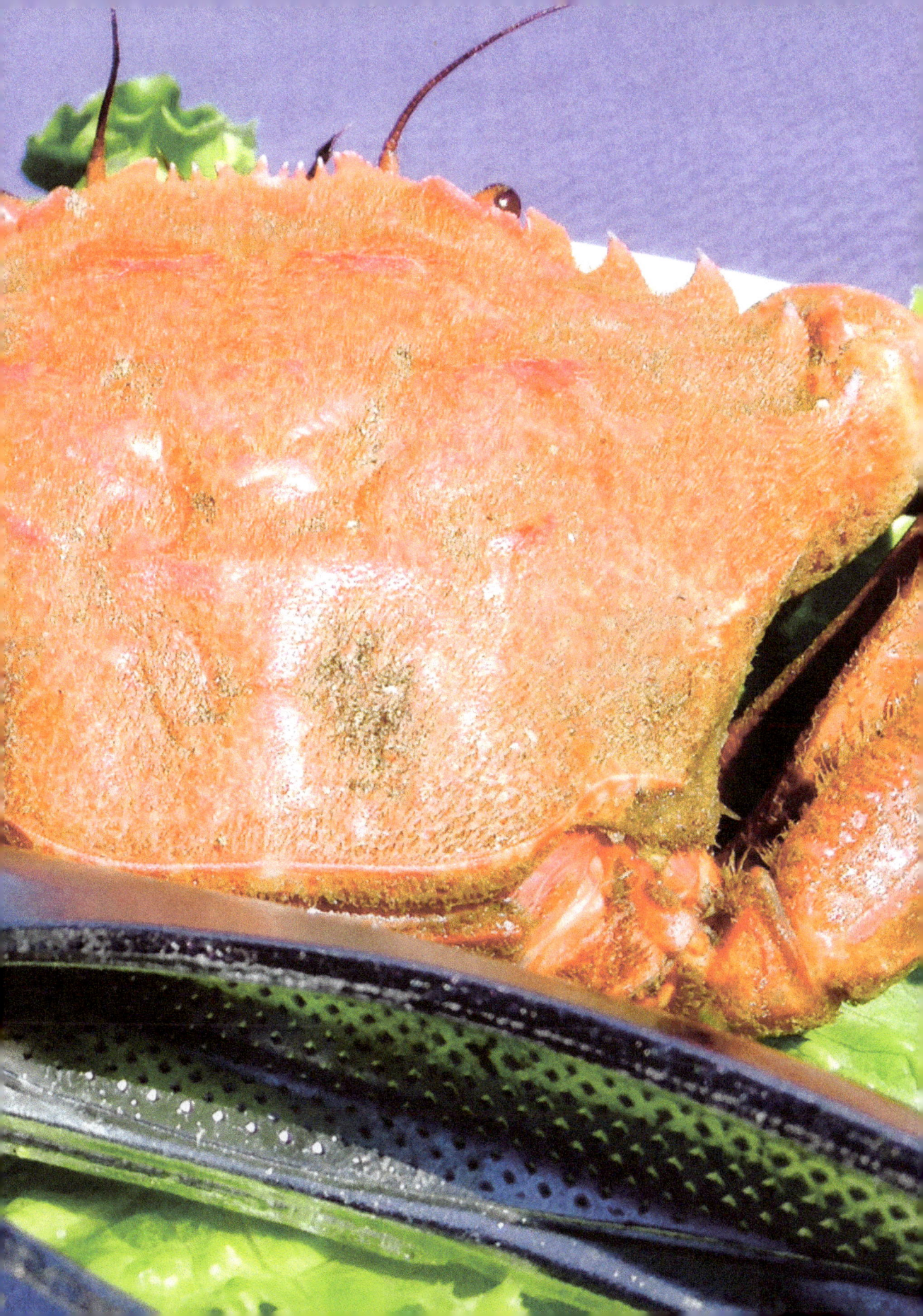

SUPERFOODS: salmon, eggs, beef, bison, lamb, shrimp, tuna, calf liver, bone broth, lemons, avocados, coconut, olive oil, garlic, parsley, basil, cinnamon, tumeric, cayenne pepper, mustard
CALCIUM: hard cheeses & canned sardines with bones
B12 & FOLIC ACID: octopus, livers, clams, fish eggs, fish

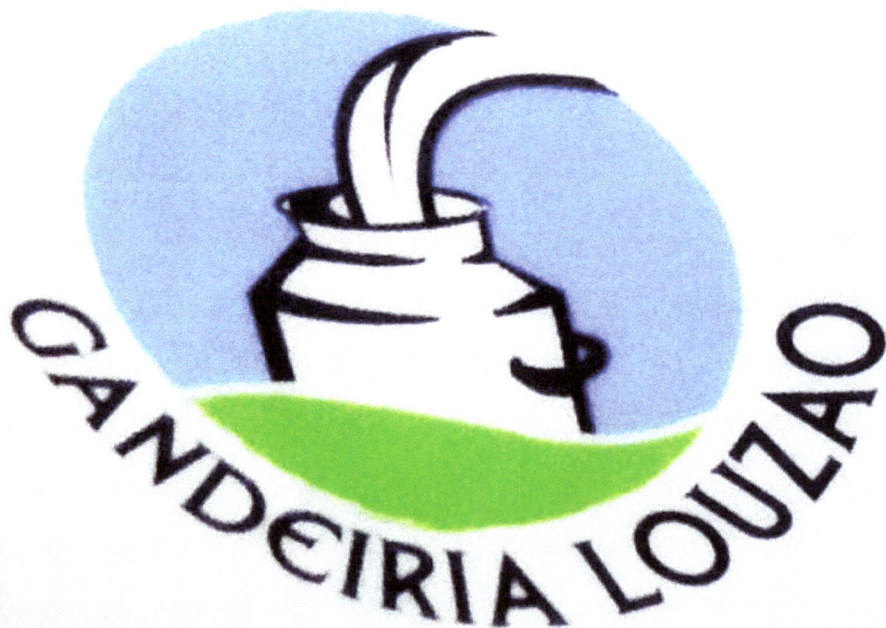

GANDEIRIA LOUZAO

A Riveira, 1 - Santeles

Tels : 673

HIGH IN MINERALS: saffron, sesame seeds, sunflower seeds, curry powder, ground ginger, ground paprika, anchovies, chili powder, cocoa, clams, cumin seeds

HIGH IN VITAMINS: anchovies, bacon, chicken livers, chorizo, clams, ground paprika

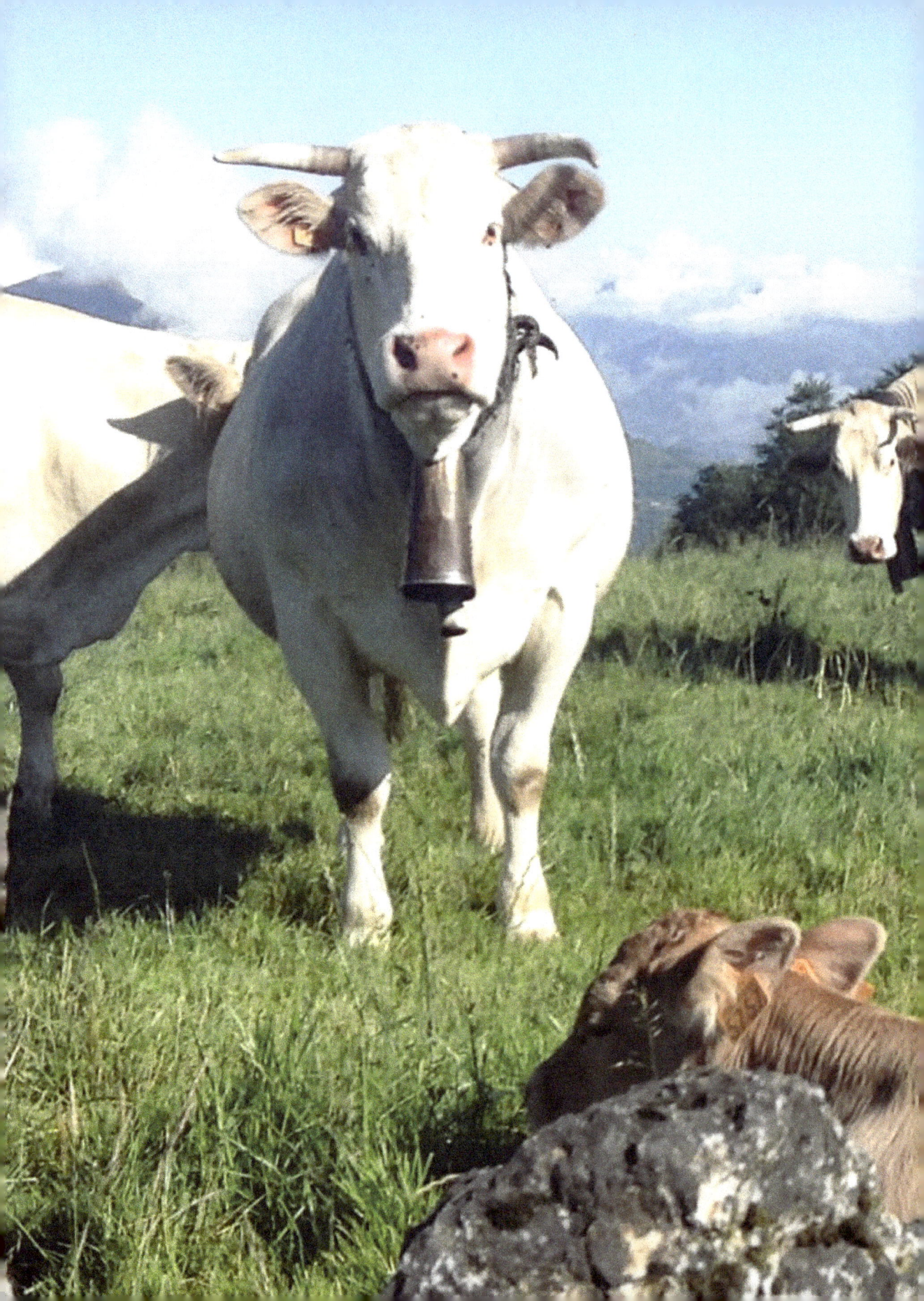

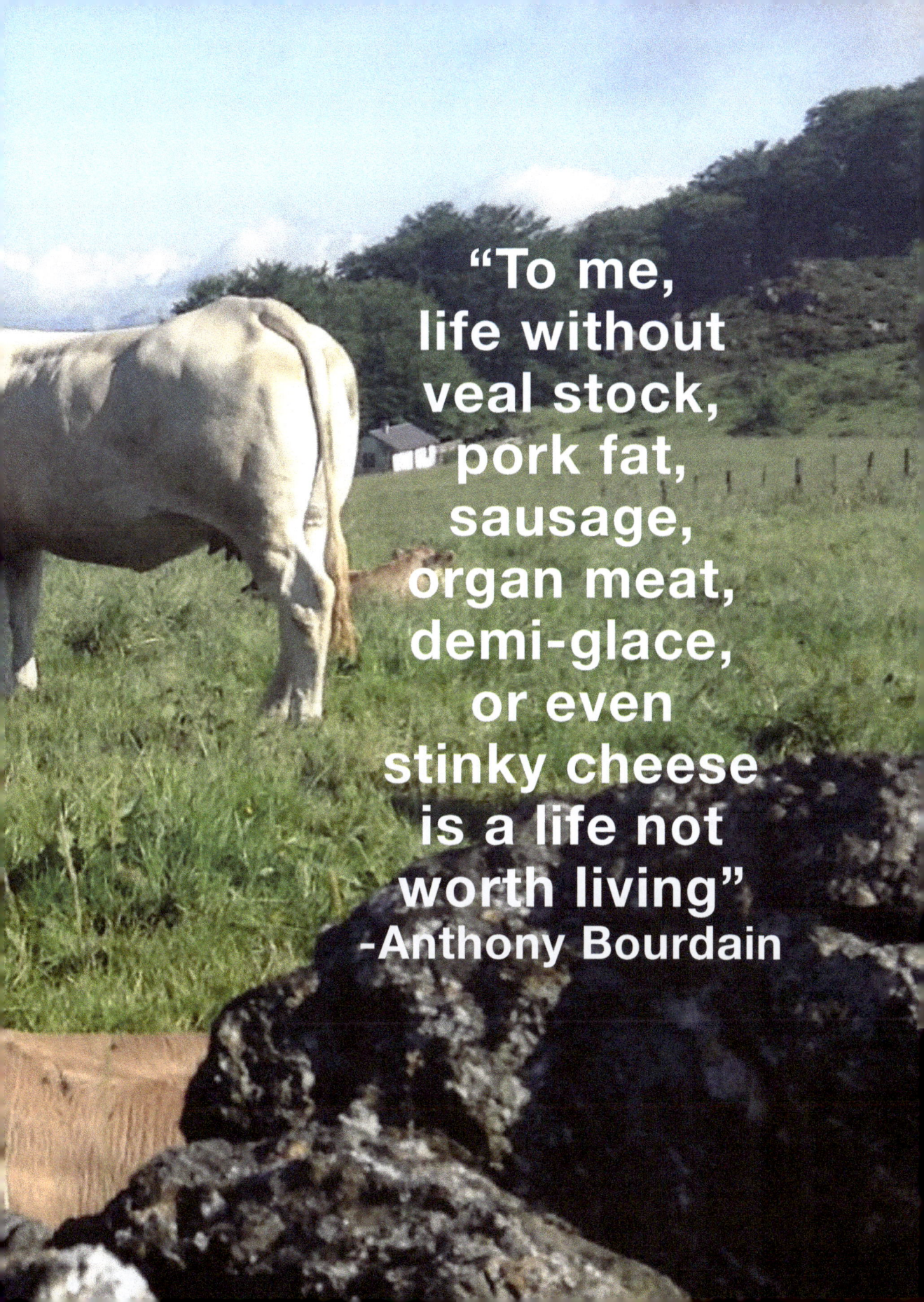

"To me, life without veal stock, pork fat, sausage, organ meat, demi-glace, or even stinky cheese is a life not worth living"
-Anthony Bourdain

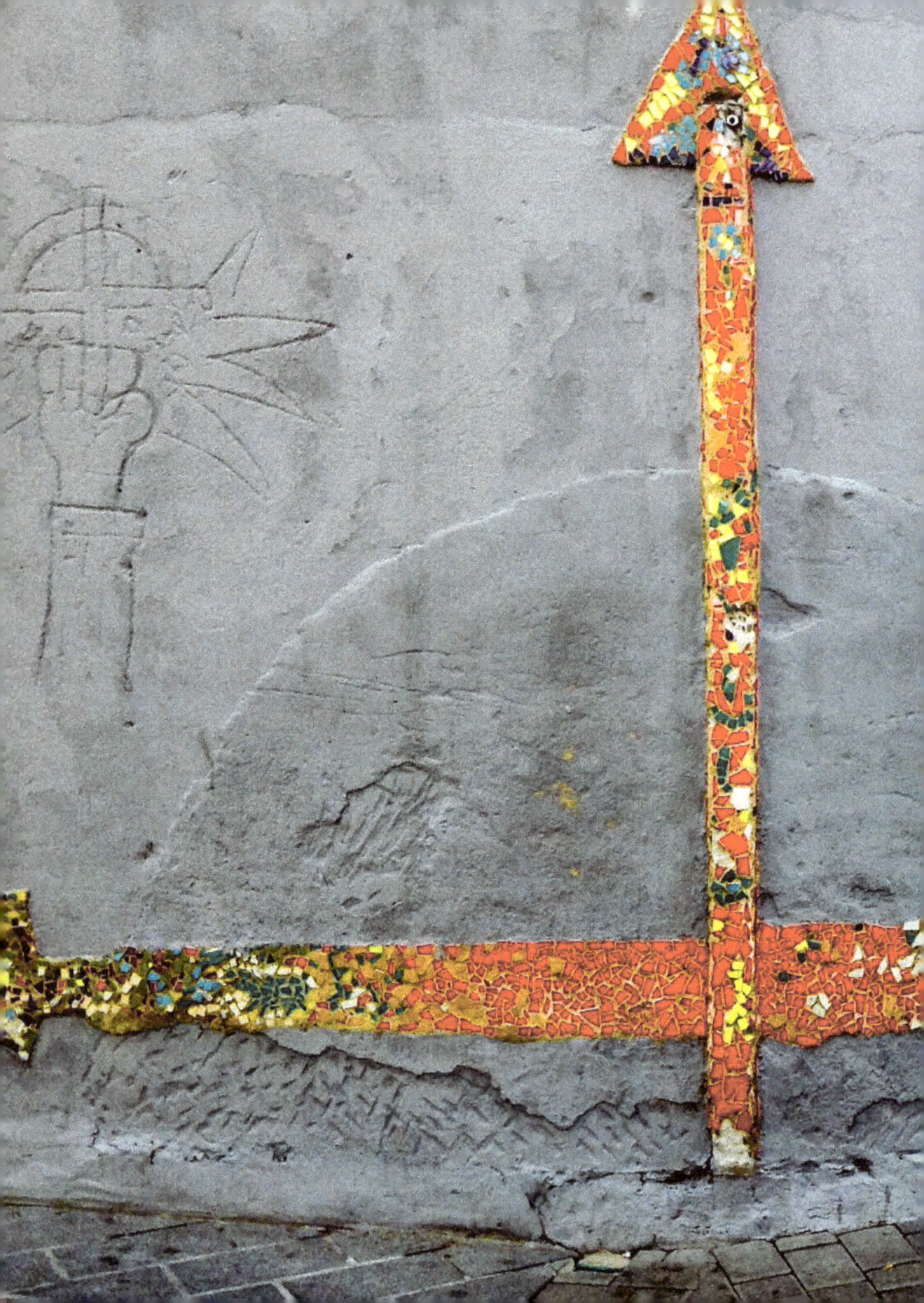

advancing

!ULTREiA! ONWARD CONTINUE

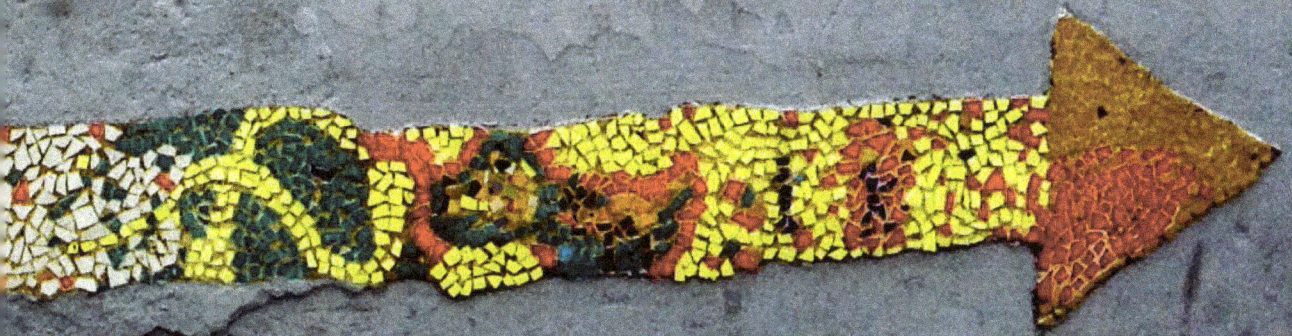

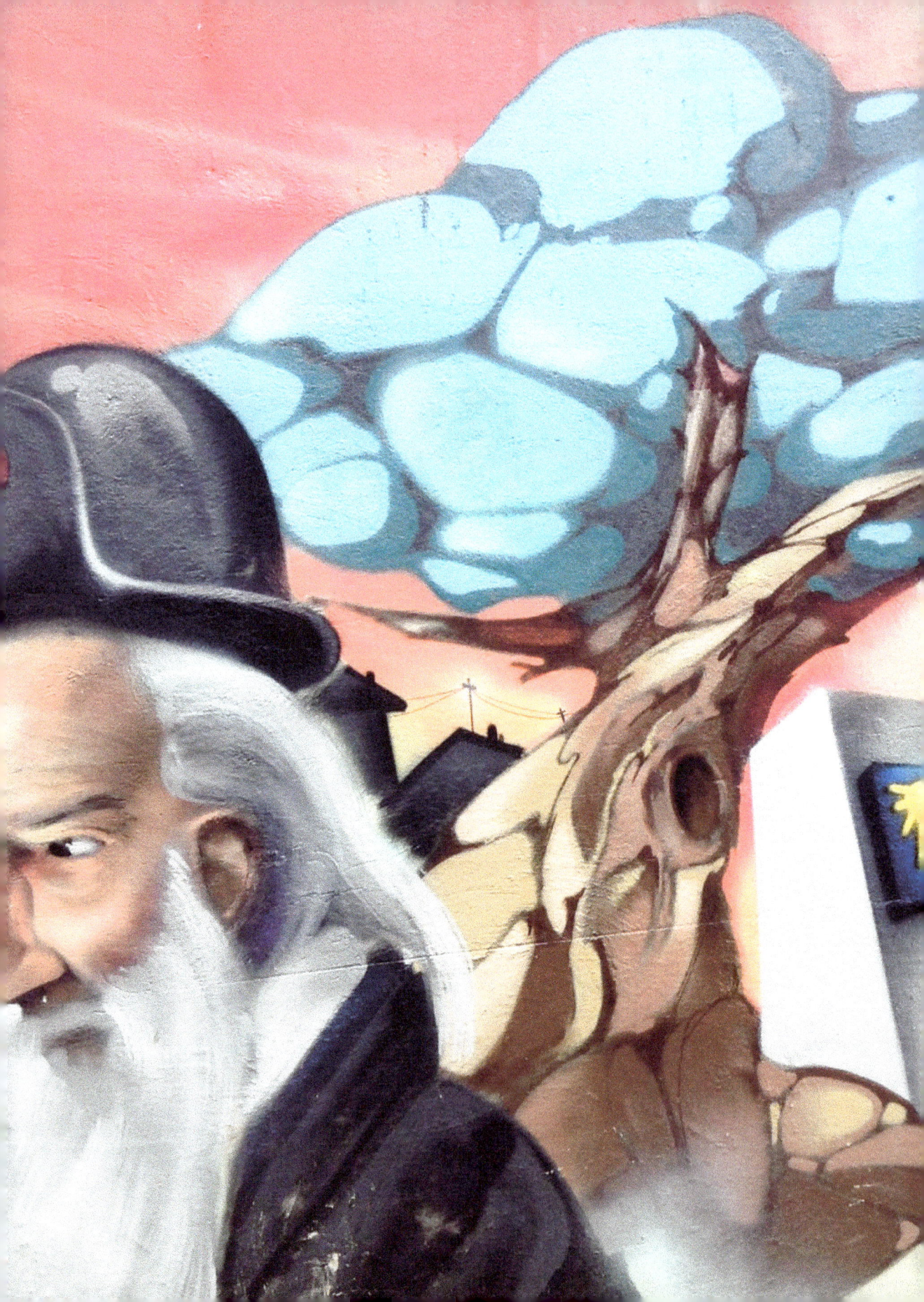

¡ULTREïA!

onward

upward

beyond

unction

keep going

to persevere

to be persistent

above and beyond

go upper, go farther

a wish of an unfailing courage

eia: a cry of joy

HALLELUJAH

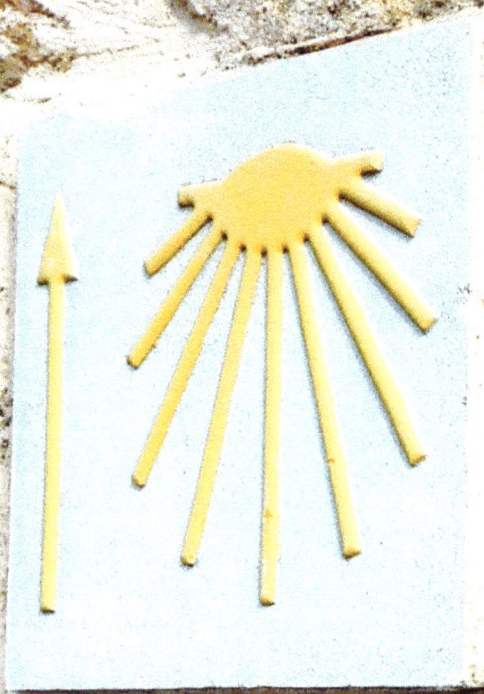

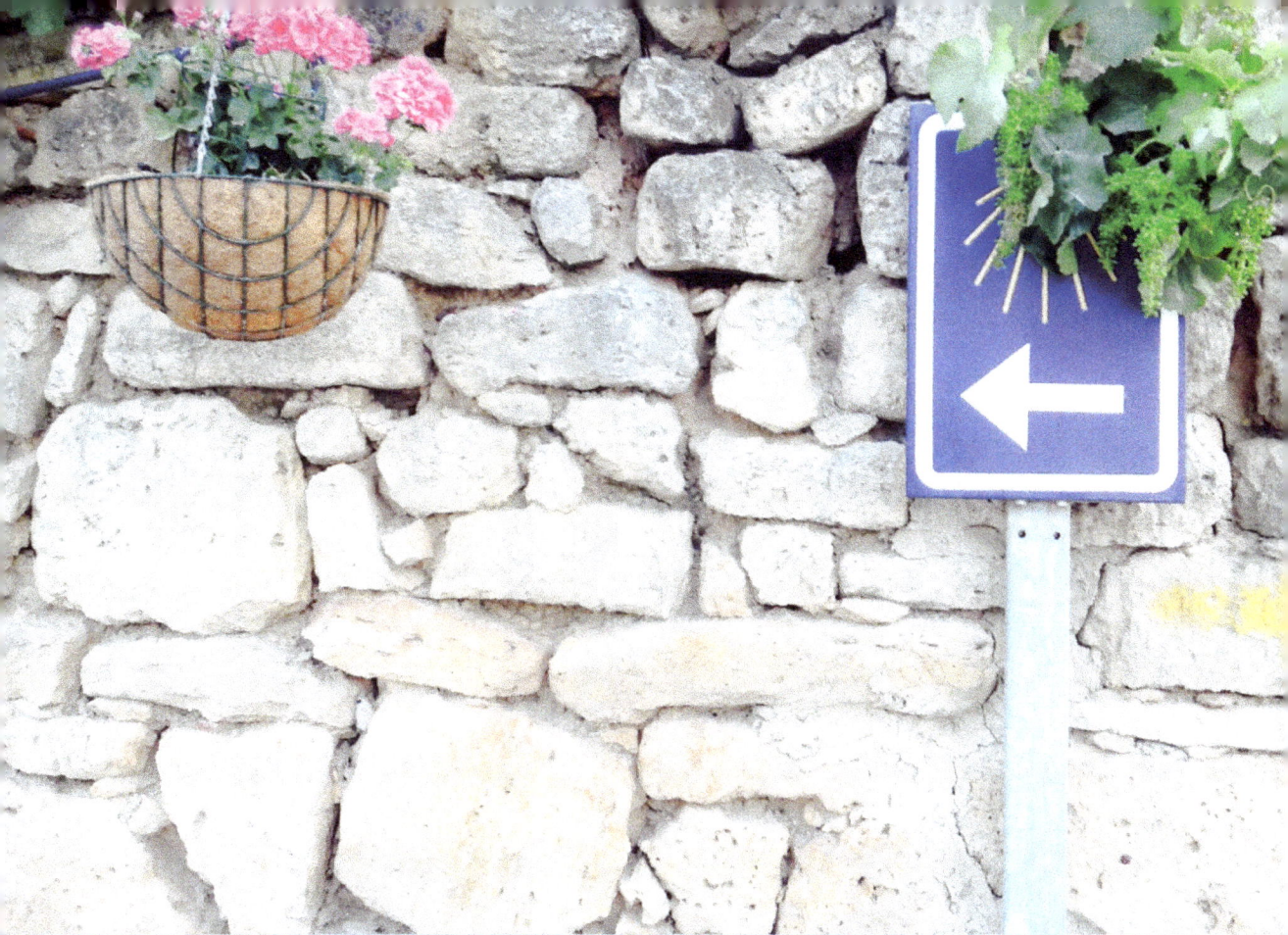

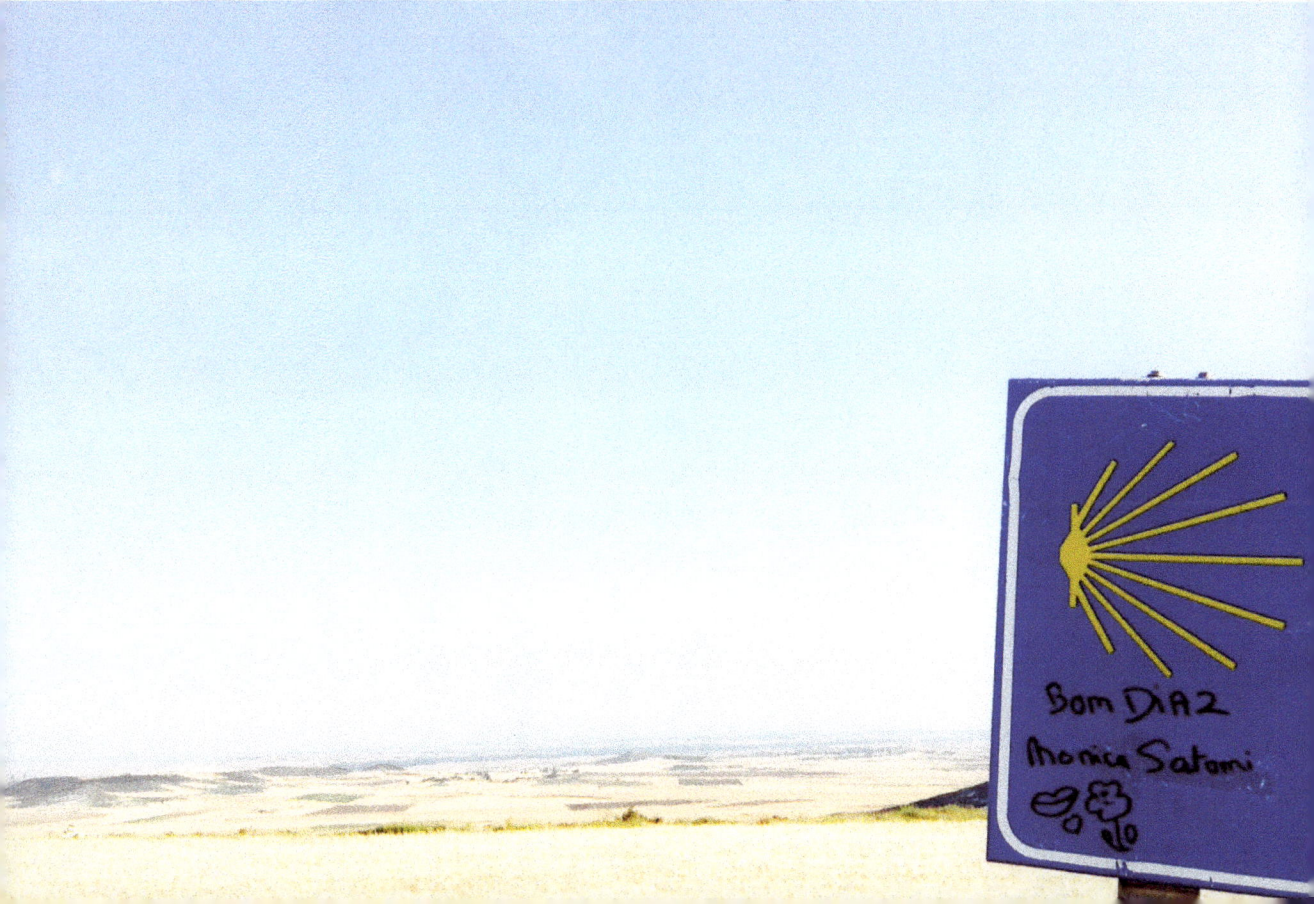

Bom DiA2
Monica Satomi

ONE MOMENT

ONE BREATH

ONE THOUGHT

ONE IDEA

ONE ACTION

ONE STEP

ONE DAY

AT A TIME

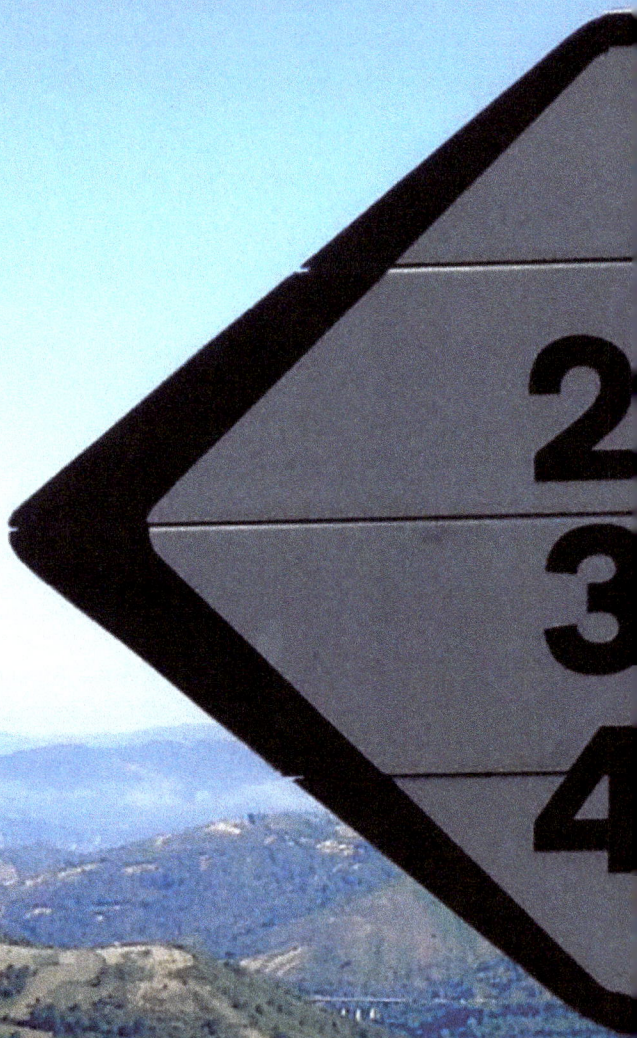

LU-633

,5 **TRIACAST**

,5 **SA**

,5 **SA**

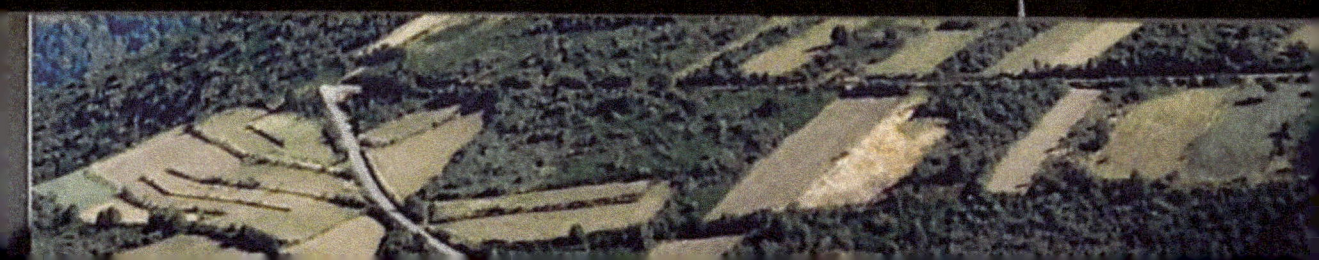

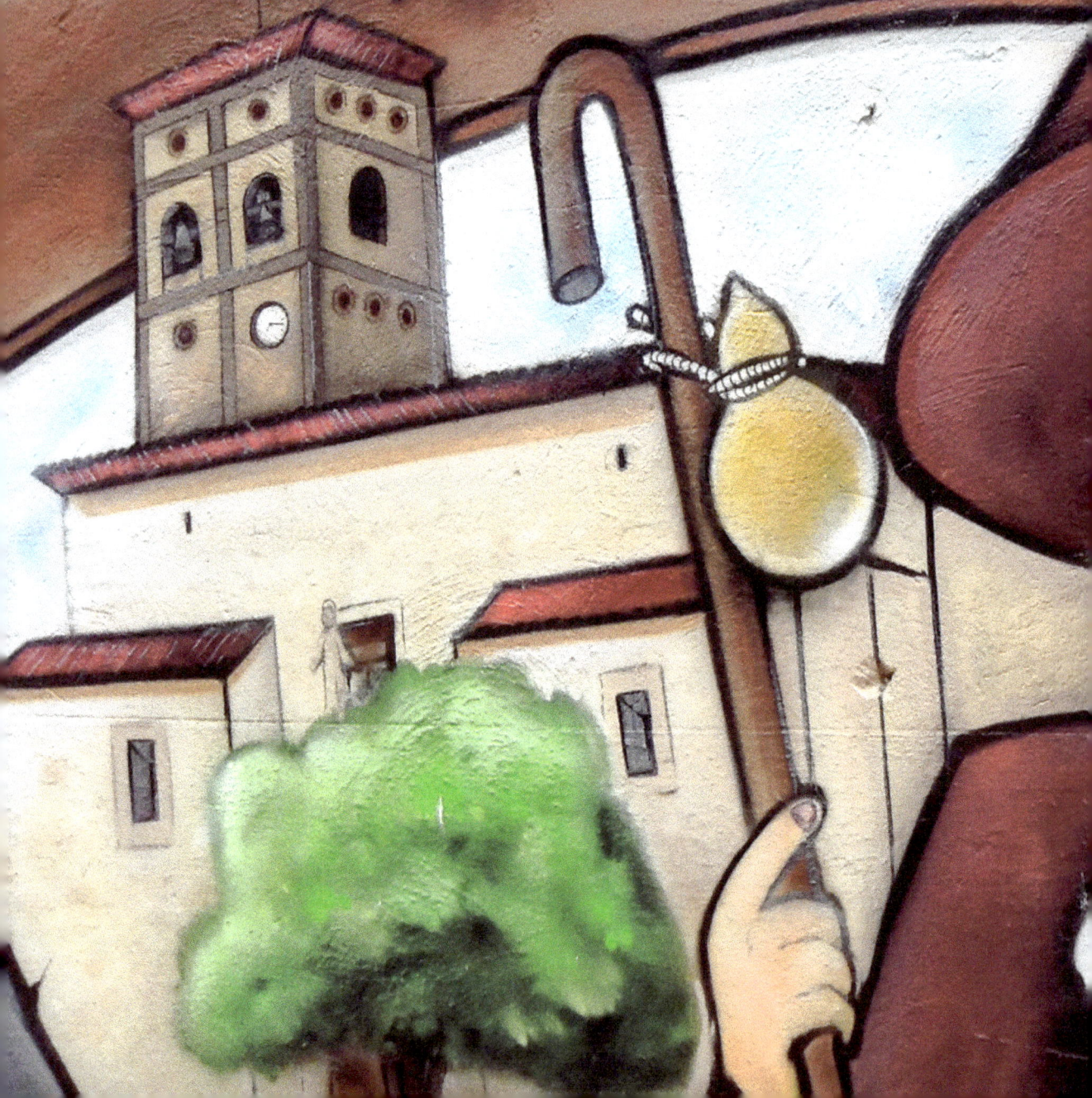

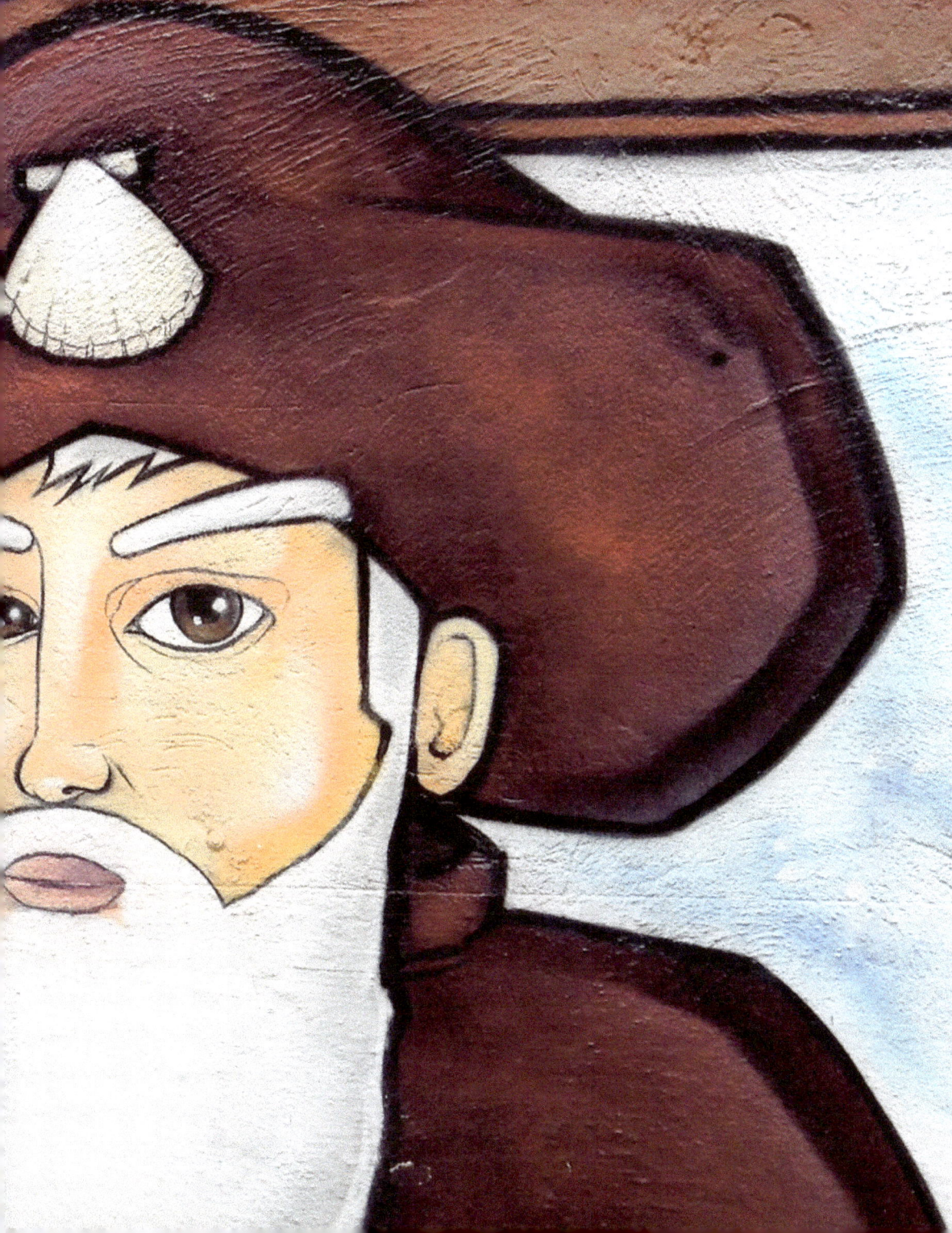

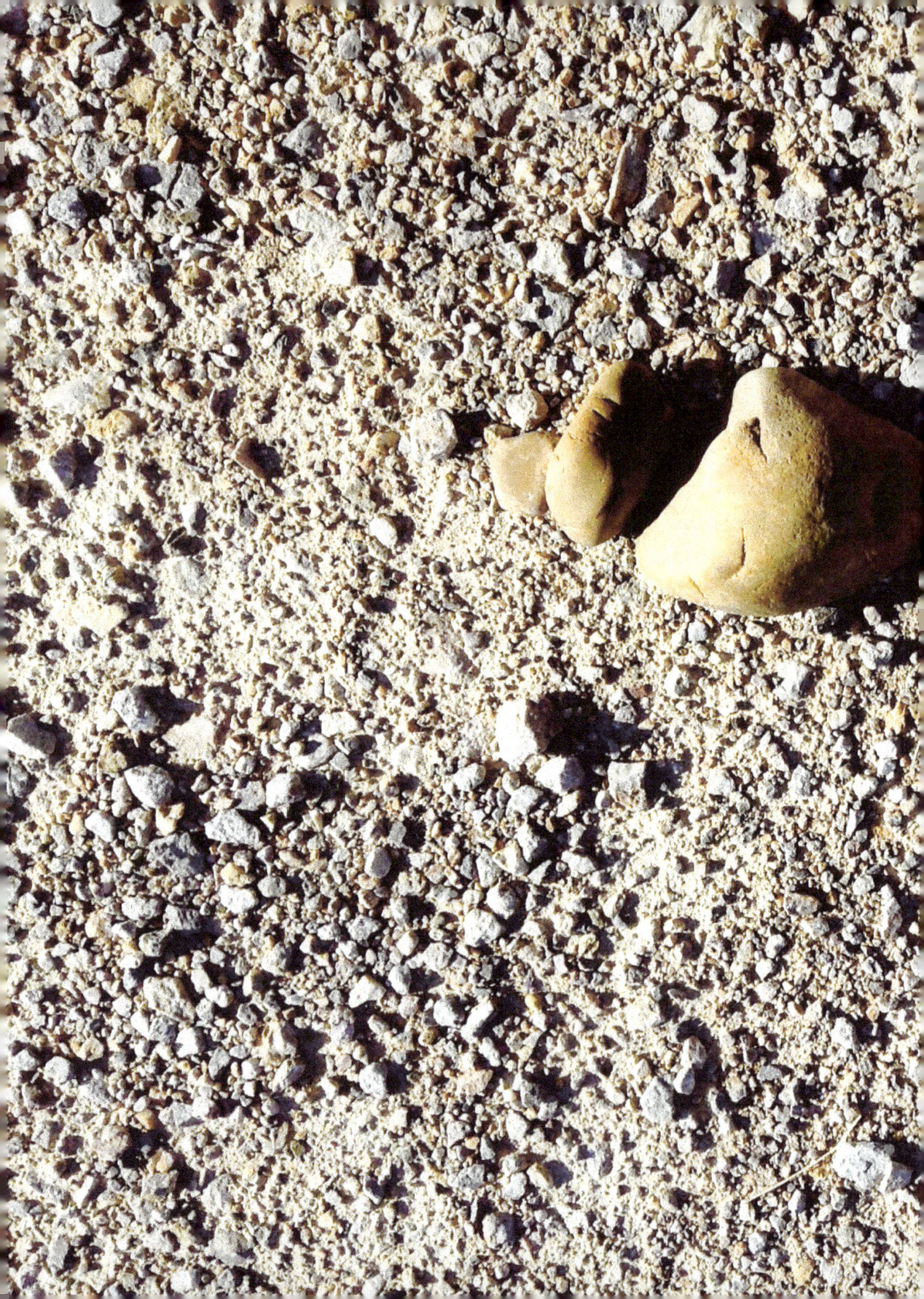

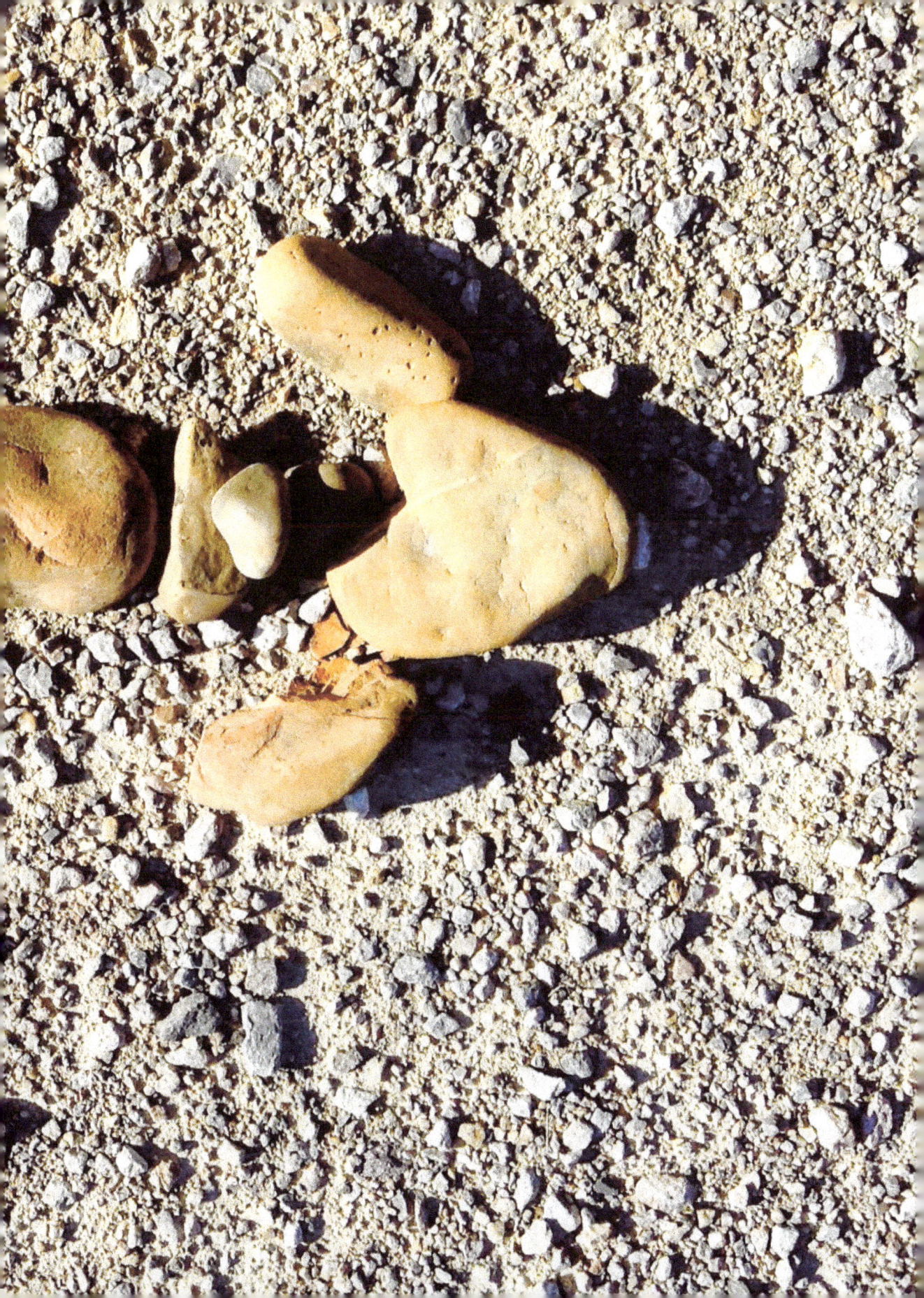

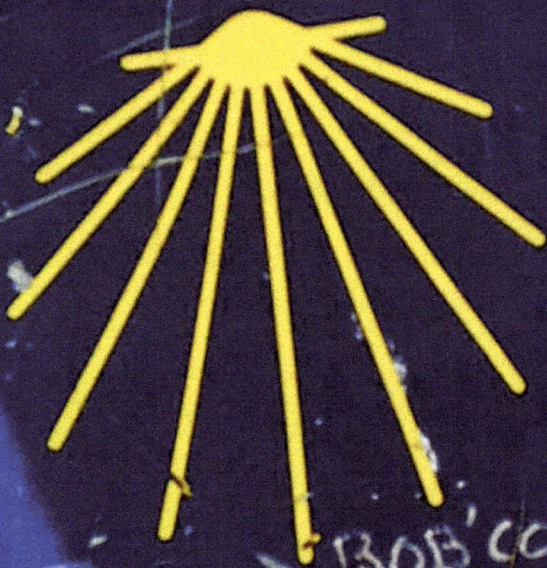

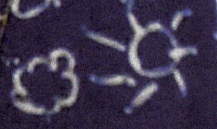

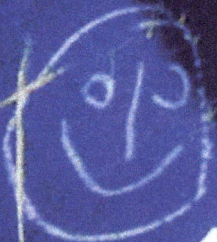

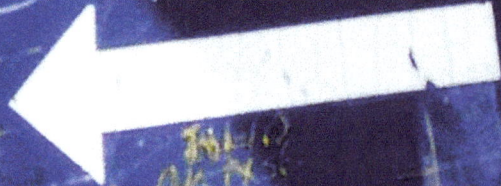

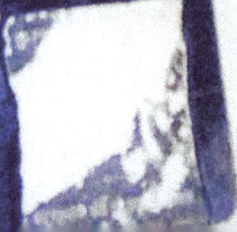

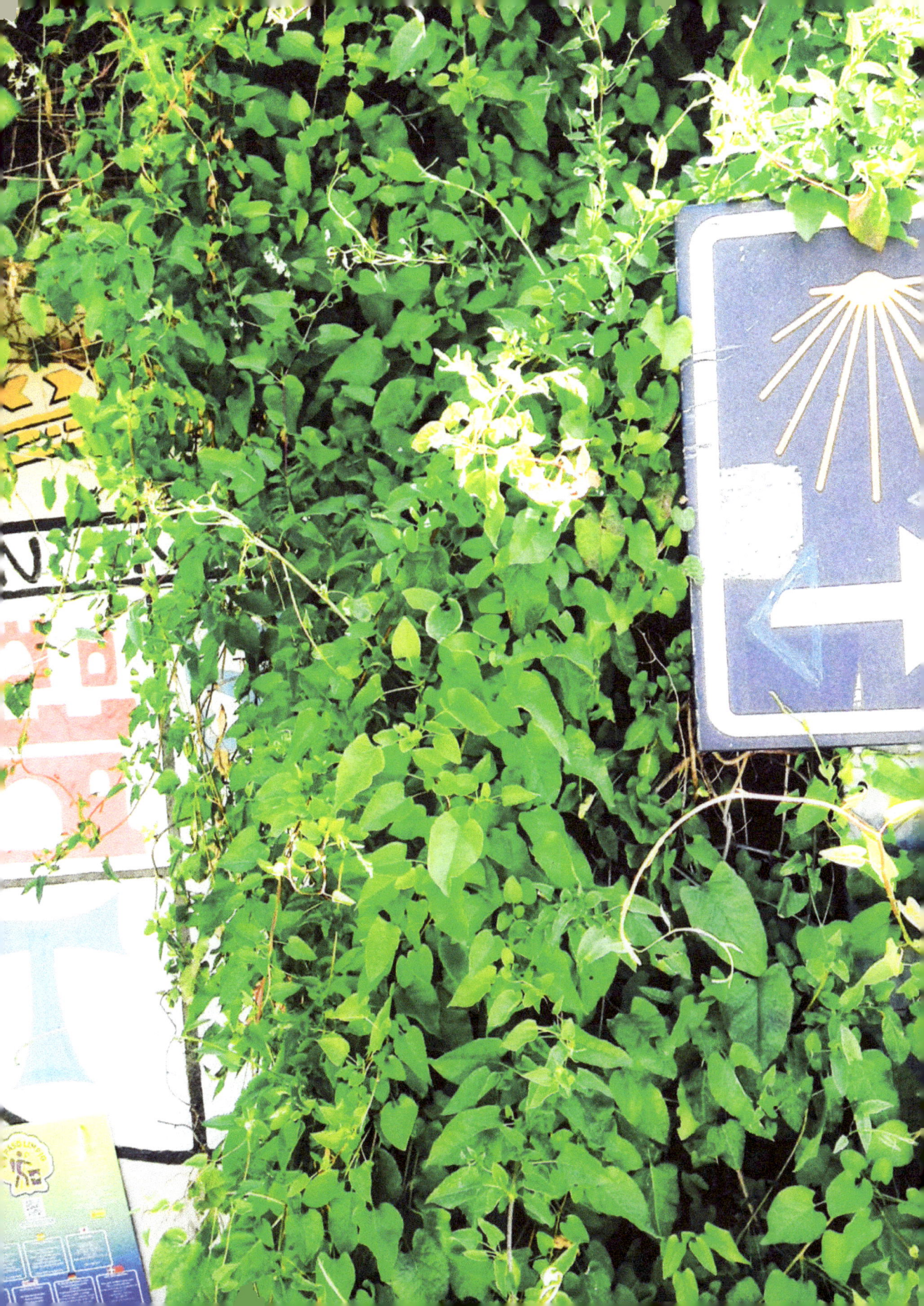

Walking the Camino was a phenomenal way for me to practice living in the moment. If I thought ahead, it caused distraction from finding my way. It also was a great lesson in faith. There were so many unknowns especially not knowing if I could make it! Back home, whenever I feel my spirit spiraling or my faith falling, I hear myself say "chin up young person!" (from the book/movie *The Object of My Affection*). It always seems to help. I am so fortunate to be a naturally happy, positive person, but there are times (almost always when I am tired) when I lose my faith. It is a very uncomfortable feeling that can often cause panic or desperation. I am so grateful that my parents taught me the dangers of abusing chemicals to alter my feelings, because I can understand the addicting lure of using them to alleviate the panic, pain and fear. I am also so grateful to them for showing me the enriching coping mechanisms (and the joys!) of nature, always being active and outside, learning and higher education, athletics, music, art, religion, spirituality and programs for living a healthy life. Because of their guidance, radiance and modeling, I know that my happiness is my responsibility. If I put positive, enlightening ingredients into my life, then I will have a positive and enlightened life! These tools, road maps and "arrows" for navigating difficult times have made my life feel truly joyful and blessed. My mom and dad: M I R A C L E S ! ! ! ! !

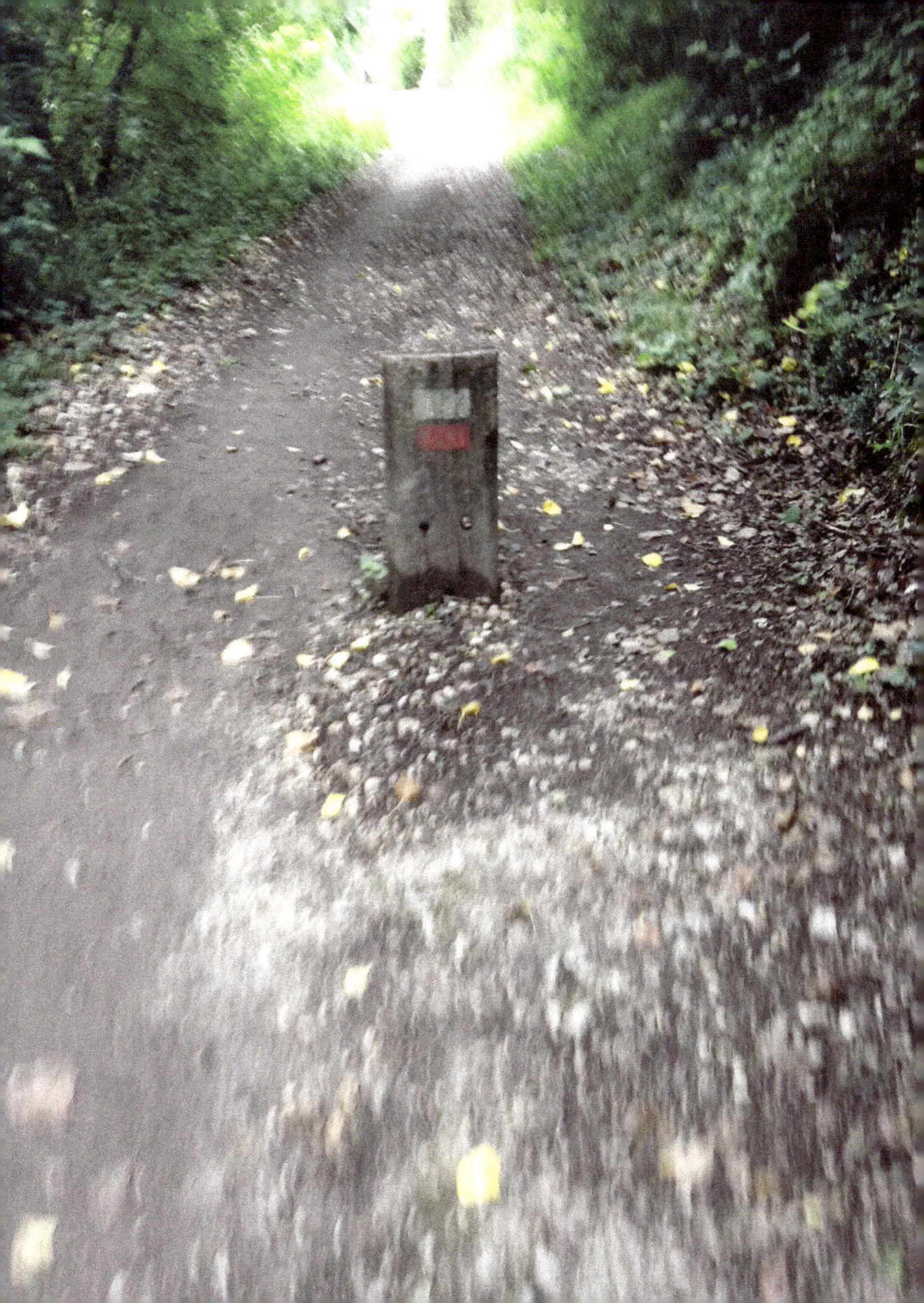

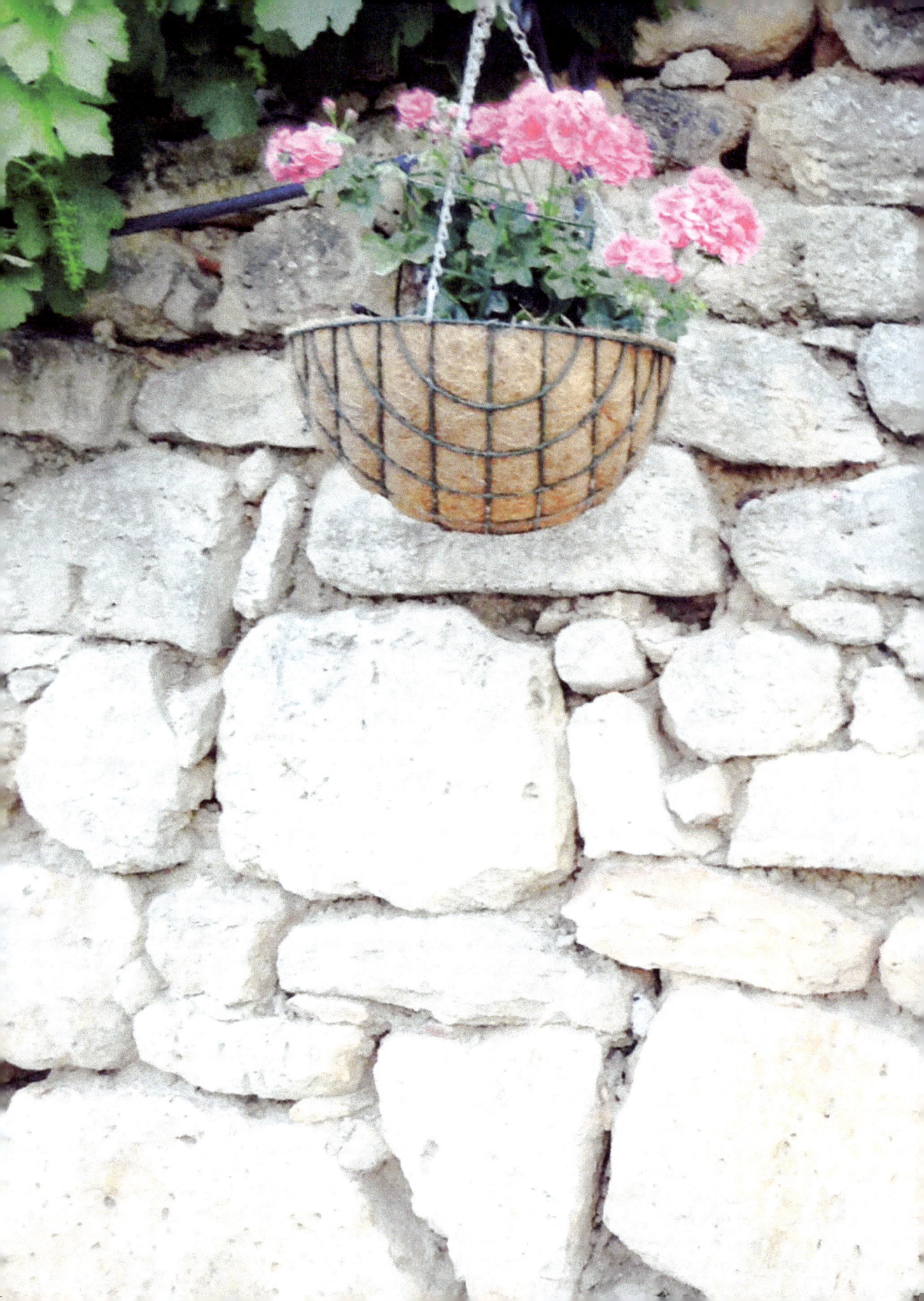

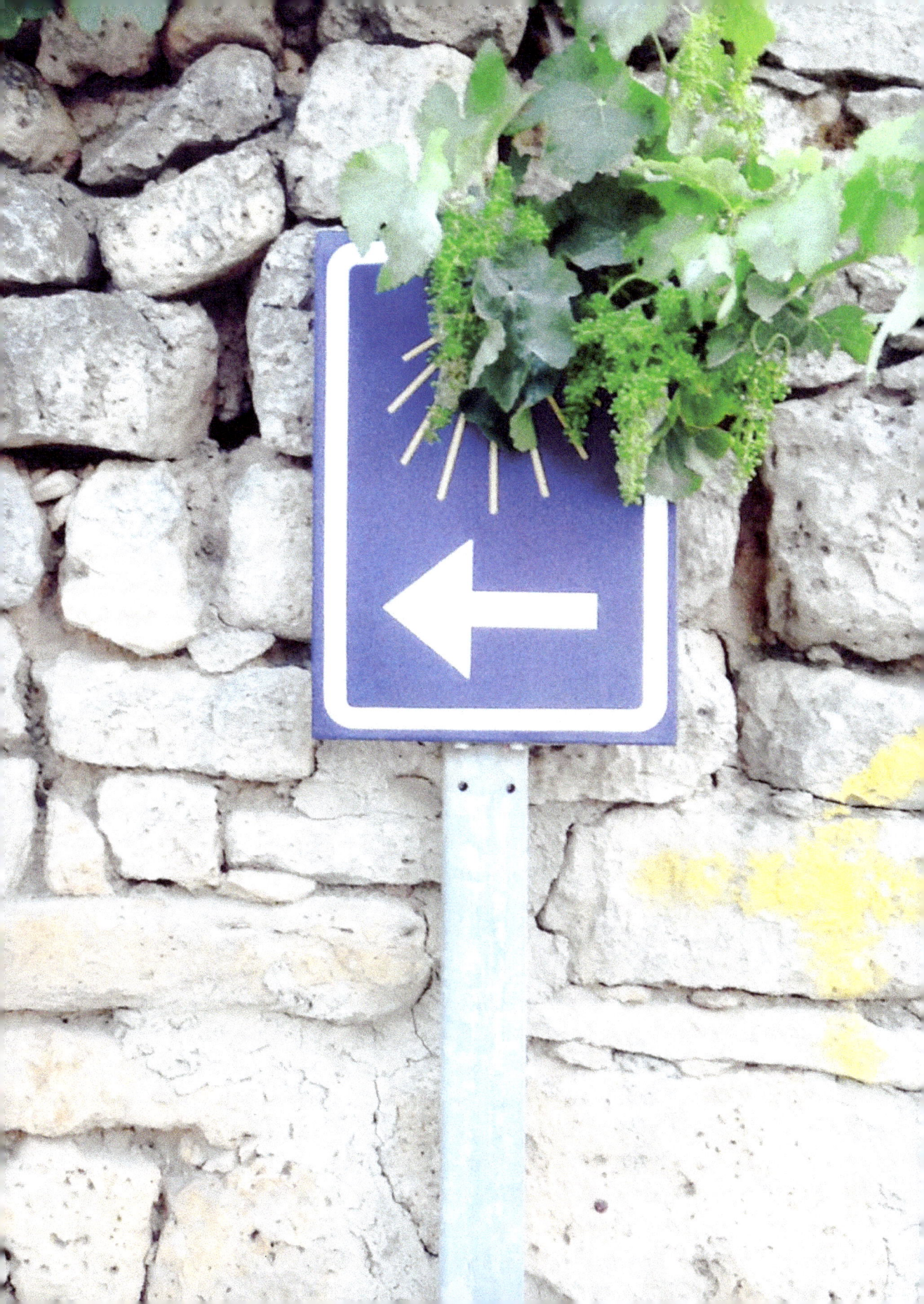

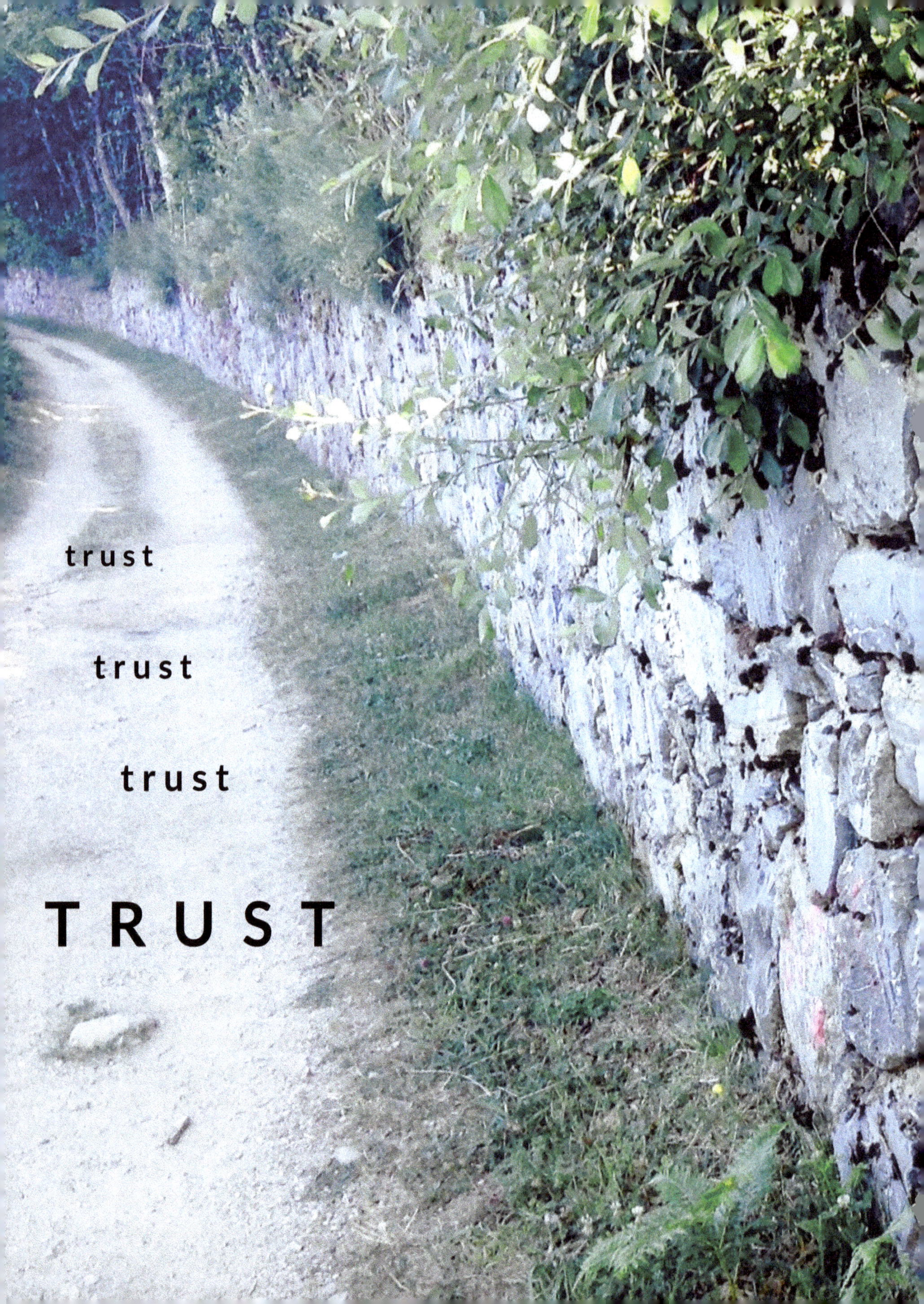

trust

trust

trust

TRUST

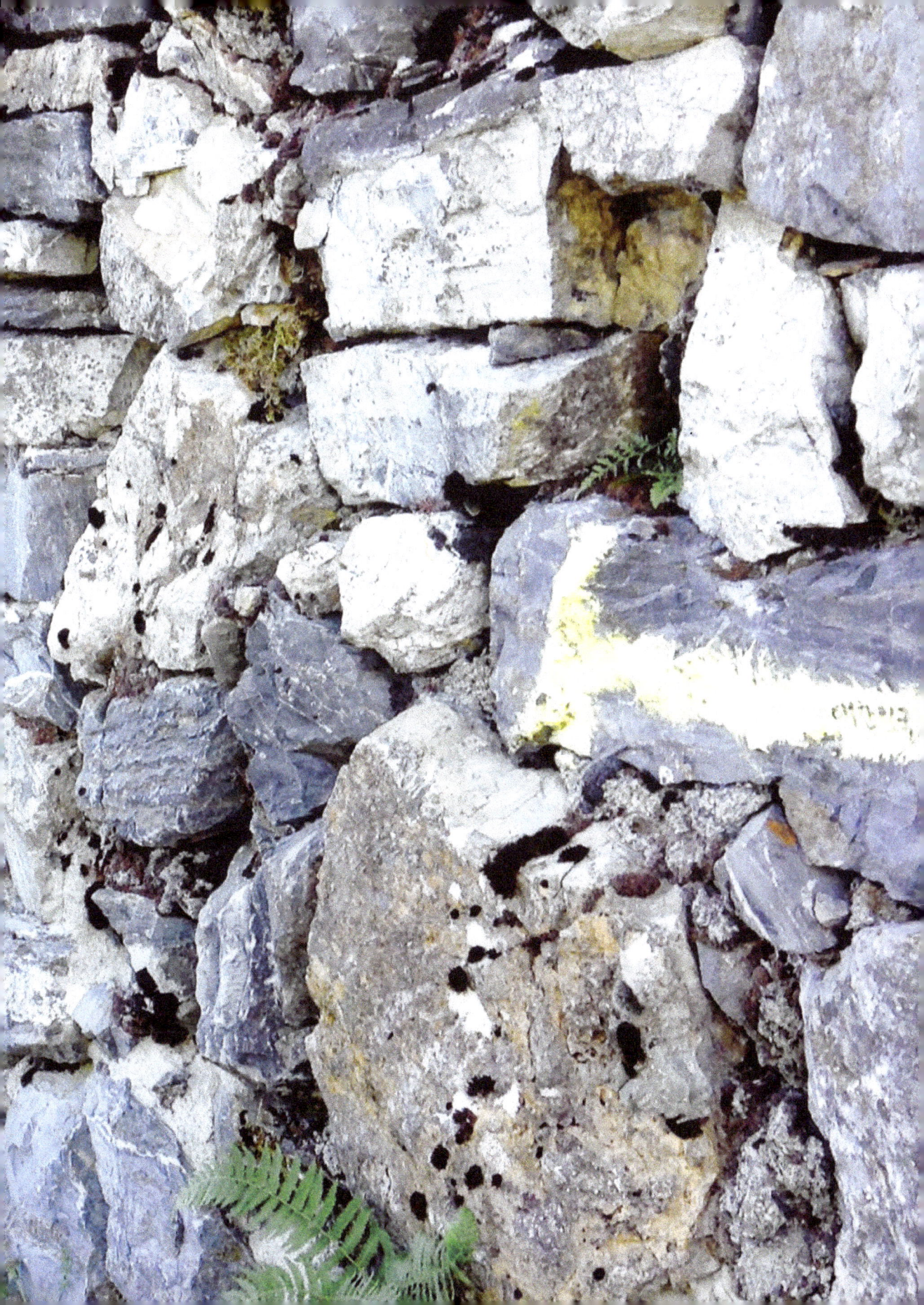

community

GREET ENCOURAGE SMILE SHARE

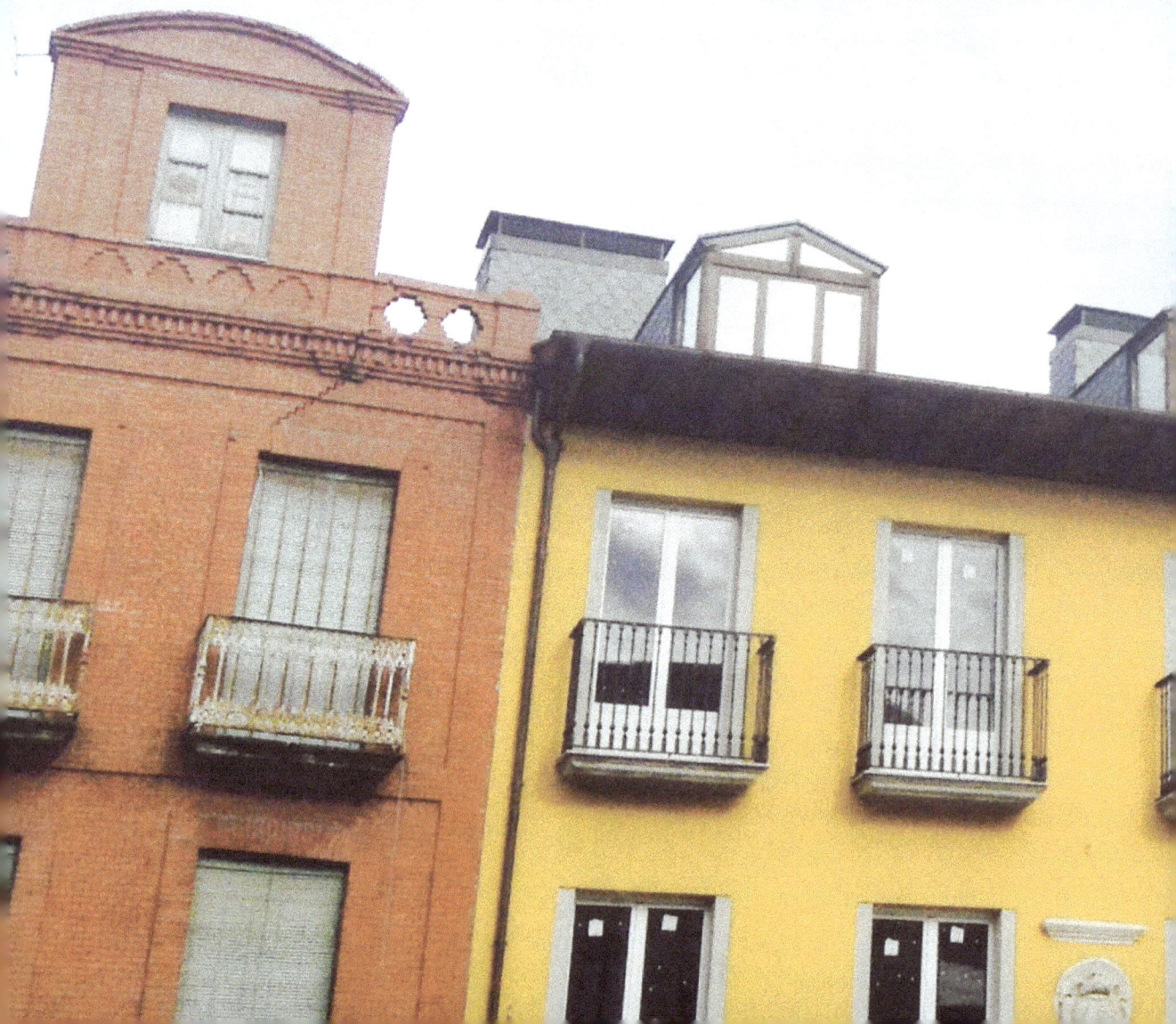

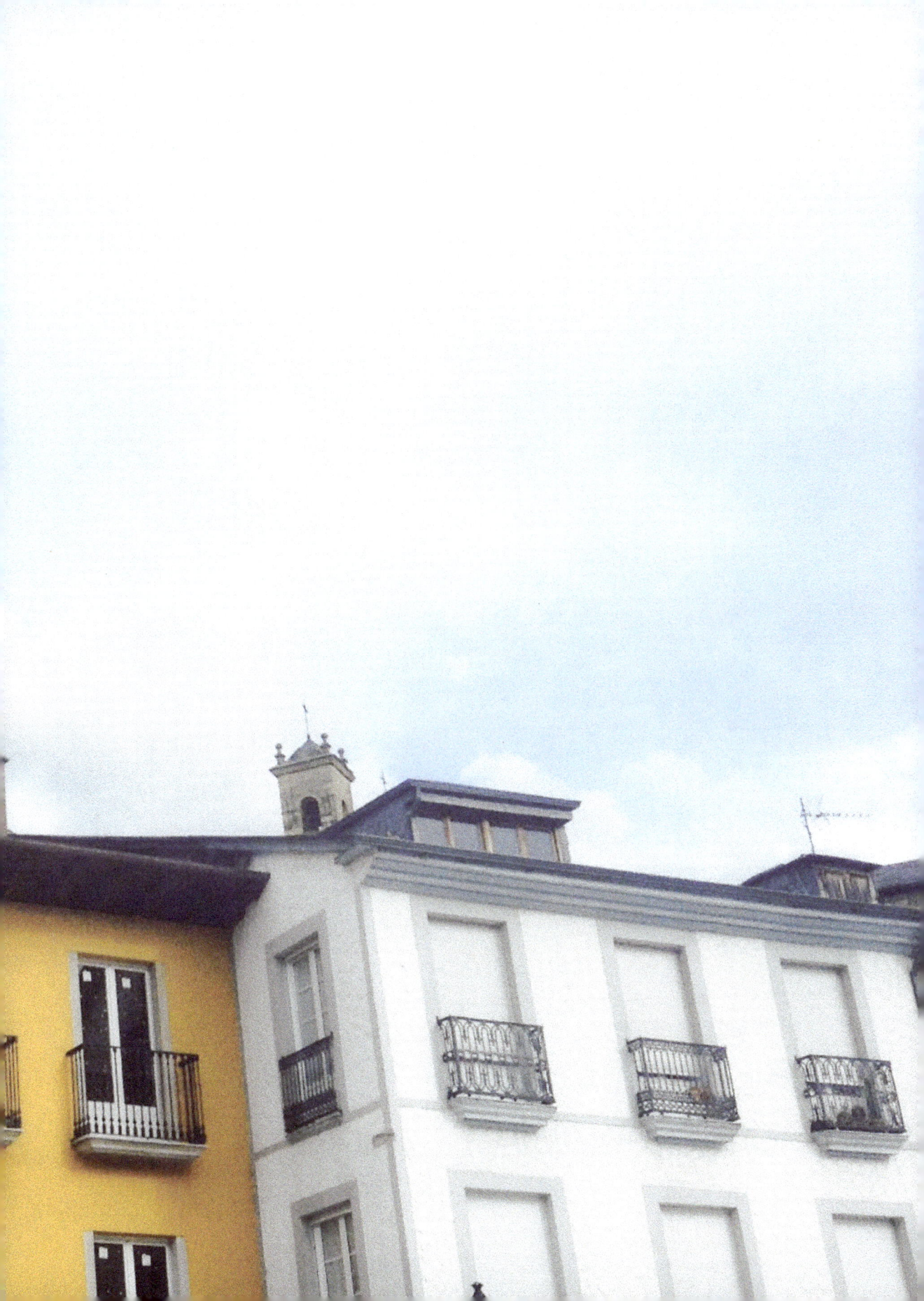

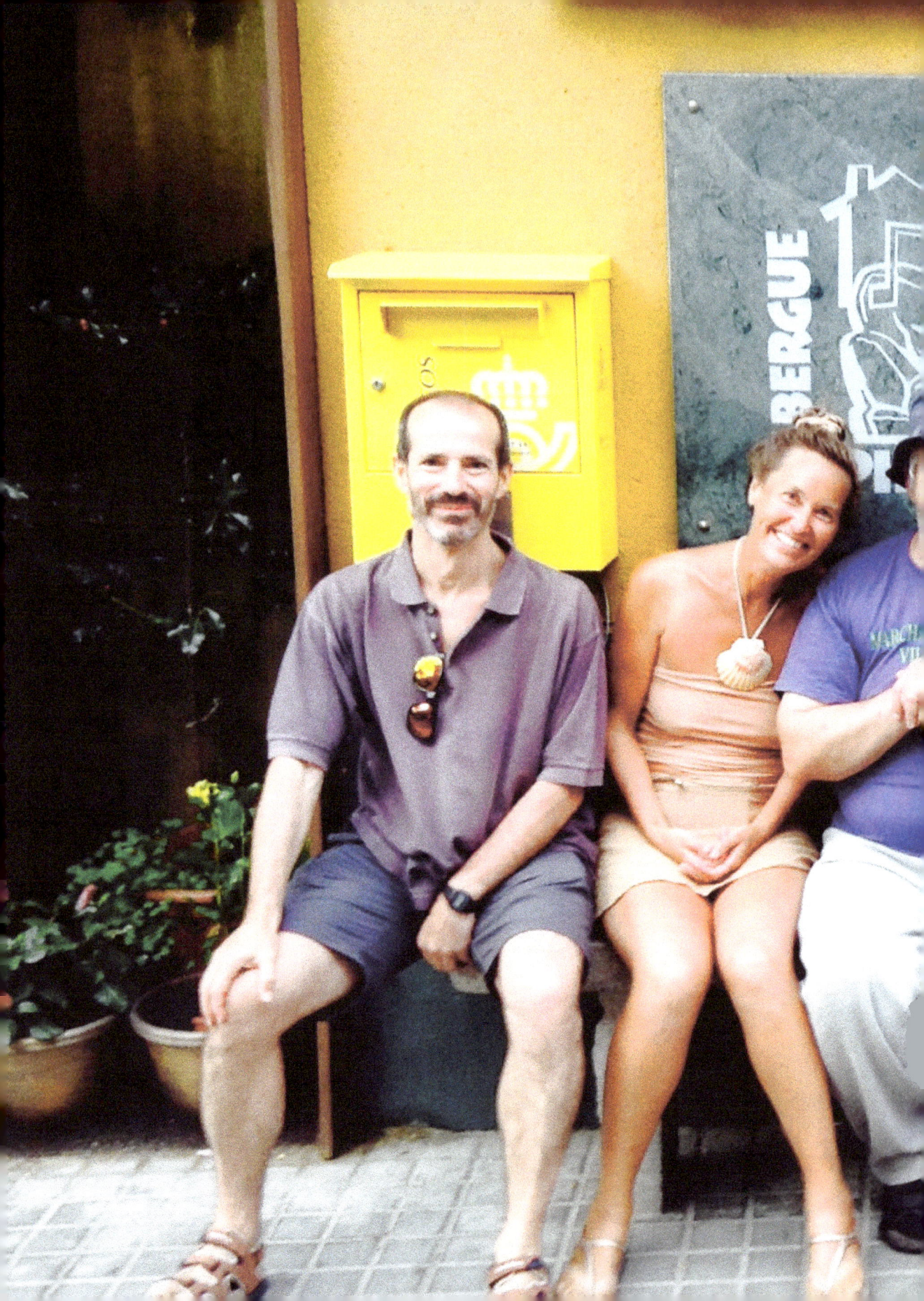

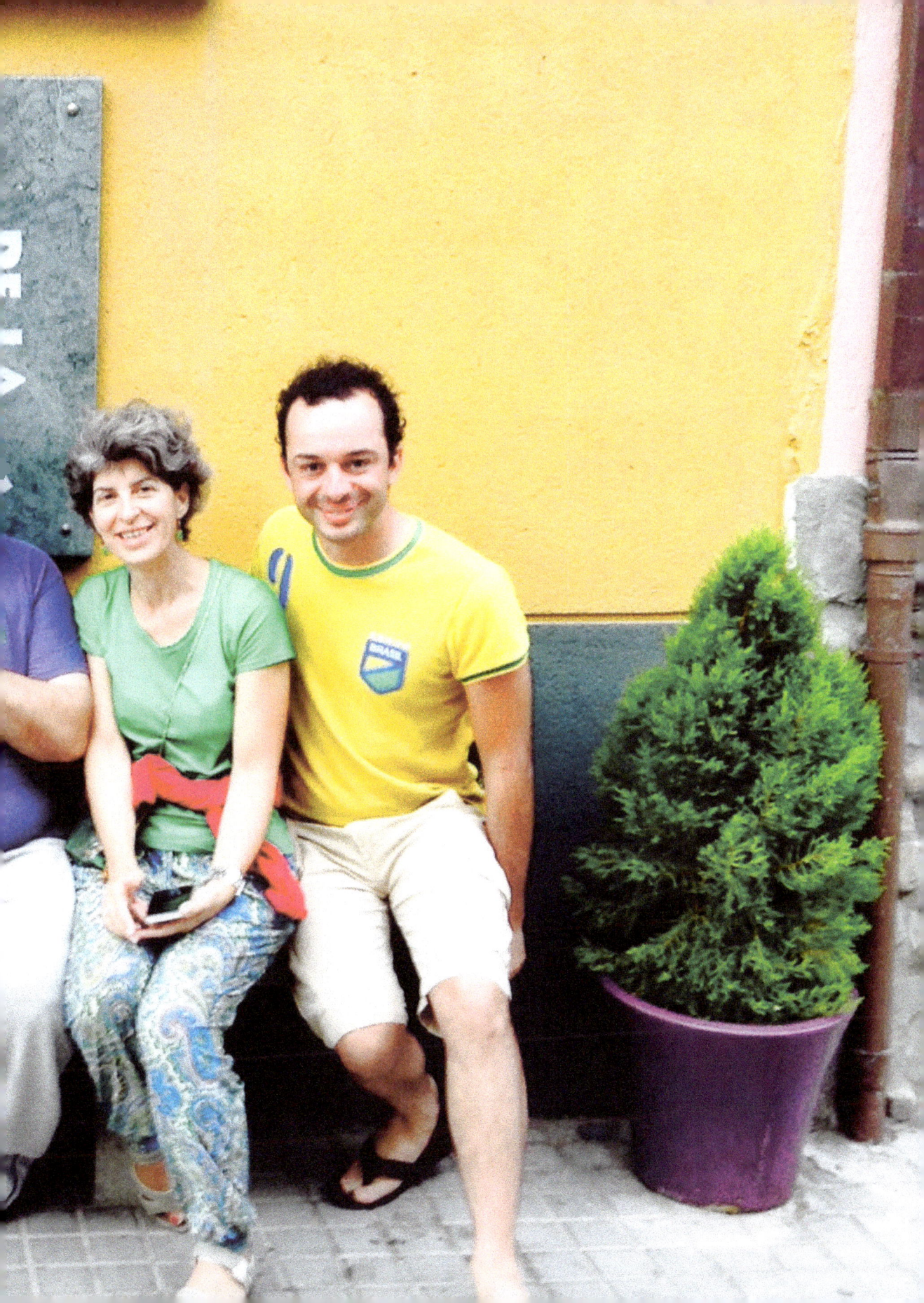

Rome Wisc

Germany DC

Mexico Pa

Romania Ca

Italy Califo

Lond

Austr

Vir

Verona

onsin

Sici

pain

apan Arizon

nplona Paris

nada

France

rnia

nBelgium

lia USA

inia

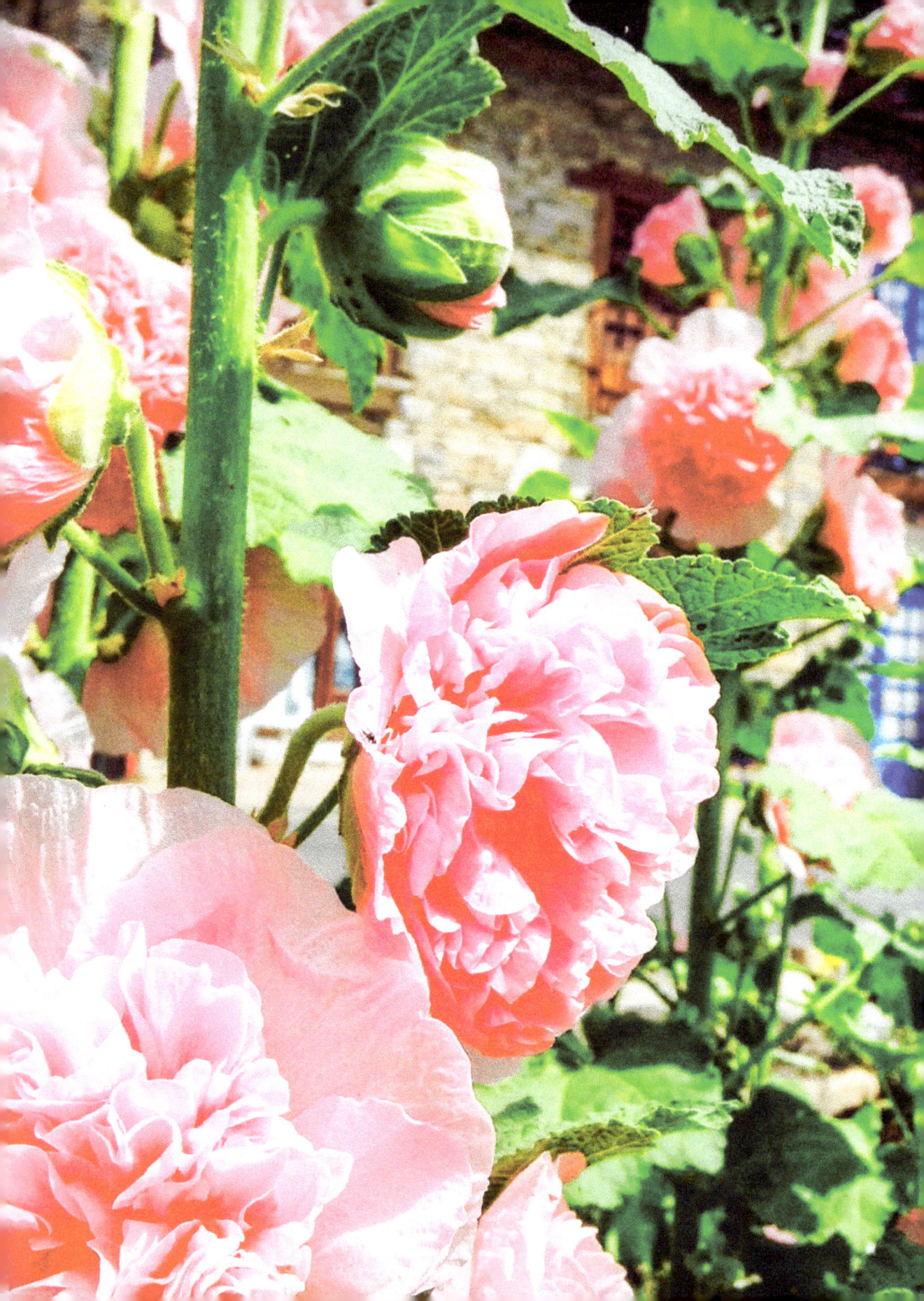

Before walking the Camino, I always had a fear of Facebook. As I started meeting people on the Camino and not wanting to lose them, I faced my fear and joined. It was also so much easier and faster to share my photos and communicate with everyone back home. I was able to immediately connect with new Camino friends (I did not have my phone), and the people back home were so encouraging and loving in their messages. I was overwhelmed with gratitude for the whole system. I also appreciated being able to use Messenger to speak individually with people as though I did have my phone. I am so grateful for joining Facebook because I still communicate with the people I met on the Camino. Facebook and Messenger offer an instant and free way of doing that!

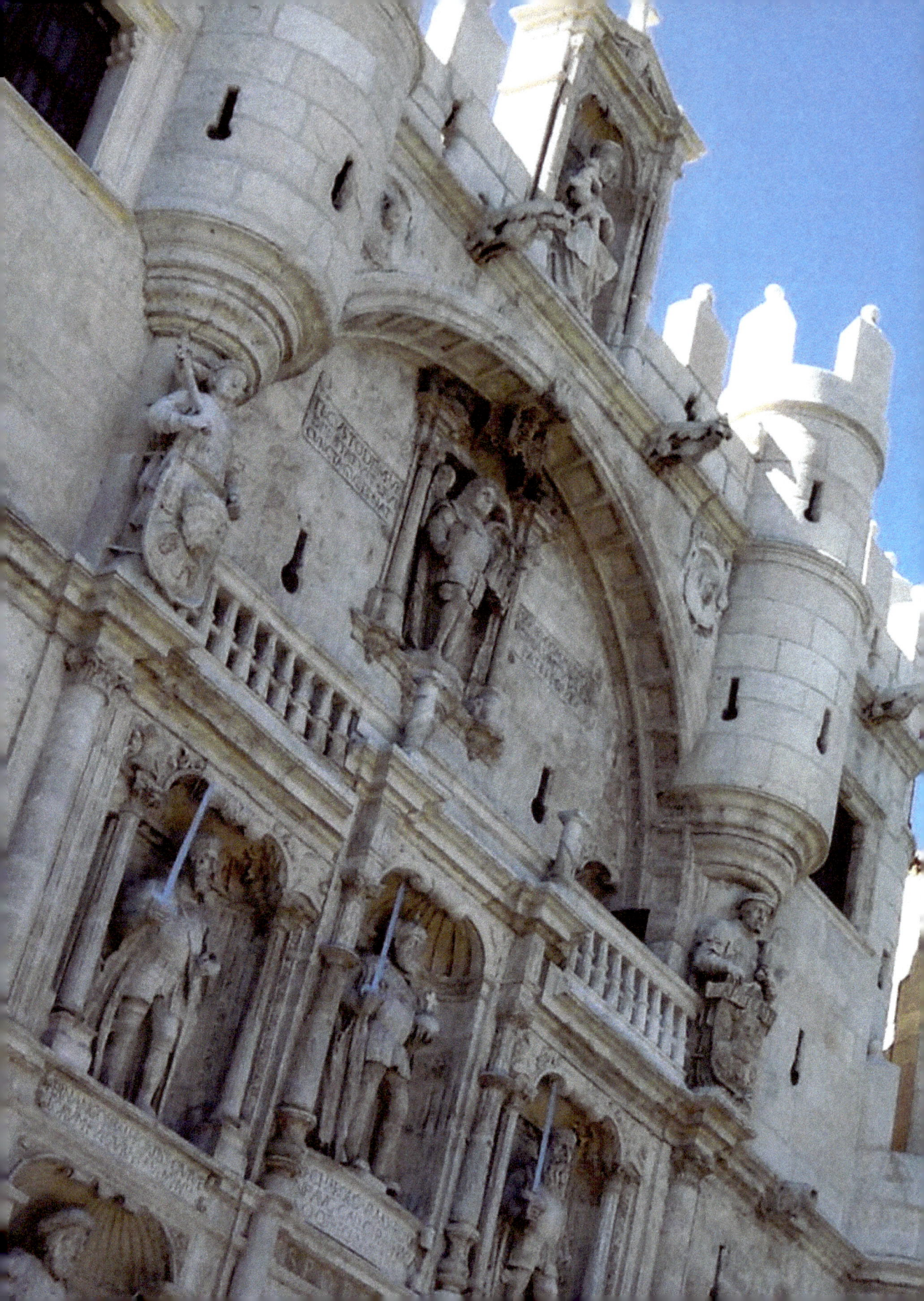

new friends ancient family

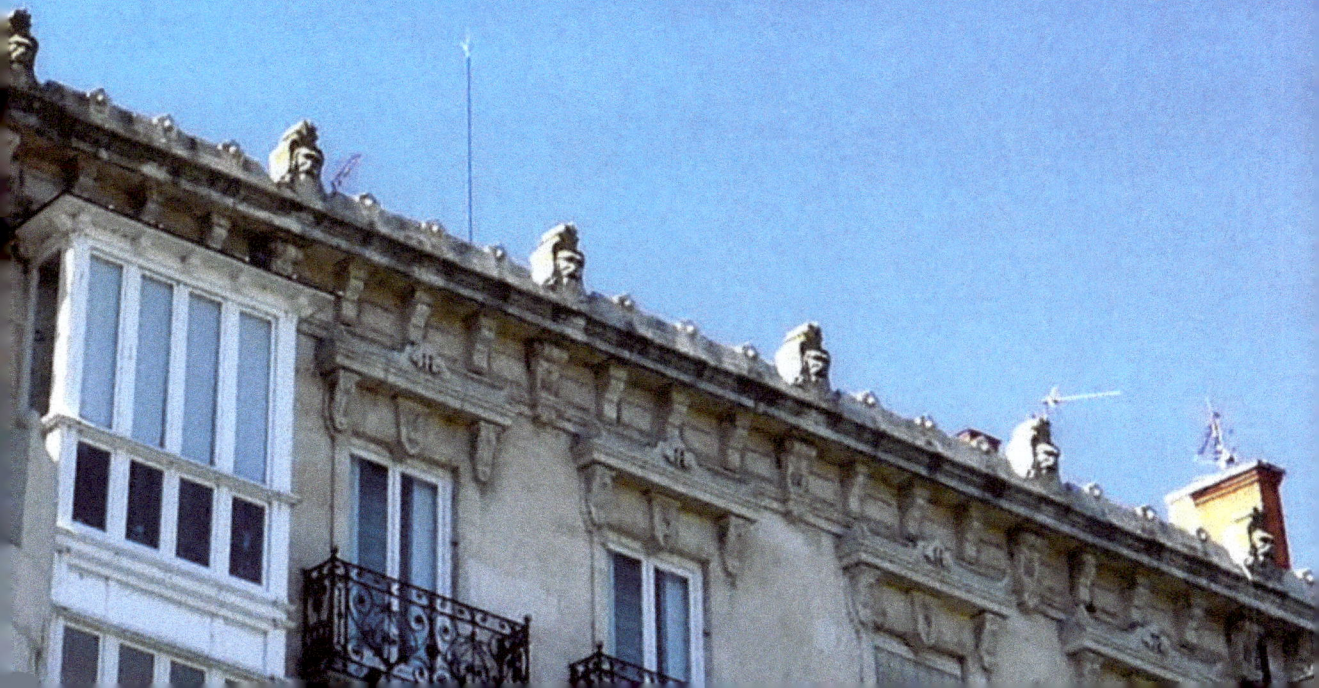

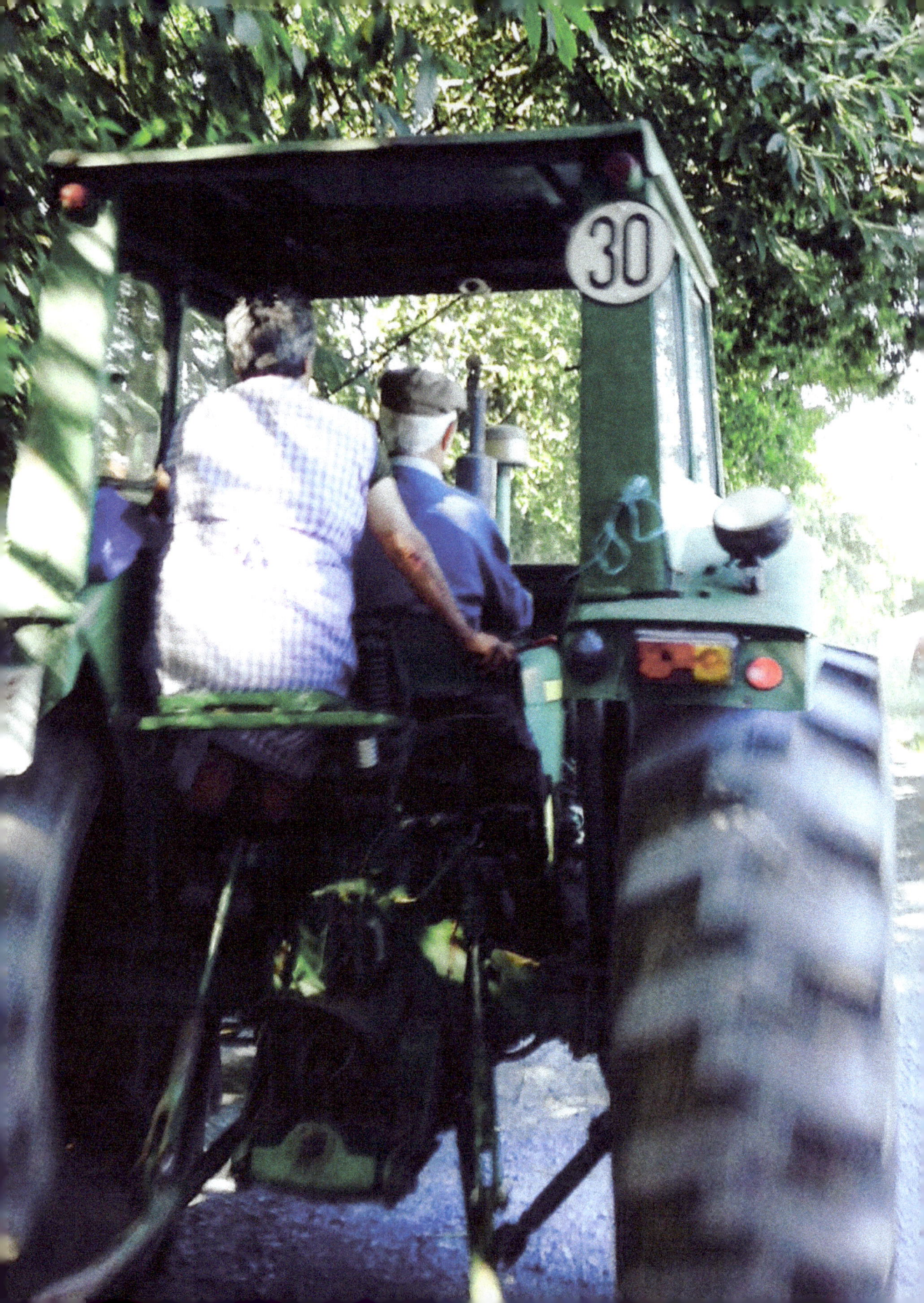

My Experience

After all of the reading and research, I knew that many pilgrims have made significant connections with people while walking the Camino. As departure time approached, I was so excited that I had spent the past five months exhaustively making all of my preparations so that now I was free to just walk and enjoy every moment of the experience. This is exactly what happened! From the moment I arrived in CDG Airport in Paris, I held sacred every person I encountered. I fell madly and deeply in love with every airport employee, hotel concierge, artisan, shop owner, museum guard, bus driver, albergue owner/volunteer, and all of the people on the Camino. Even if I did not ever speak to them, I felt a deep bond of sharing all of the same miraculous Camino steps. There really are no words to describe it, but I felt as though I would "take a bullet" for all of my fellow pilgrims. To share in this divine experience is a miracle I will take with me always.

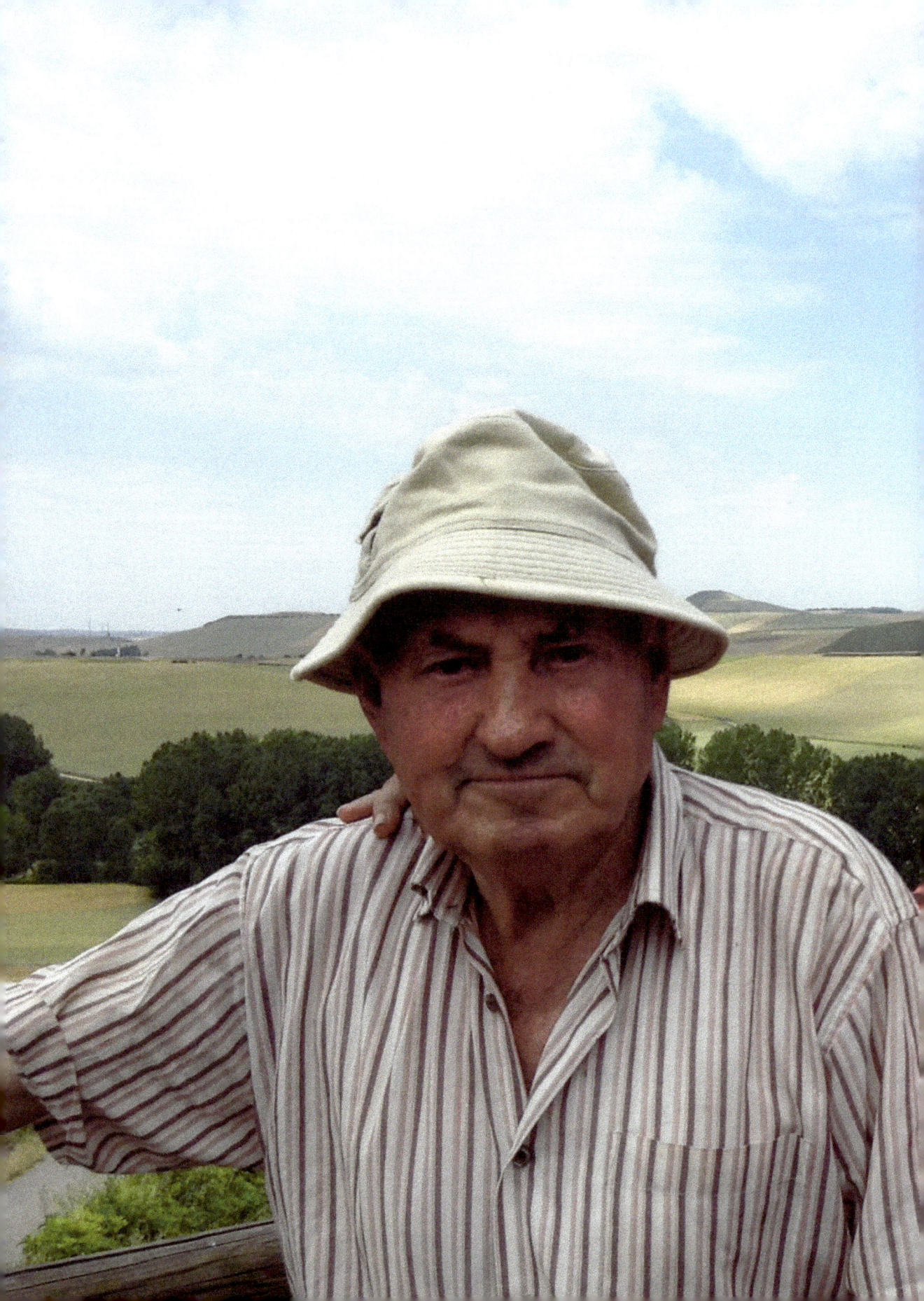

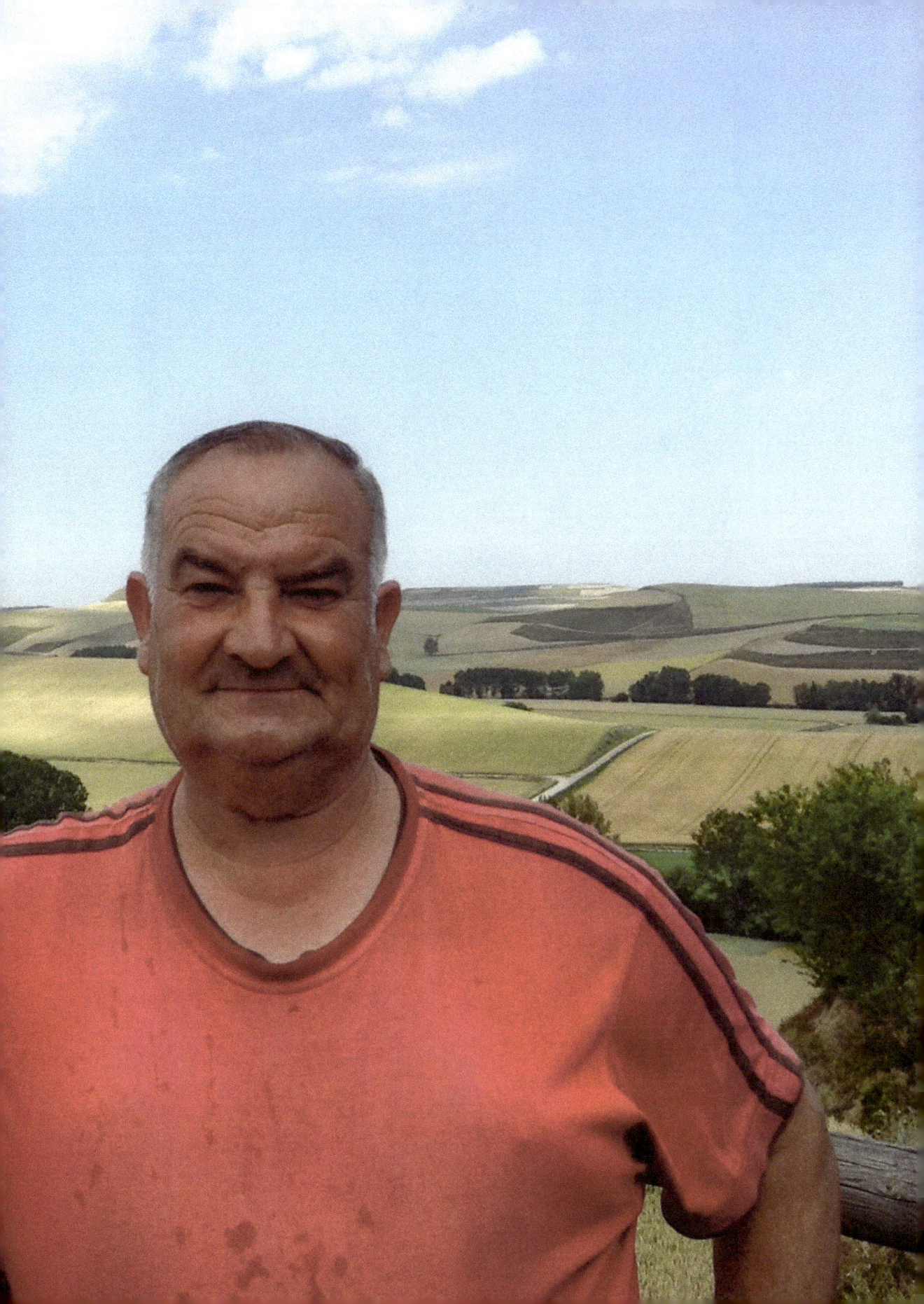

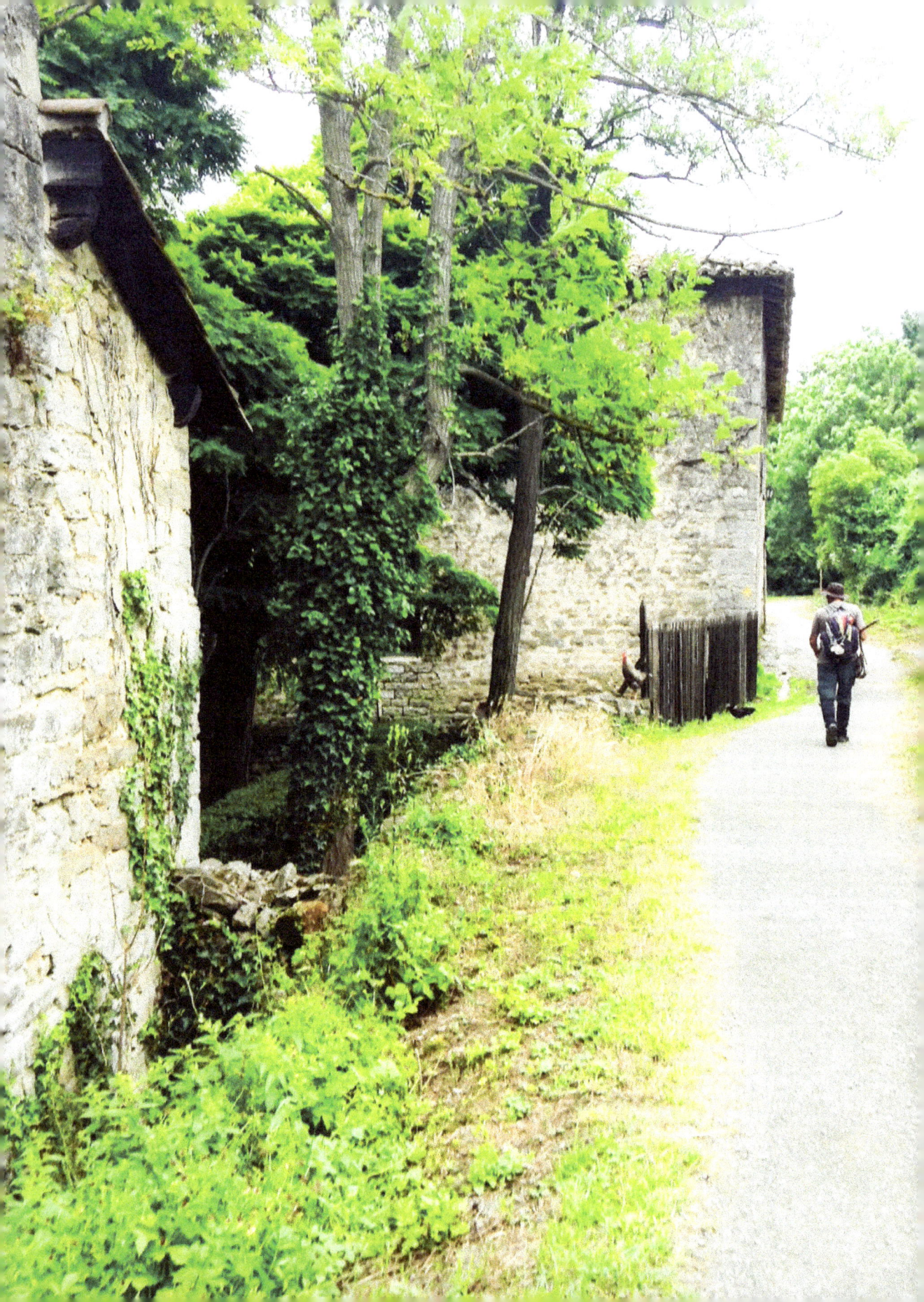

"he that walketh with wise shall be wise"
-proverb 13:20

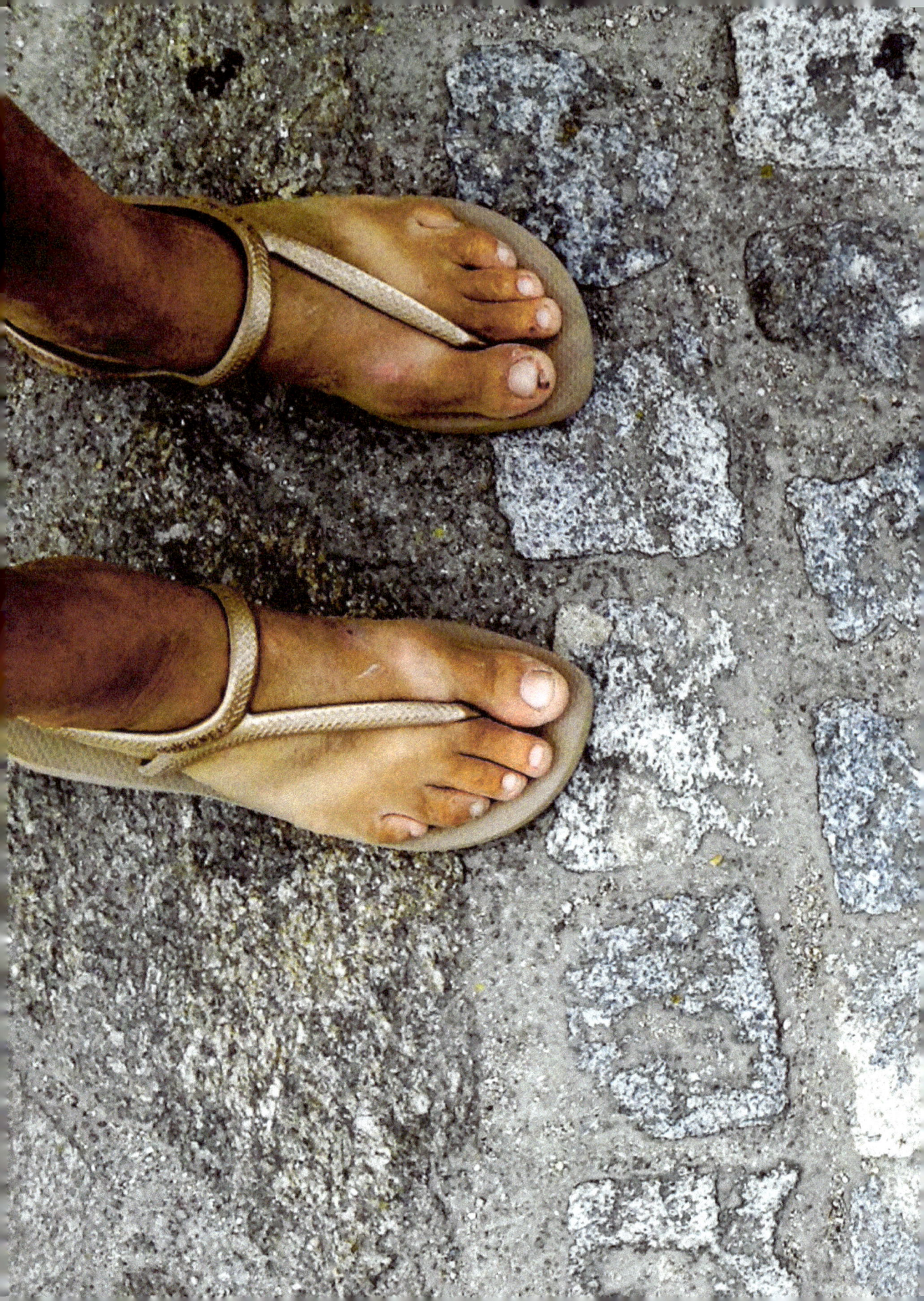

accepting

ACCEPT ACCEPT ACCEPT ACCEPT

I tell the world how I feel about myself with every word and every action.

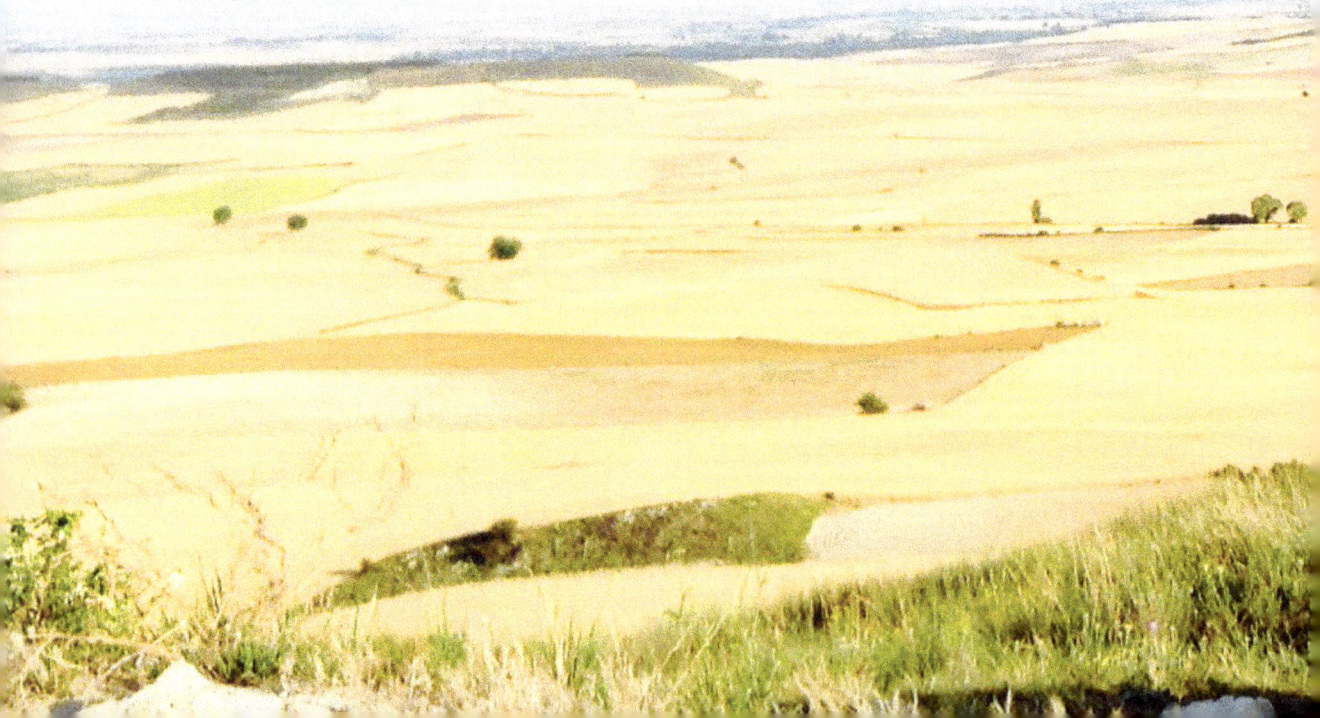

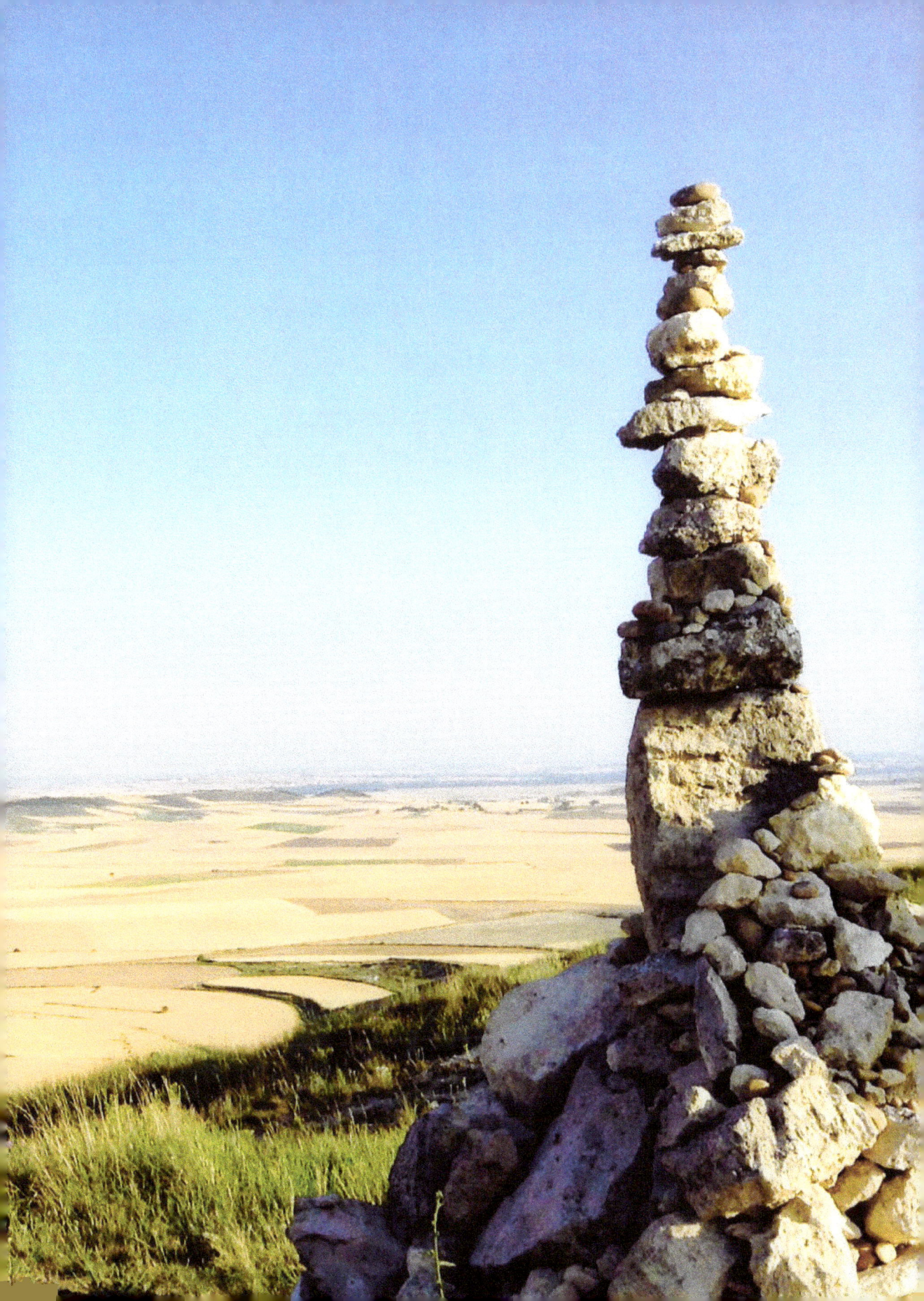

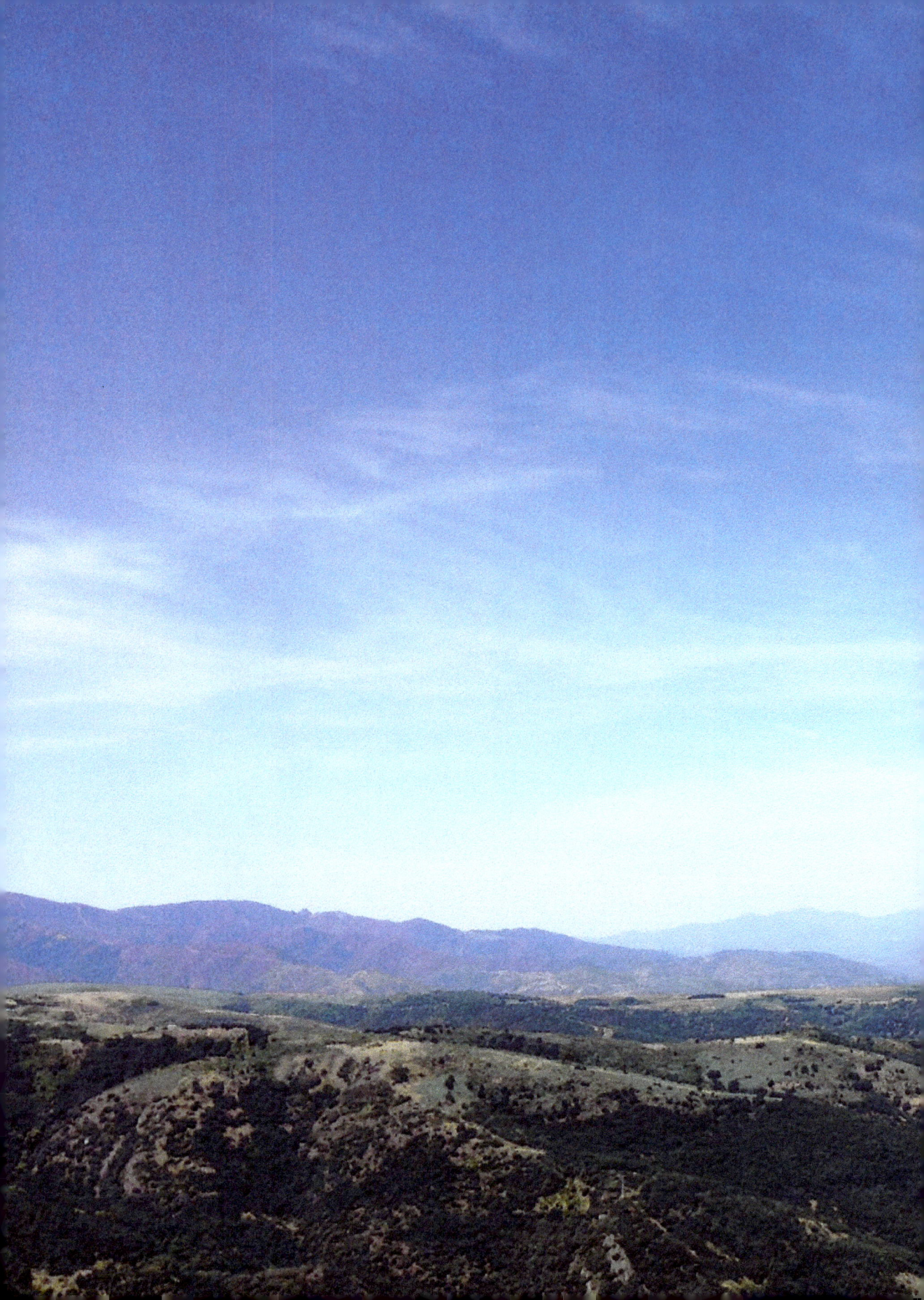

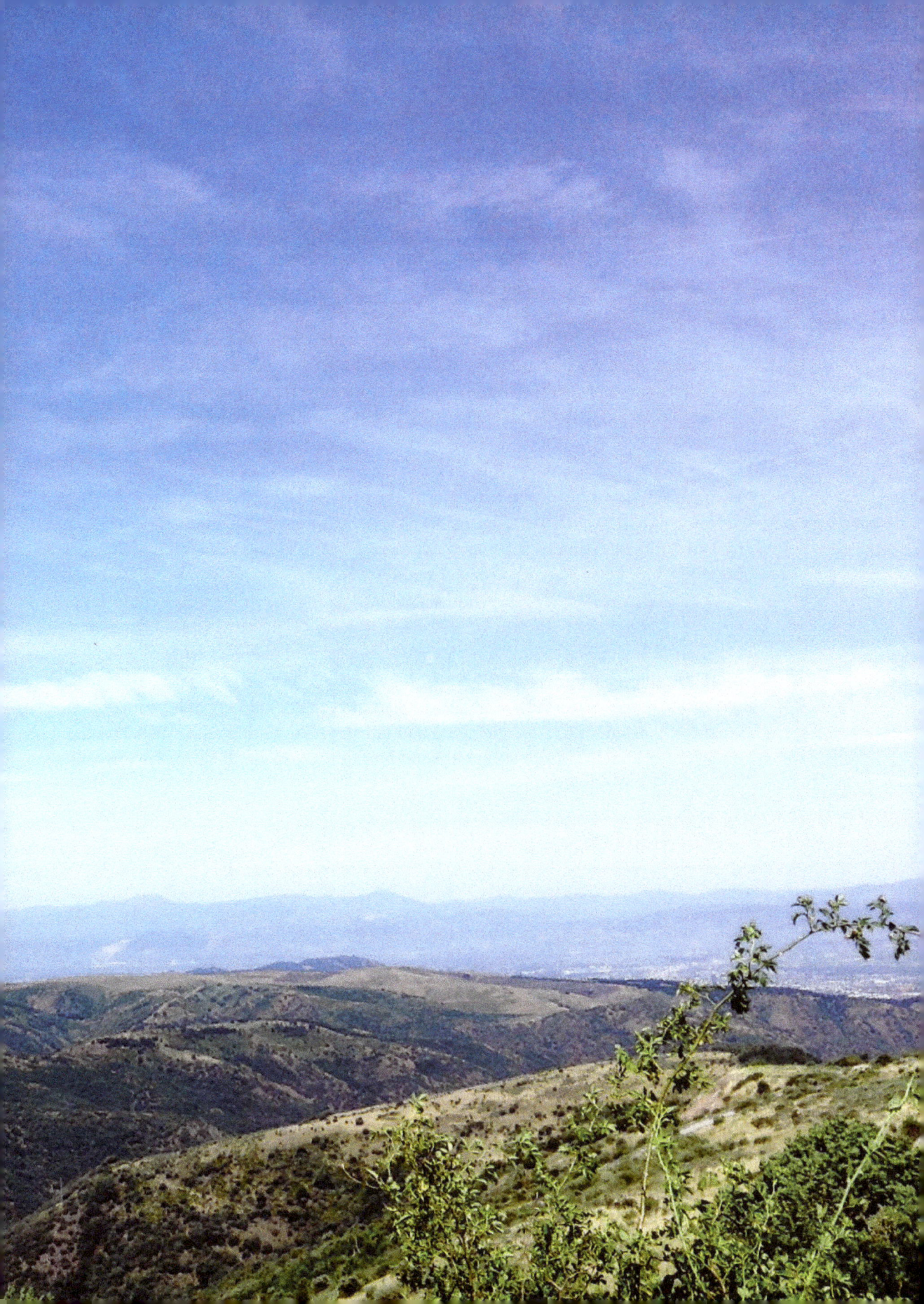

Challenges

Learning to accept has been one of my greatest learning experiences and accomplishments. Growing up the daughter of two alcoholic parents (both of whom have been in sober recovery for 40+ years!), some very early formative years were quite chaotic. Although both of my parents are beautiful, loving, highly educated, intelligent and successful people, because of their disease they were unable to always provide healthy nurturance and protection during early childhood. I adore both of my parents! They are light-hearted, loving, smart and fun, and yet I couldn't understand their behaviors. After many years of learning, I now understand that a disease like alcoholism does not allow for healthy intimate personal relationships. It is just simply one of the effects and nothing I did "wrong." Learning to not question the actions of loved ones and to not take anything personally has been one of the greatest challenges and accomplishments (when I can do it!) of my life. It has allowed me a personal freedom so great that I literally feel elevated! On the Camino, I also overcame many obstacles and achieved something I wasn't sure I could accomplish. I lived every day not knowing where exactly I was going, what would happen, who I would meet along the way, and if I could make it to the next town. The arrows and physical demands required staying focused and not letting fear control my thoughts. Facing seemingly endless, empty trails, not having replacement shoes, not being able to see any sign of a town in any direction when I was ready to be there, I had to keep my chin up and continue even though at times I felt like giving up and quitting. The Camino gave me a lifetime gift of accomplishment, acceptance and perseverance that will always be a part of me. M I R A C L E !

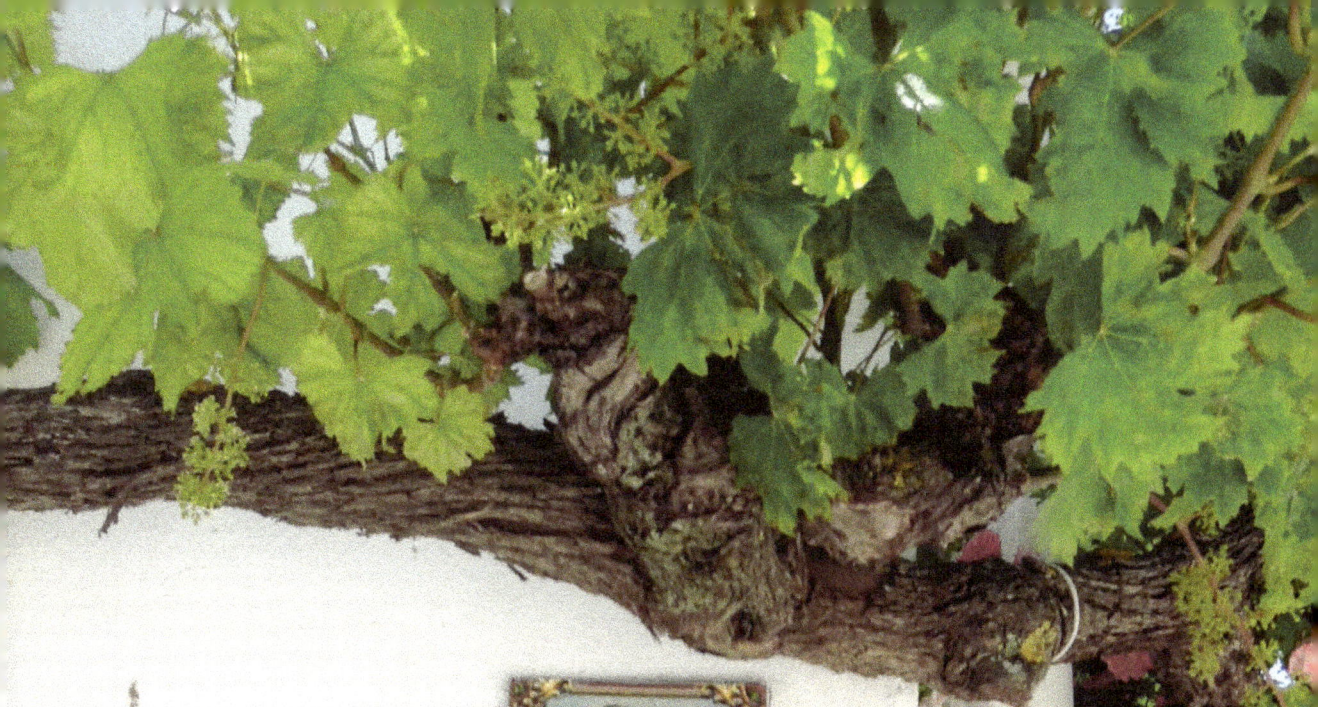

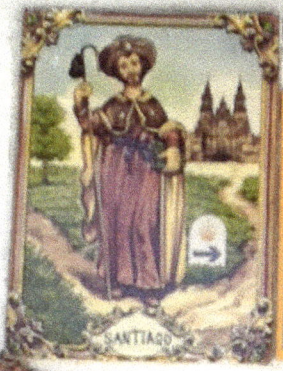

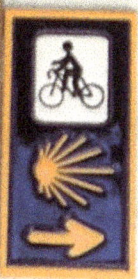

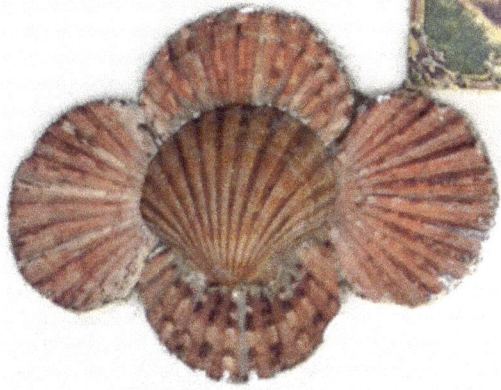

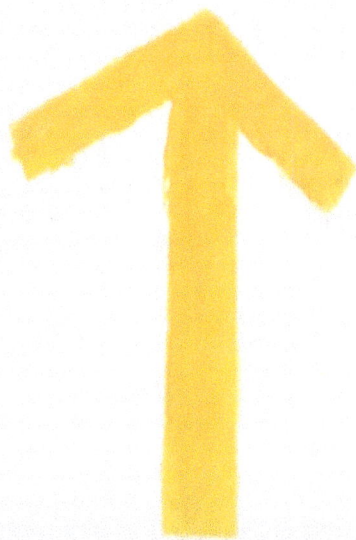

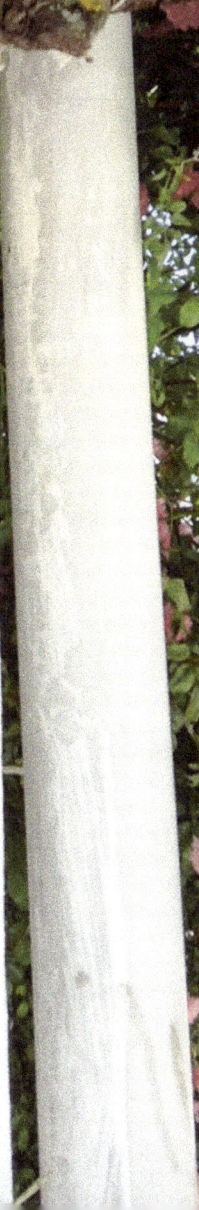

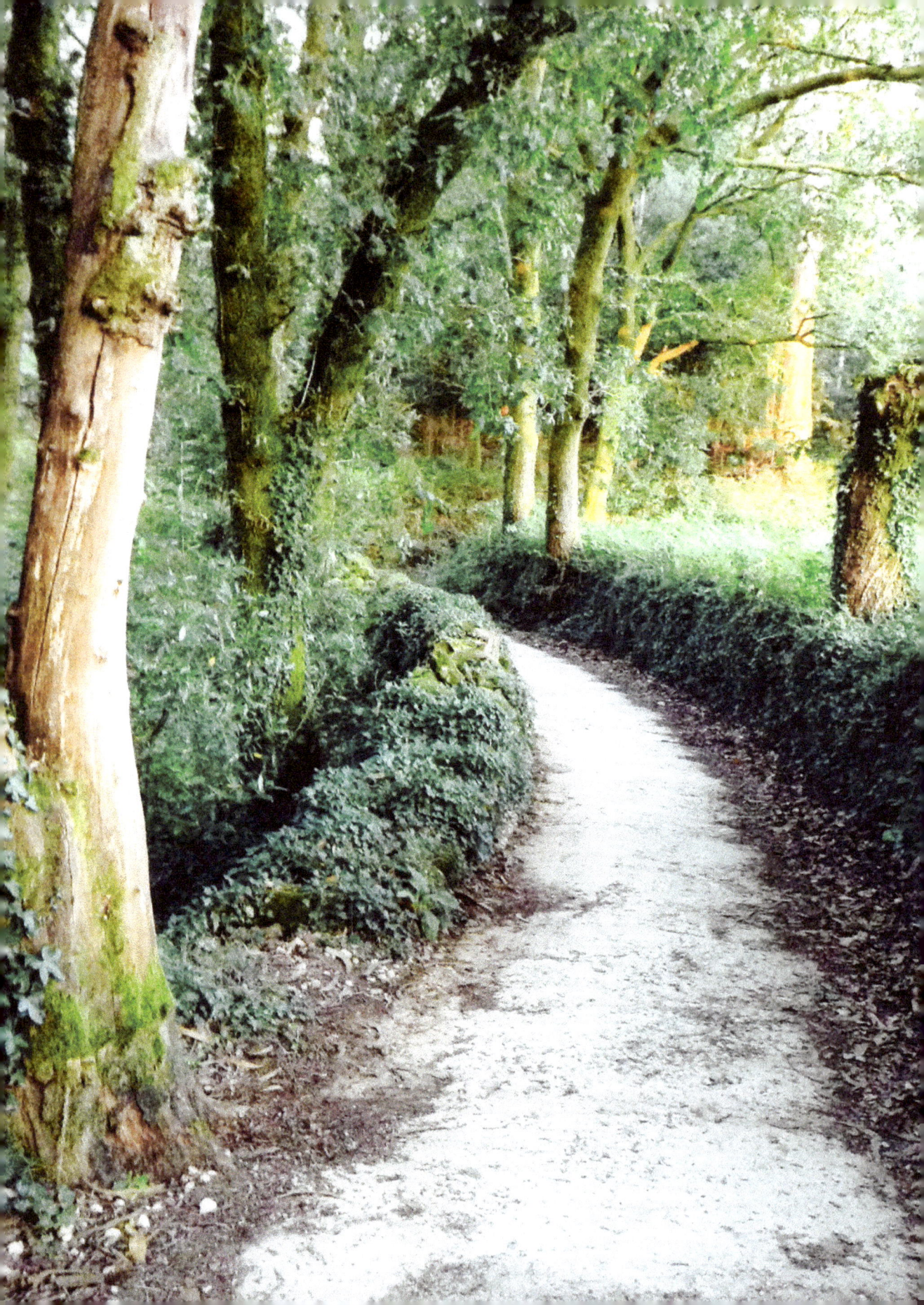

"None of us knows what might happen
even the next minute, yet still we go forward.
Because we trust.
Because we have Faith."
-Paulo Coelho

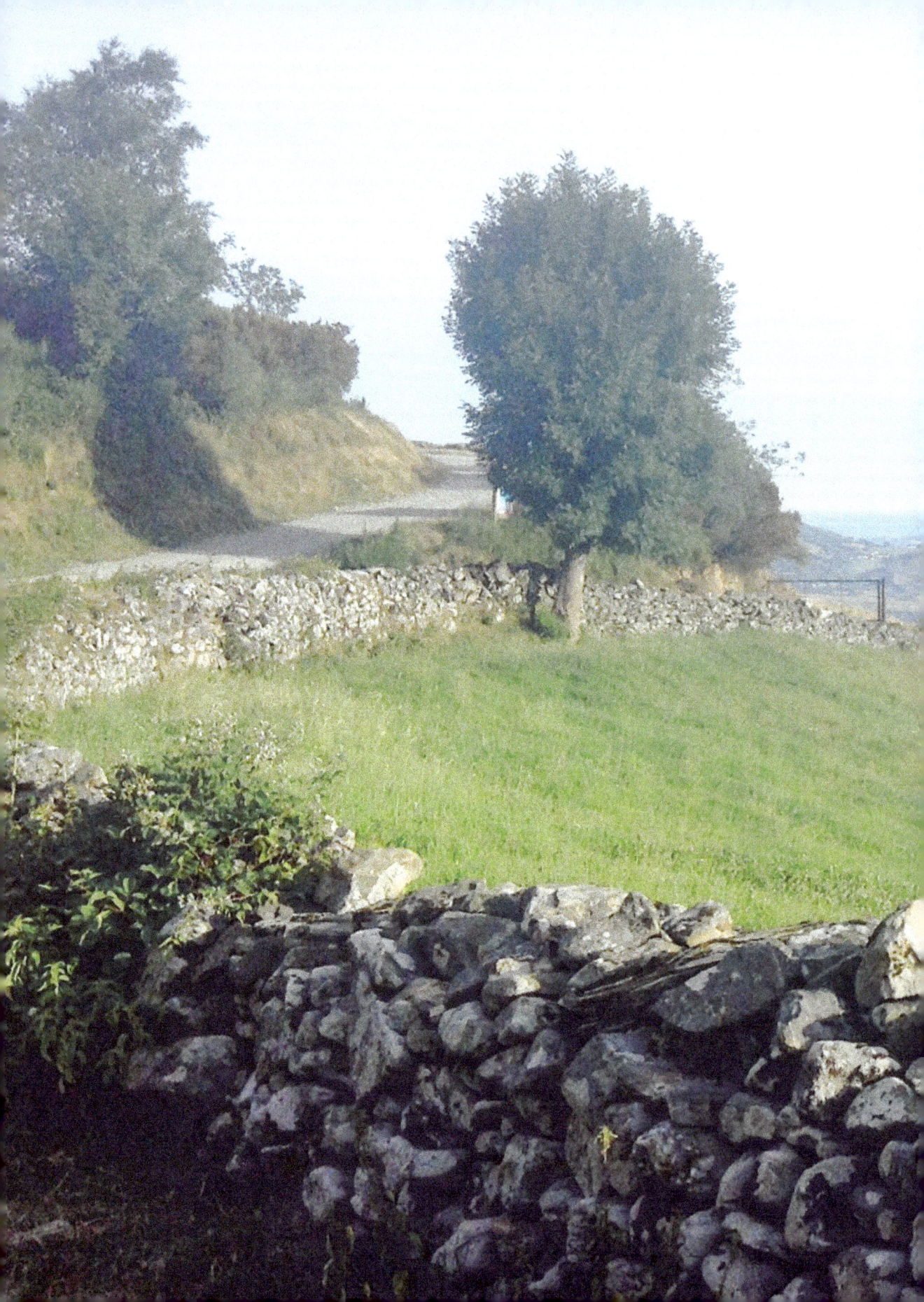

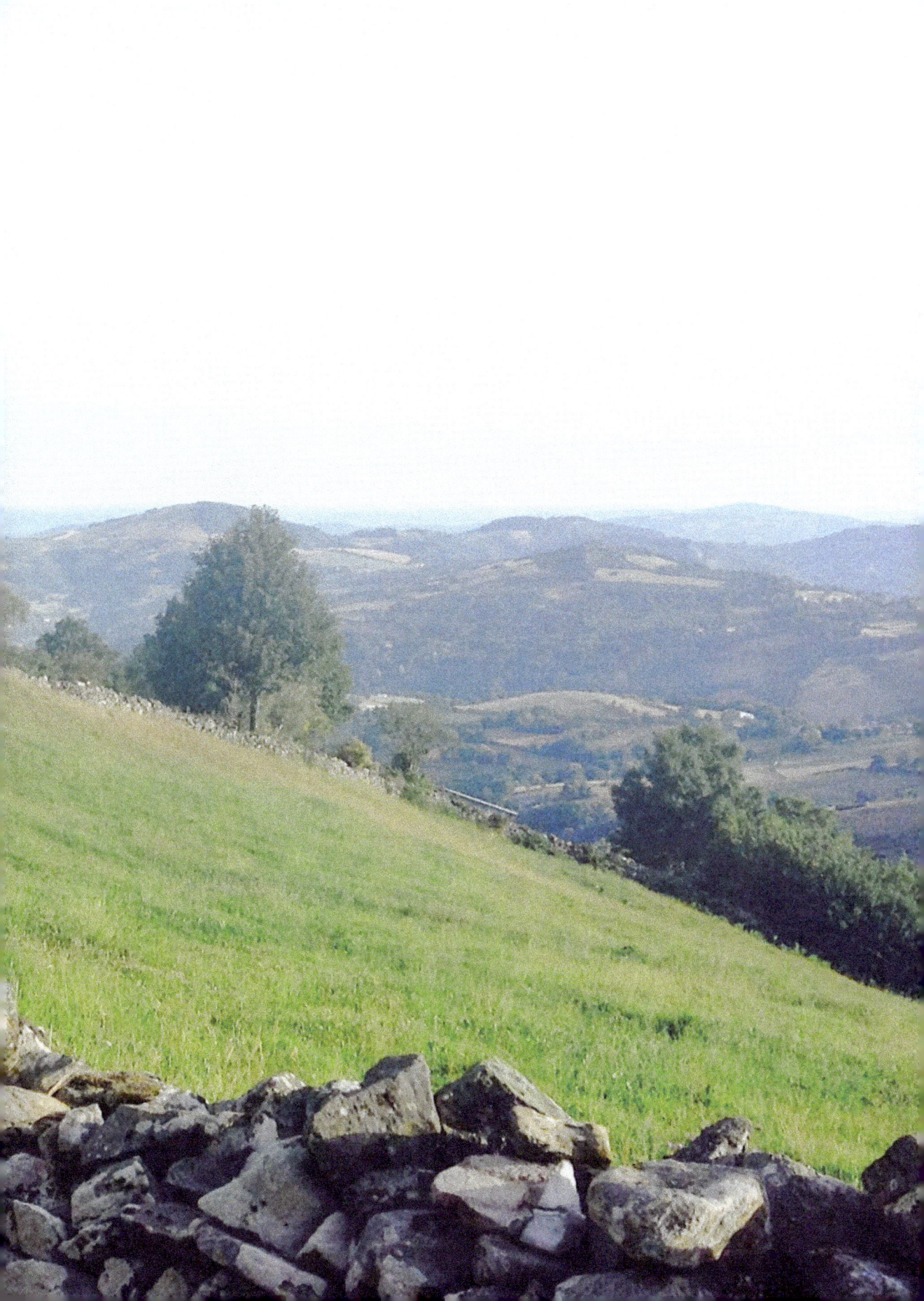

I WALK THE CAMINO LIKE I WALK IN LIFE
always accepting without exception

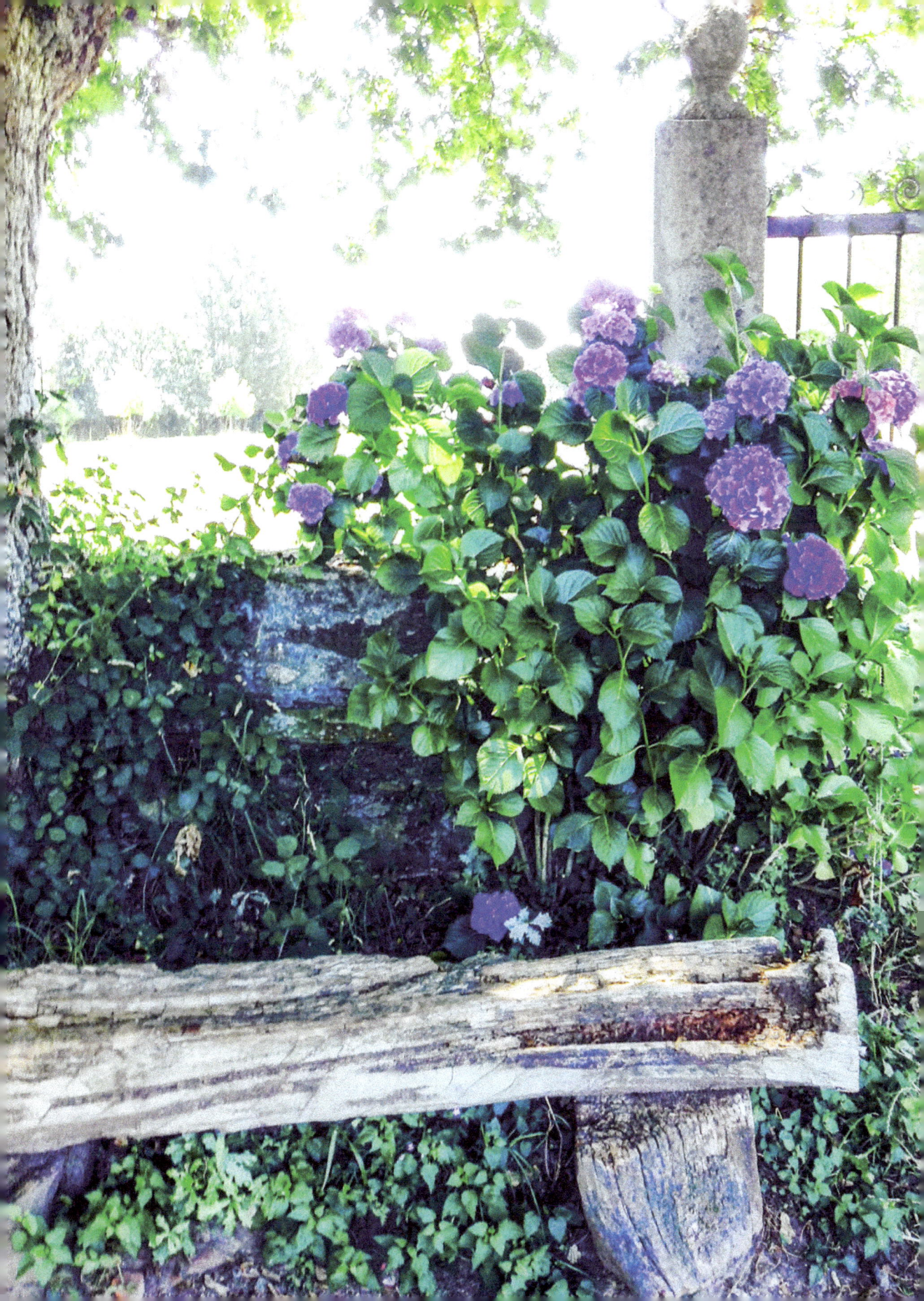

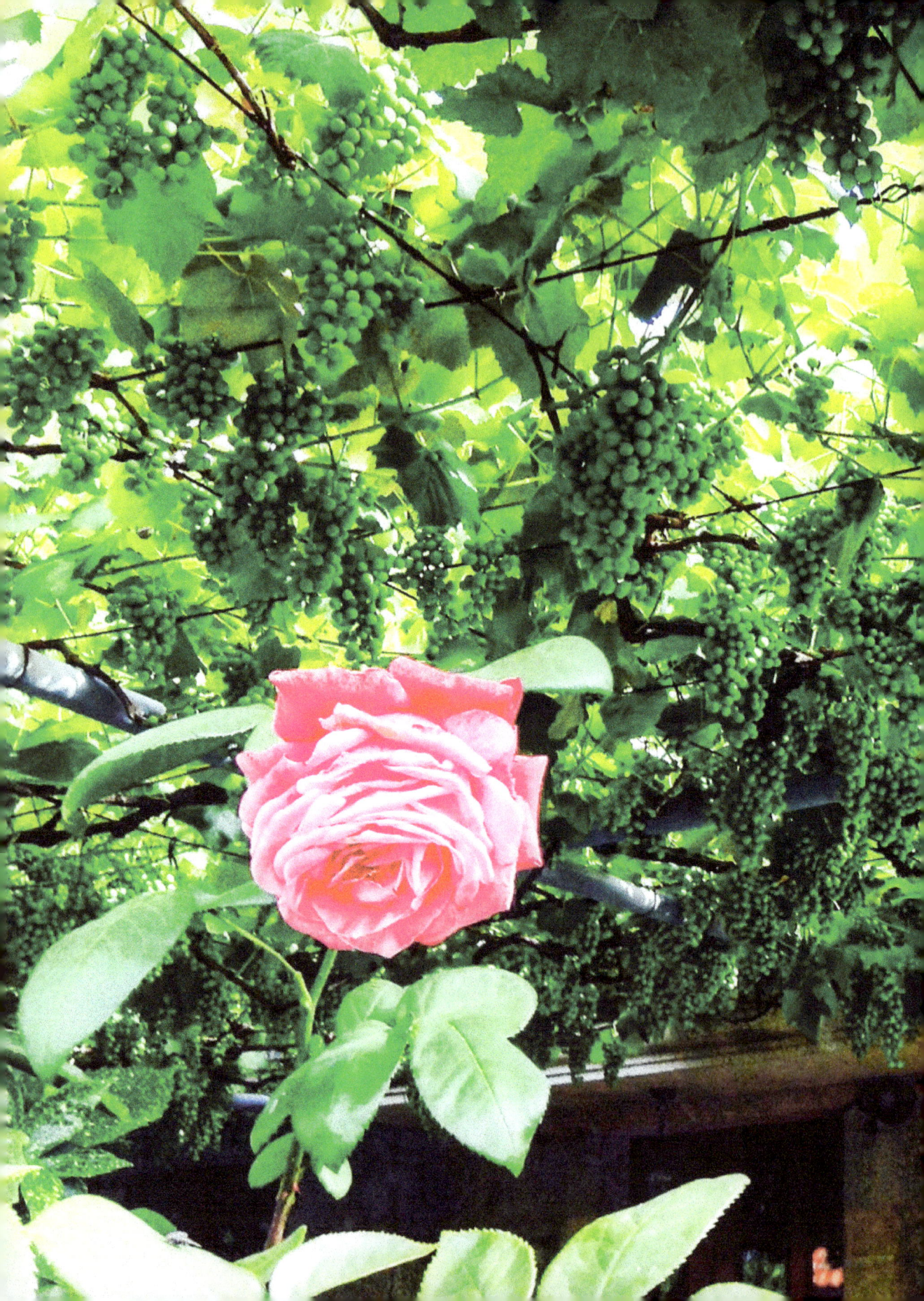

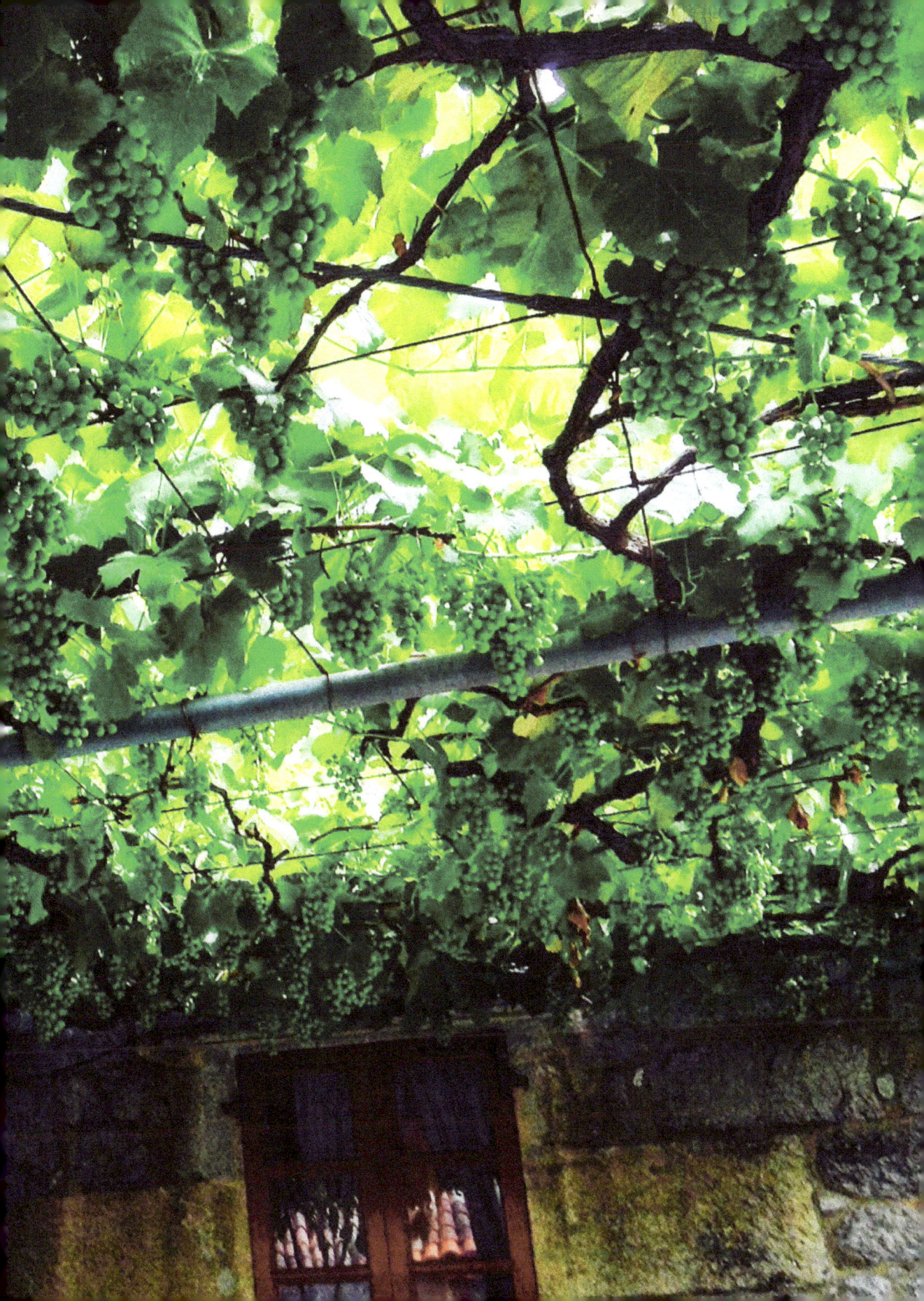

miracles

MIRACLE MIRACLE MIRACLE MIRACLE

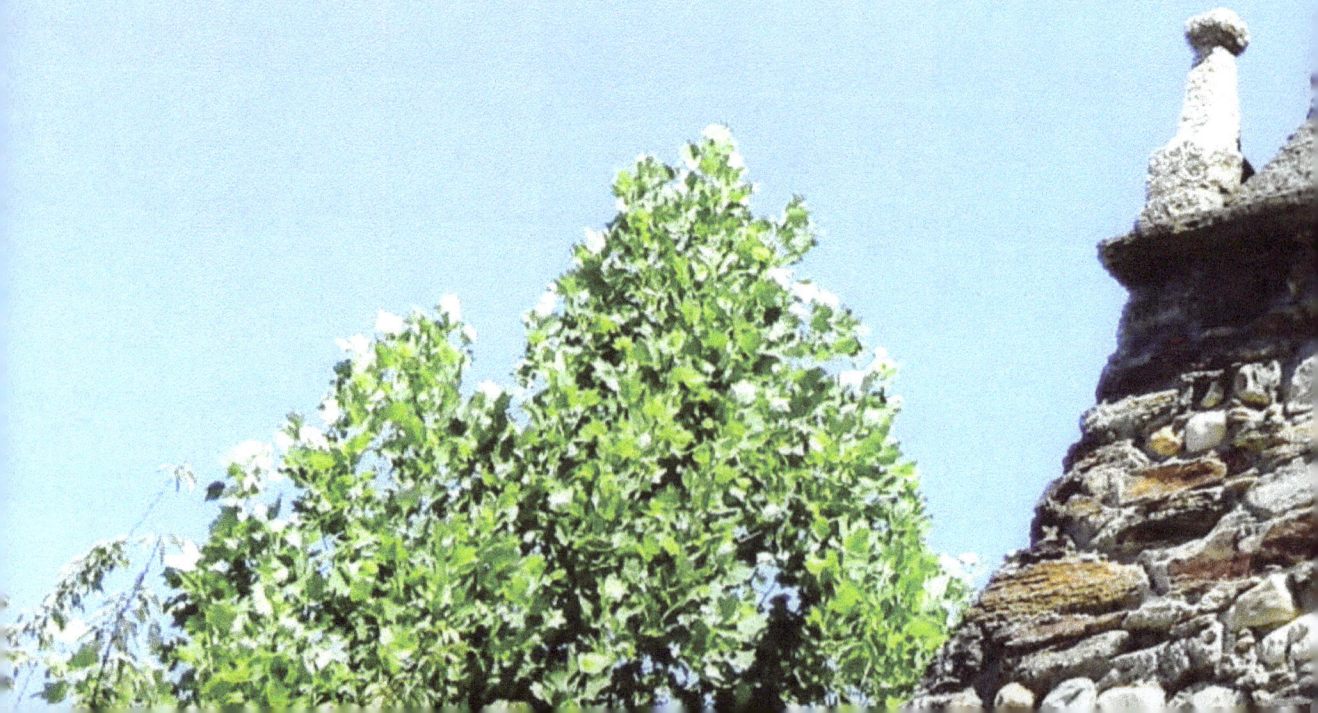

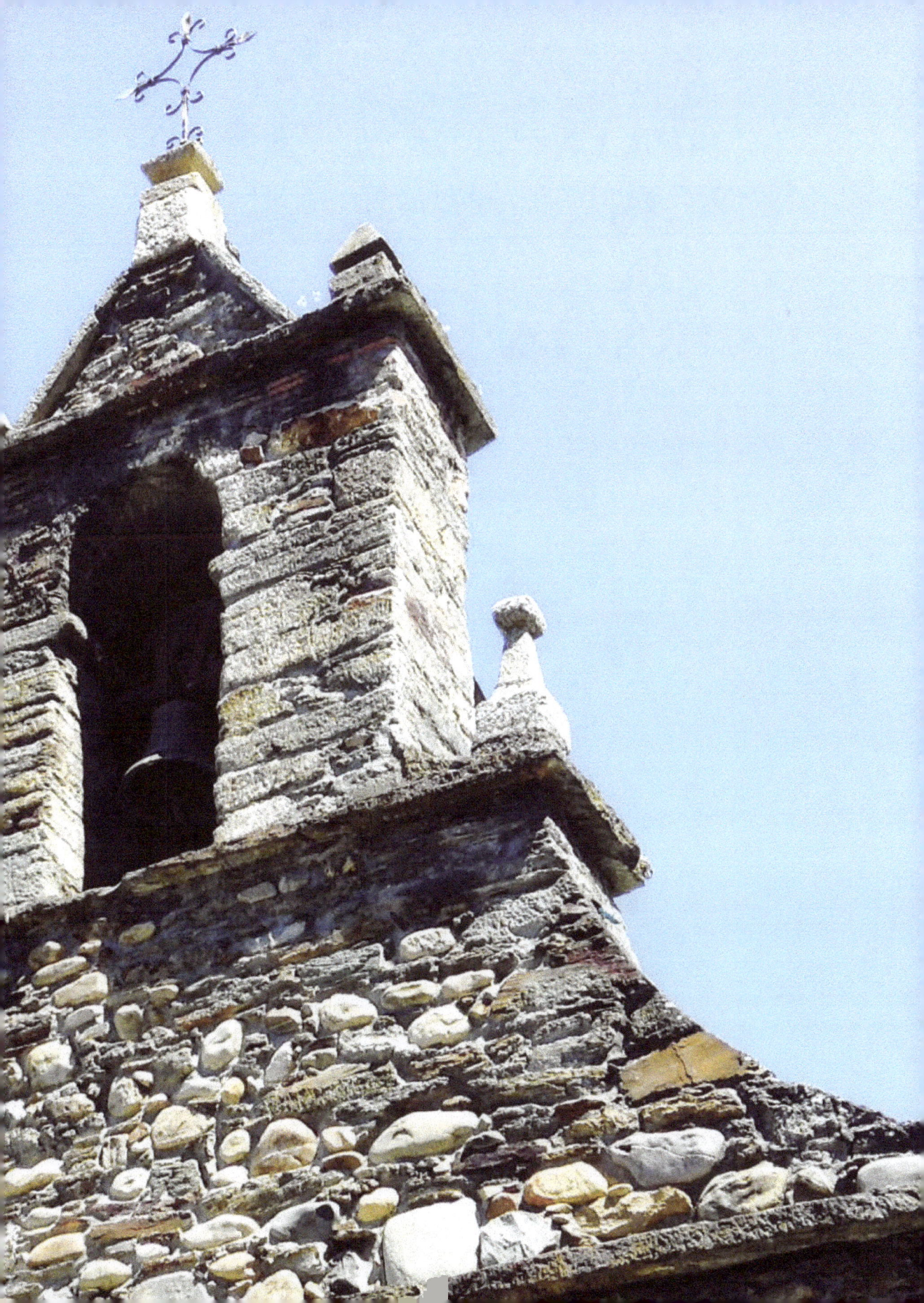

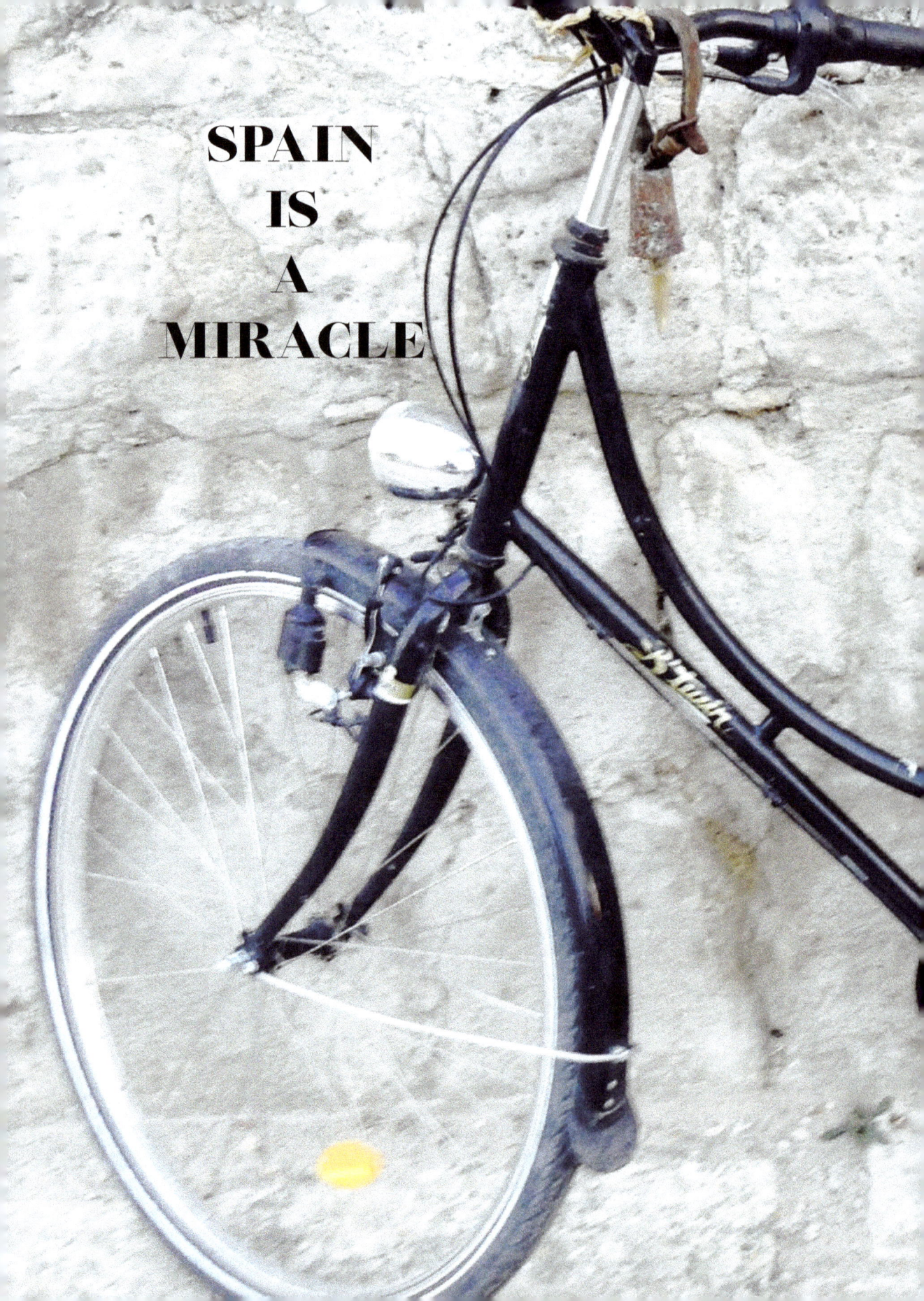

SPAIN

IS

A

MIRACLE

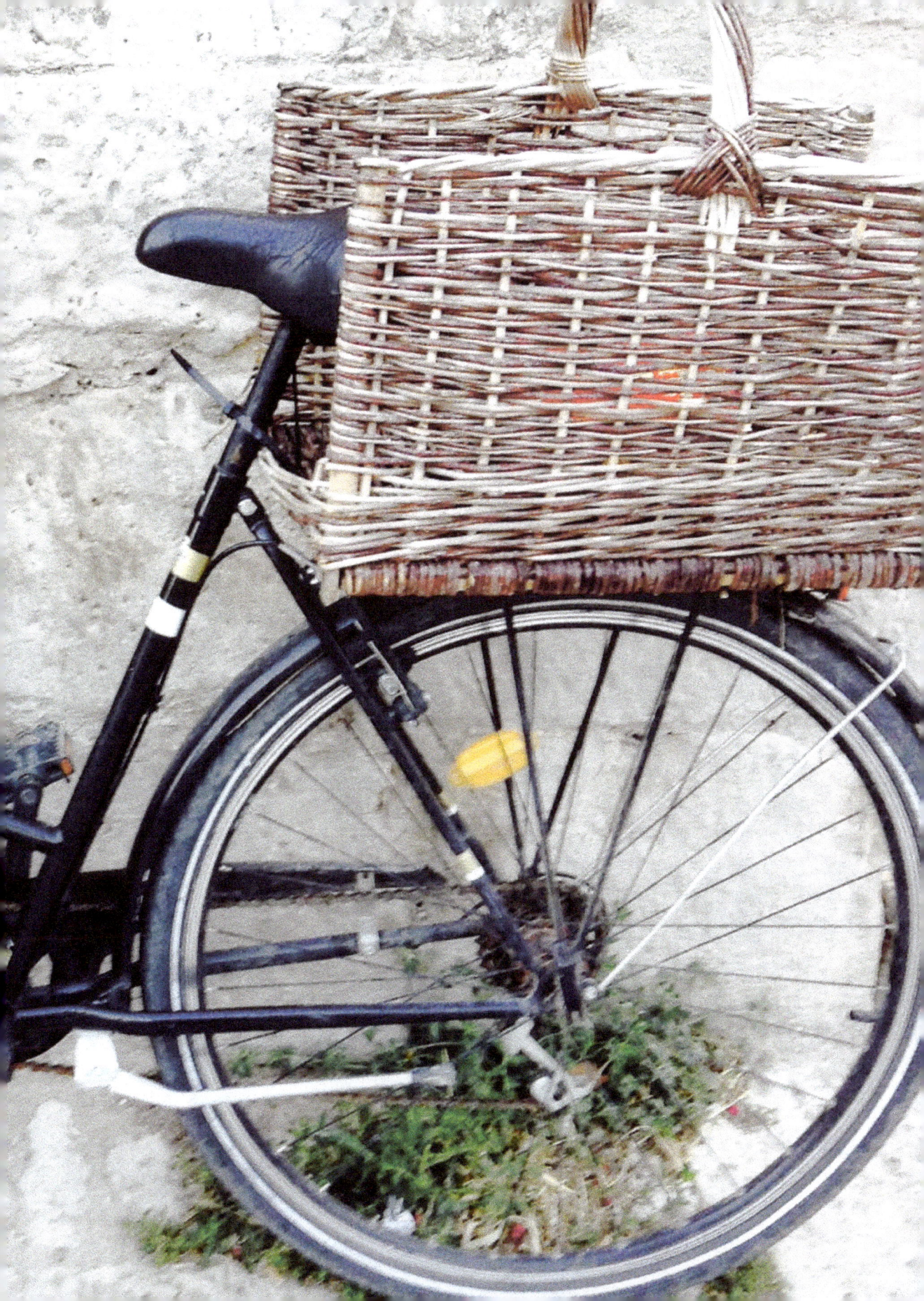

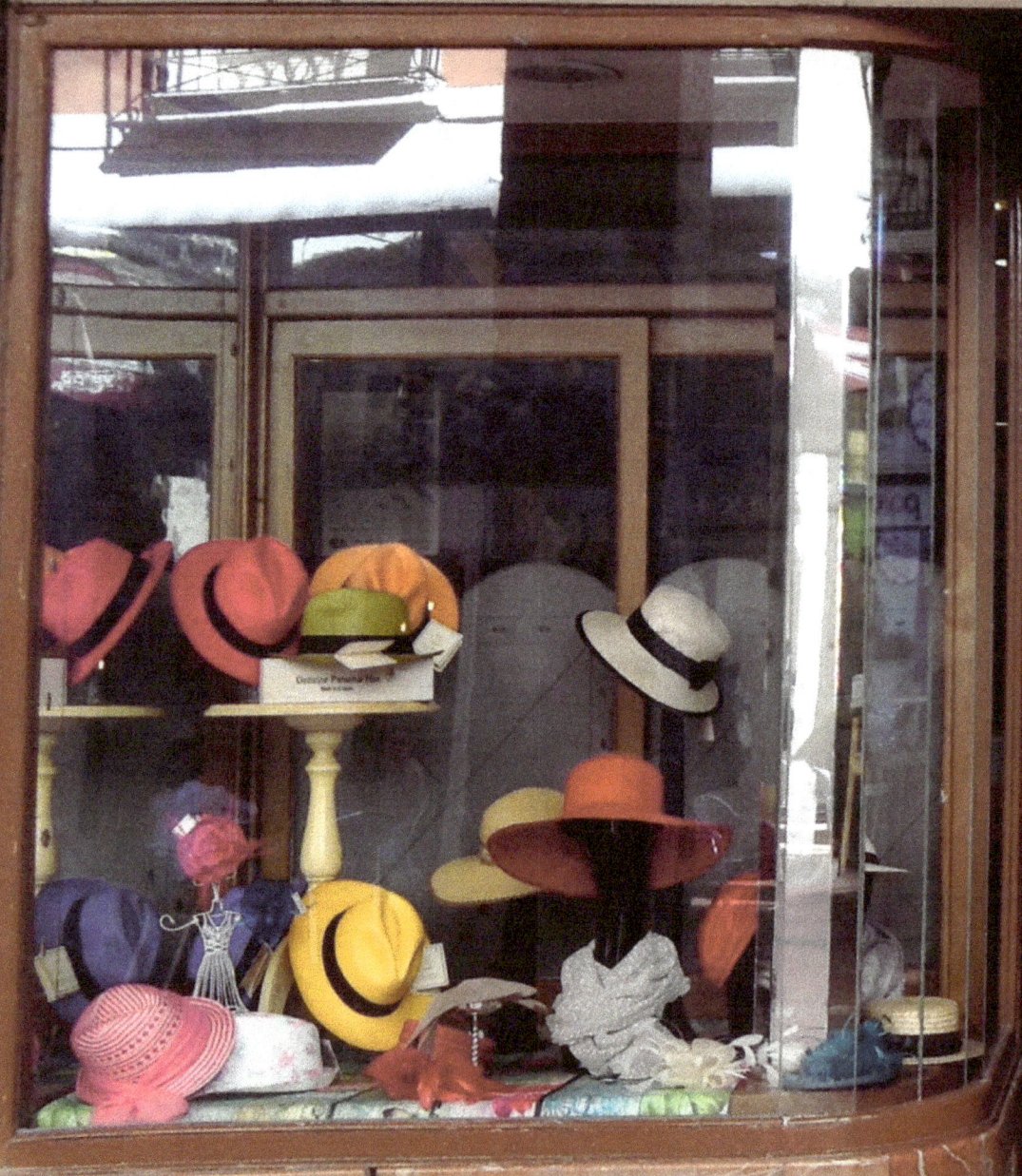

SOMBRERERIA

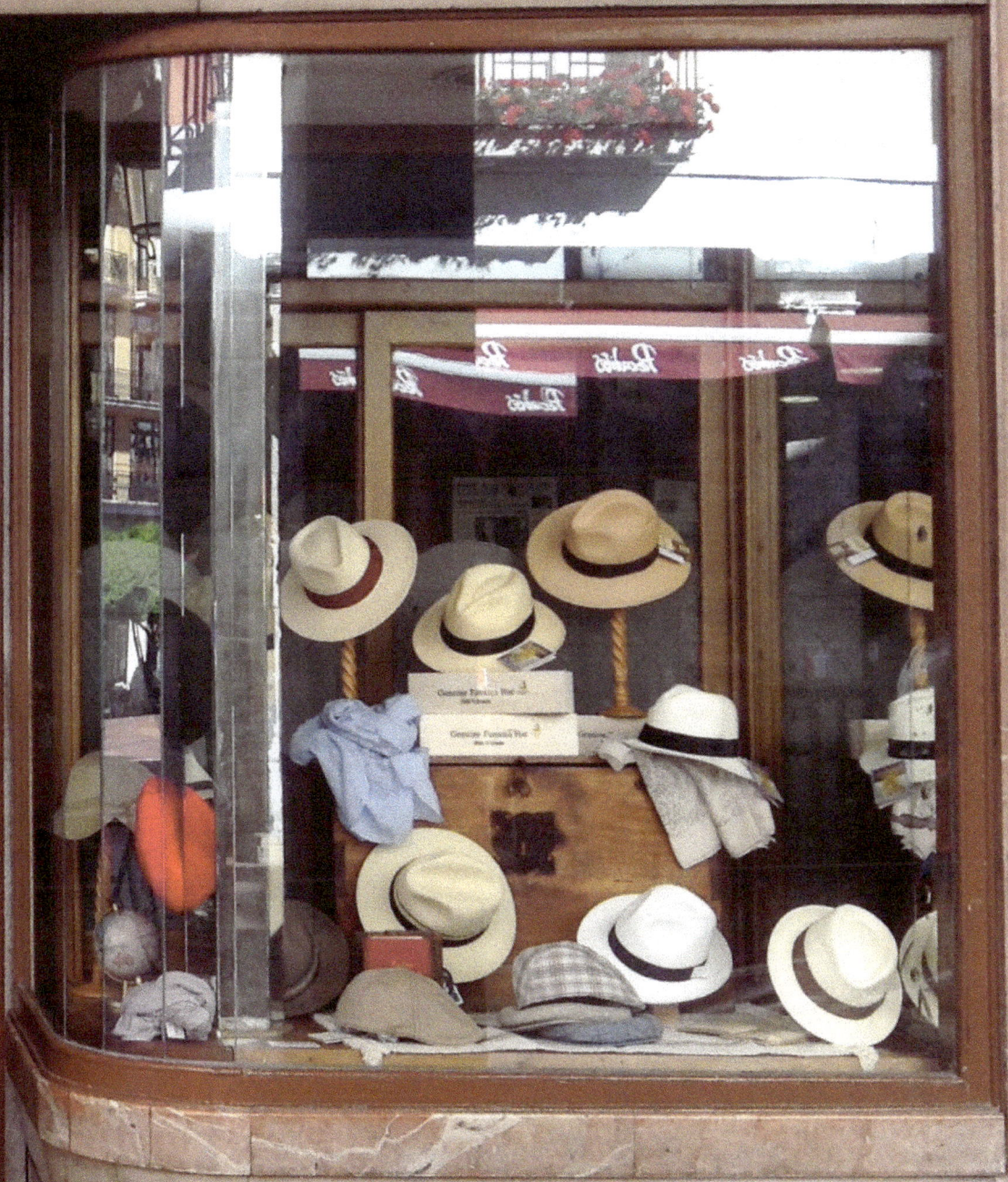

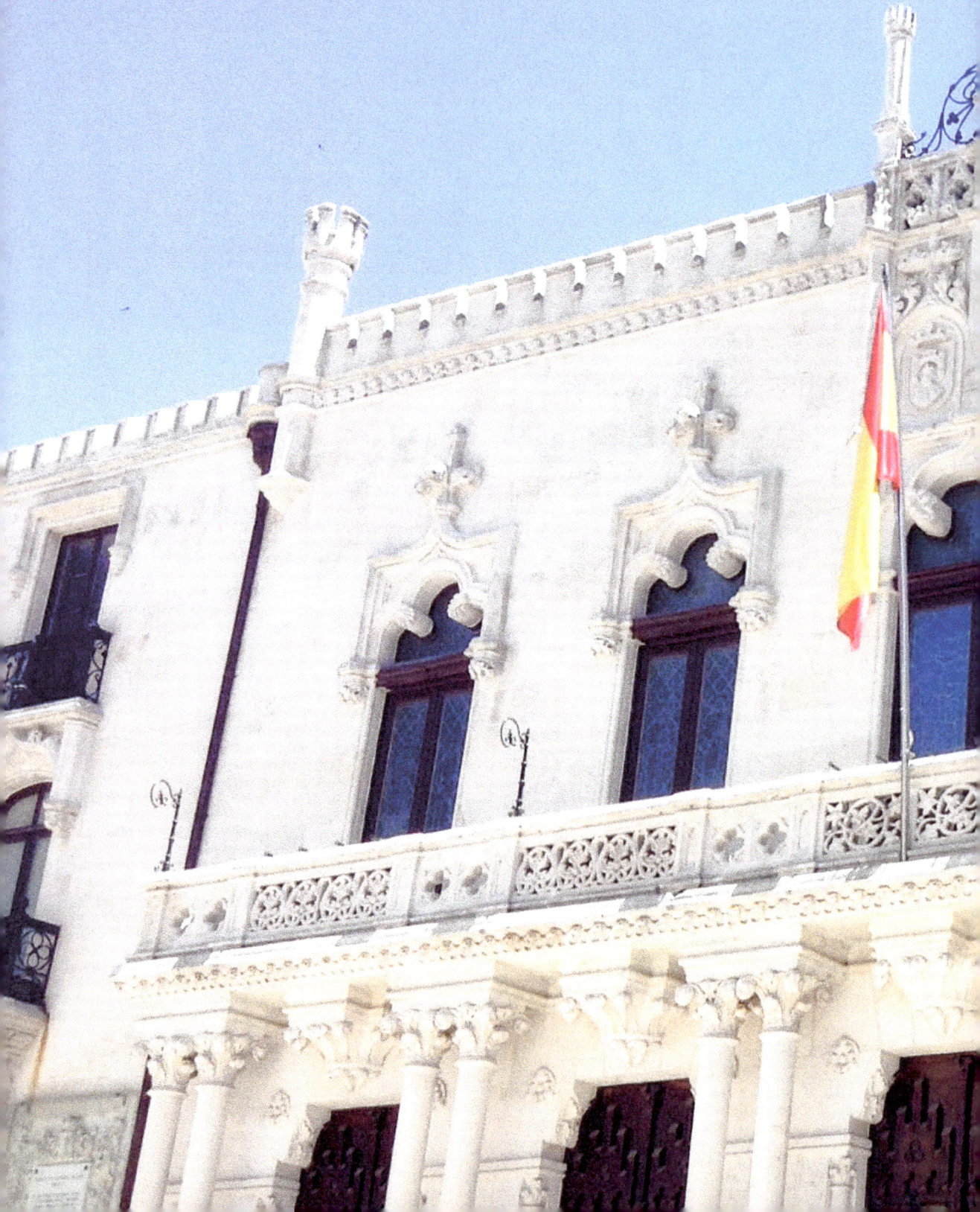

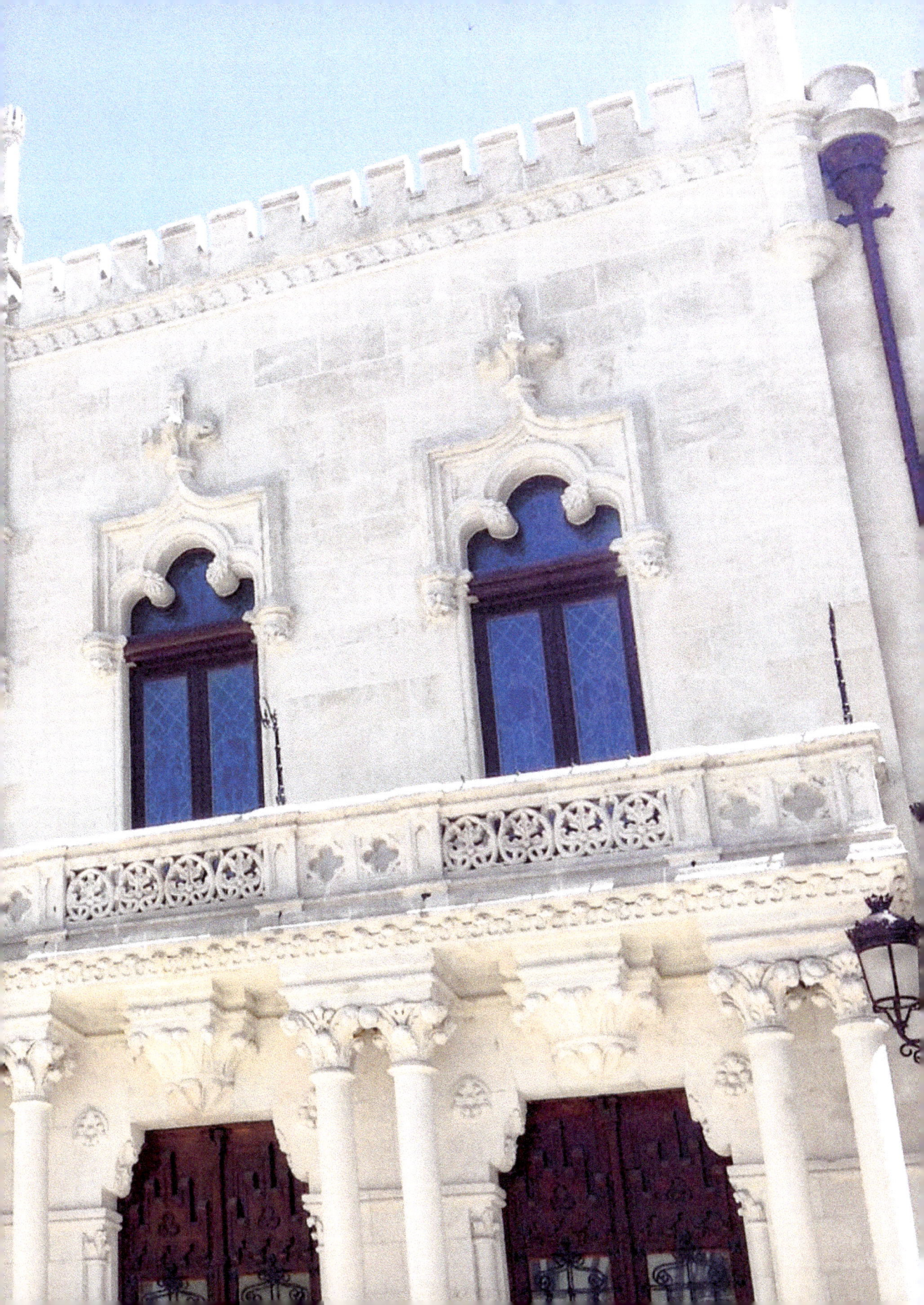

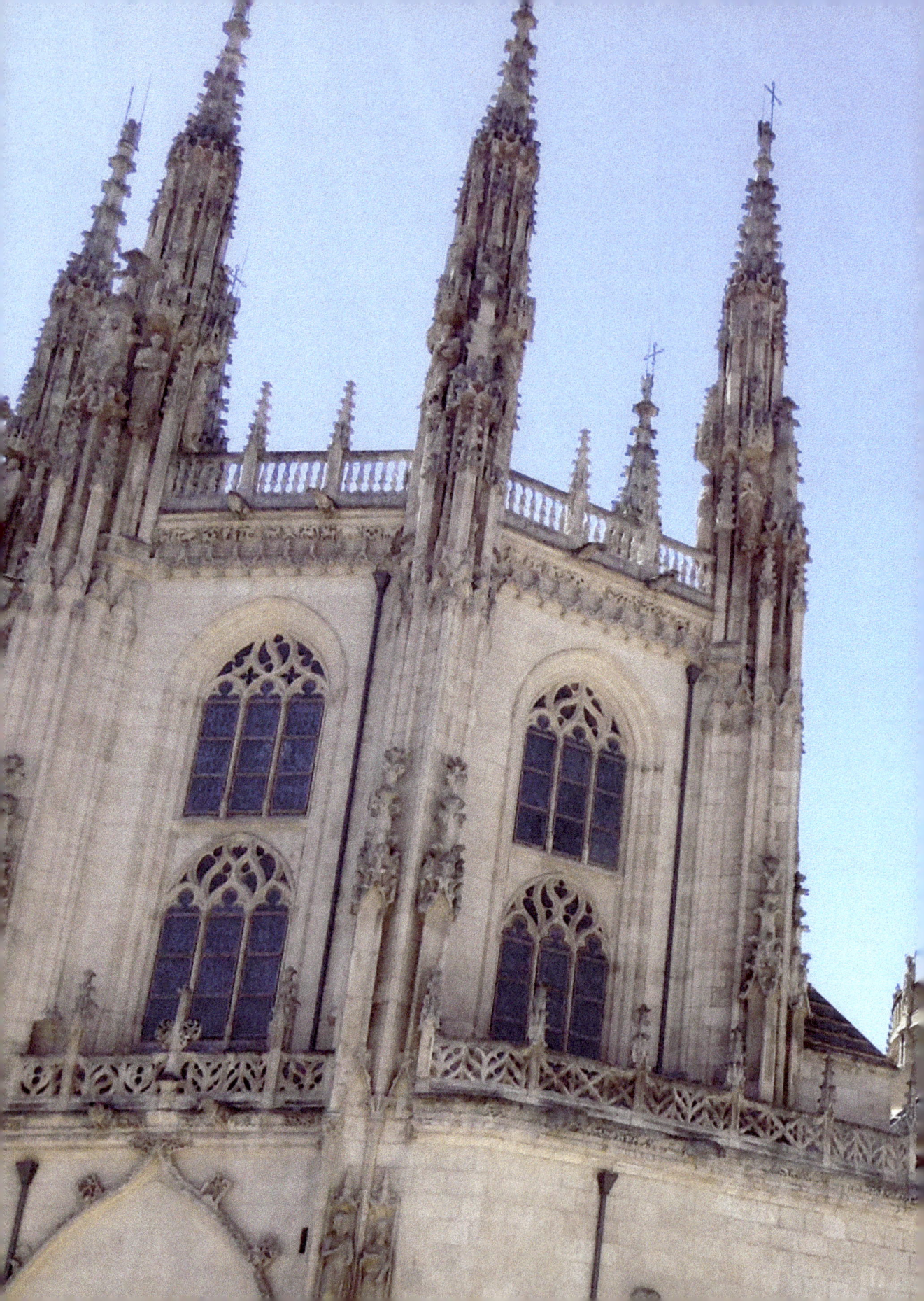

EVERYTHING IS A MIRACLE

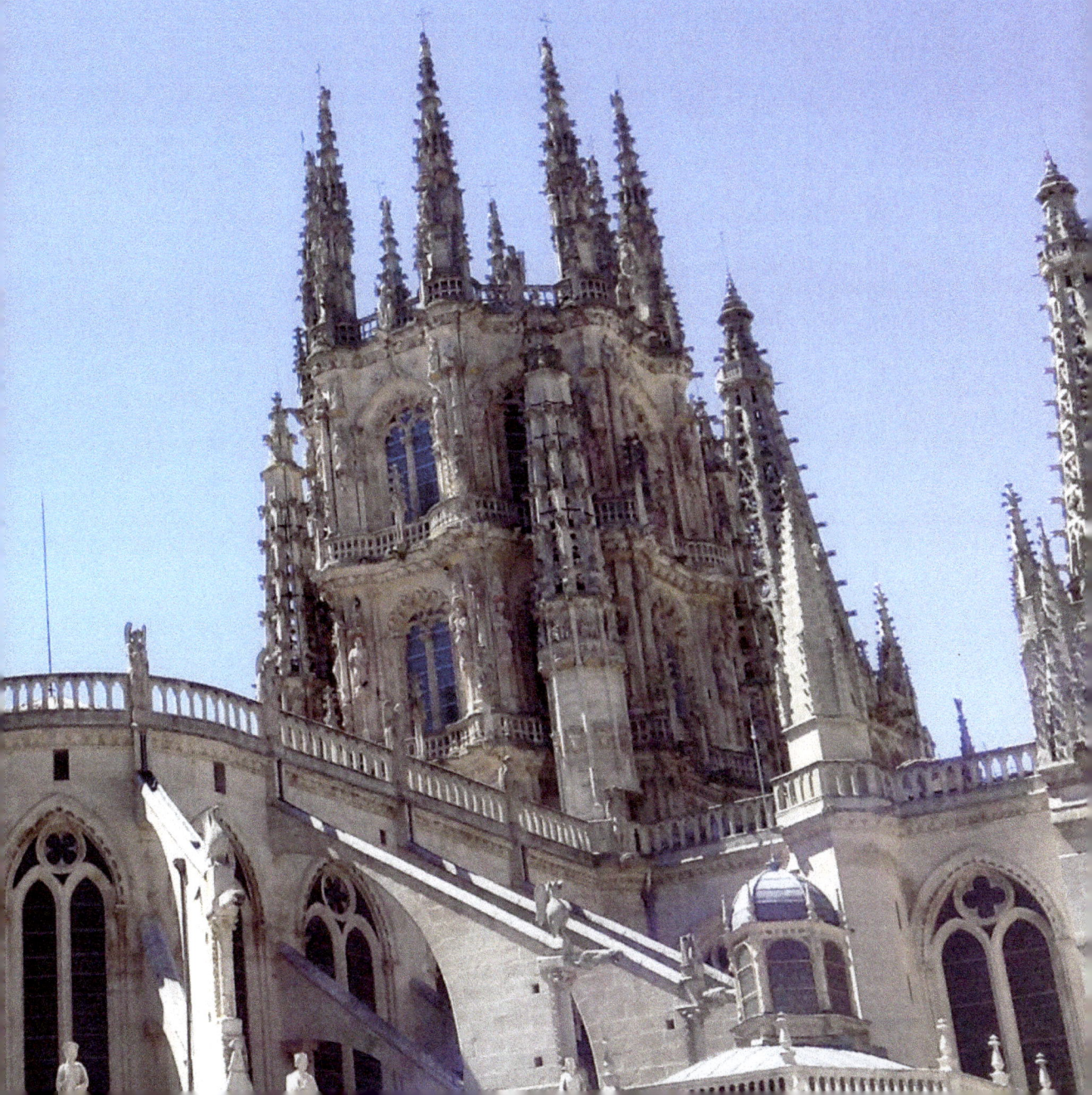

They say northern Spain/the Camino Francés abounds with miracles.
Here's to miles and miles of many more miracles!

*I had always been drawn to the idea of pilgrimages but didn't know why...
then completed one!

*I did not know about the Camino and then serendipitously discovered it!

*I had no money for travel, no plans for travel and then suddenly was going traveling!

*I had not been to Europe and did not know if I could travel there alone and then
did it!

*I did not know if I could walk every day in a row for 7-12 hours for a month
and then did it!

*I did not know if I could walk every step from one end of Spain to the other,
550 miles, 31 days without stopping and then did it!

*I did not know anyone else on the trip and then met so many.

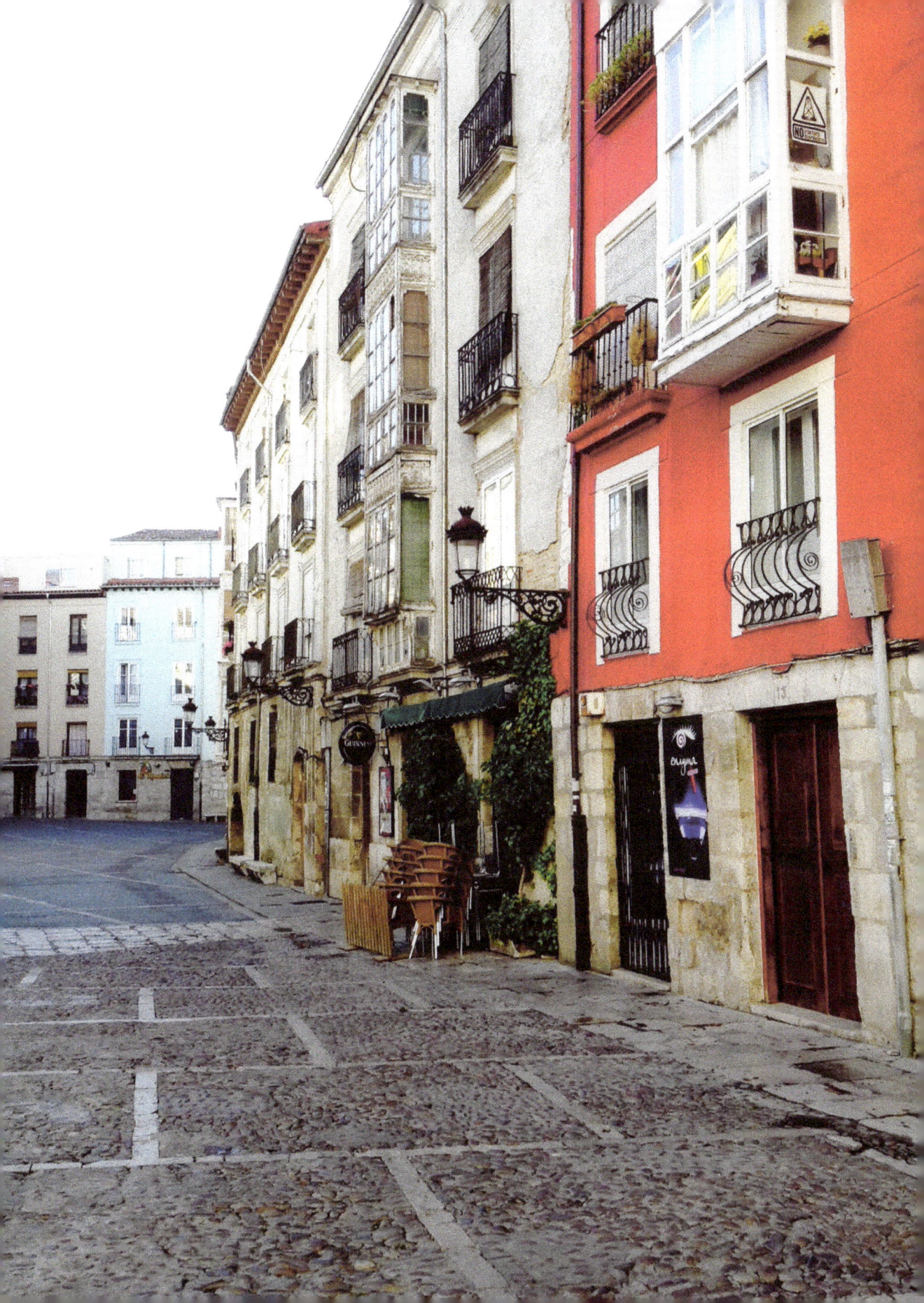

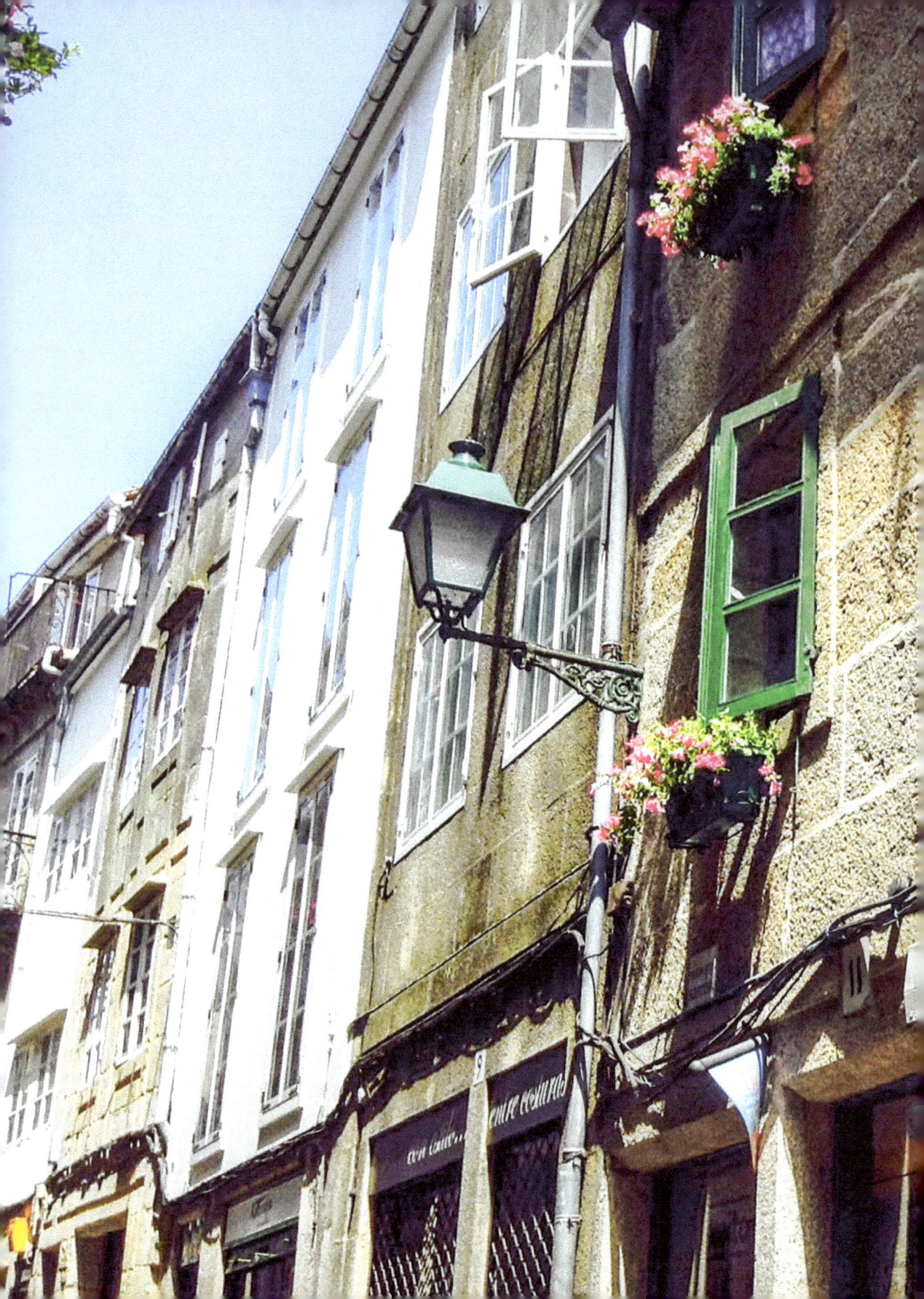

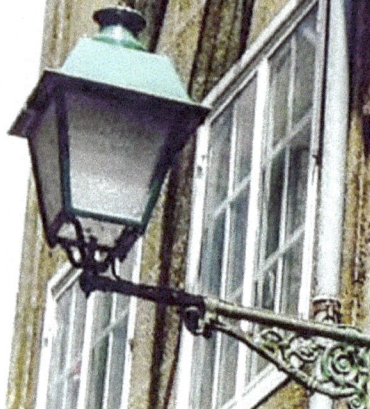

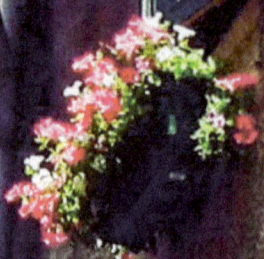

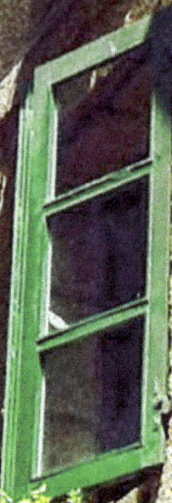

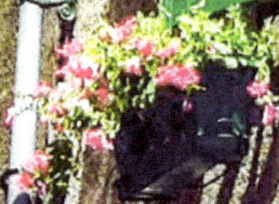

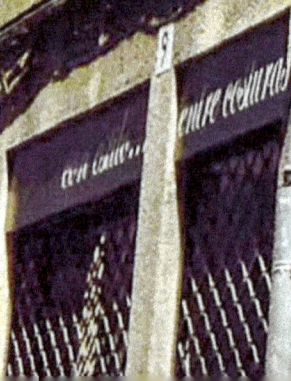

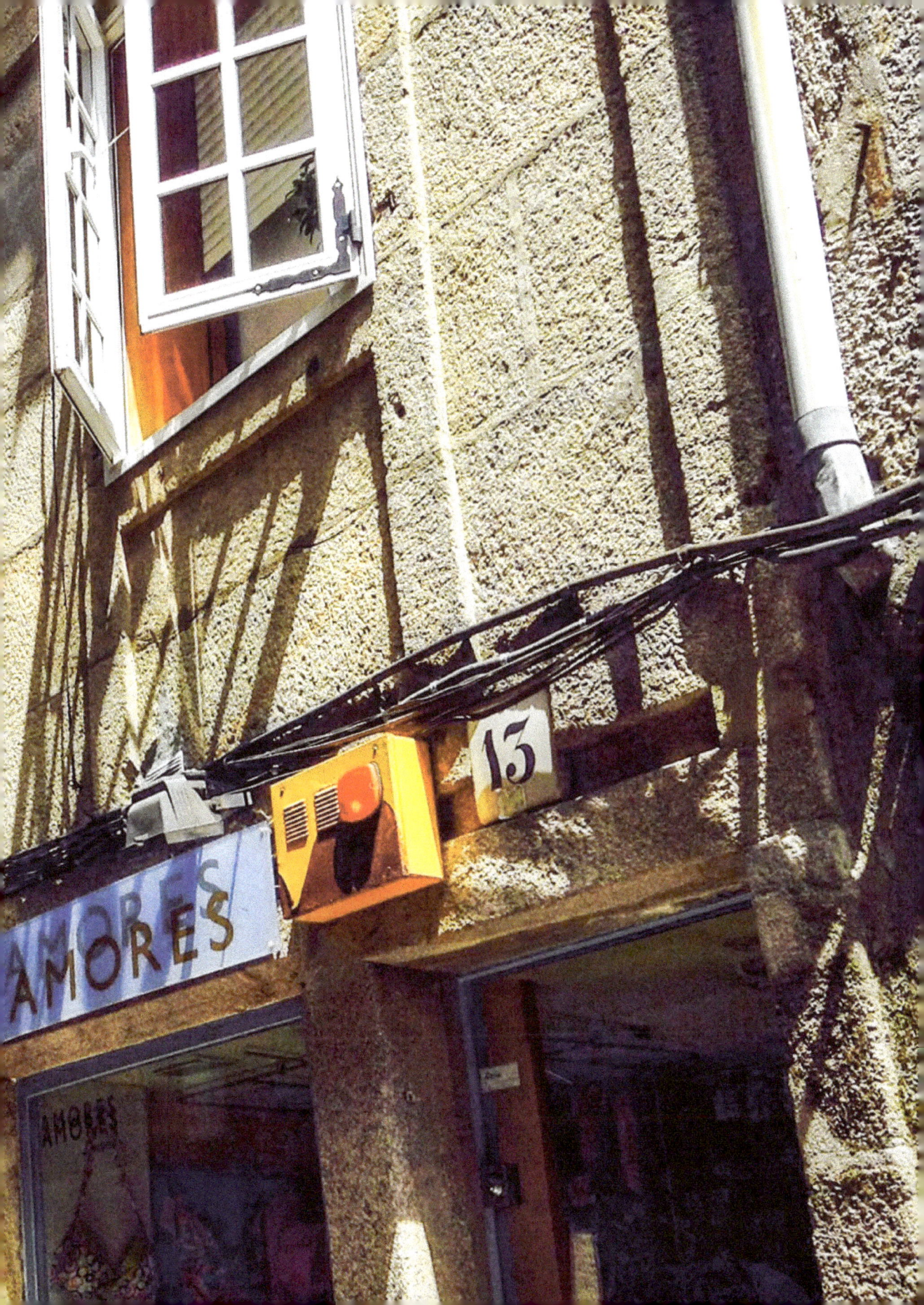

AMORES

13

AMORES

More MIRACLES

*always being able to walk again the next day! (even if the exhaustion caused me to have no idea if it would be possible)

*falling so deeply in love with Spain

*As the Camino approached, I remember feeling like it would be so much easier and so nice to stay home, but I knew I would not NOT go...(ticket had been purchased, reservations had been made, etc). I could not stay home! I would somehow figure it out/make it/face fears.

*MOMENTUM! it is easier to keep moving than to stop and start again

*cowbells

*shepherds

*wooden shutters

*orange soil

*slate stone rooftops

*beaded door curtains

*grapevines

*paper flowers

*Queso Oveja en Aceite de Oliva Trufa Blanca (Sheep Cheese in White Truffle Olive Oil)

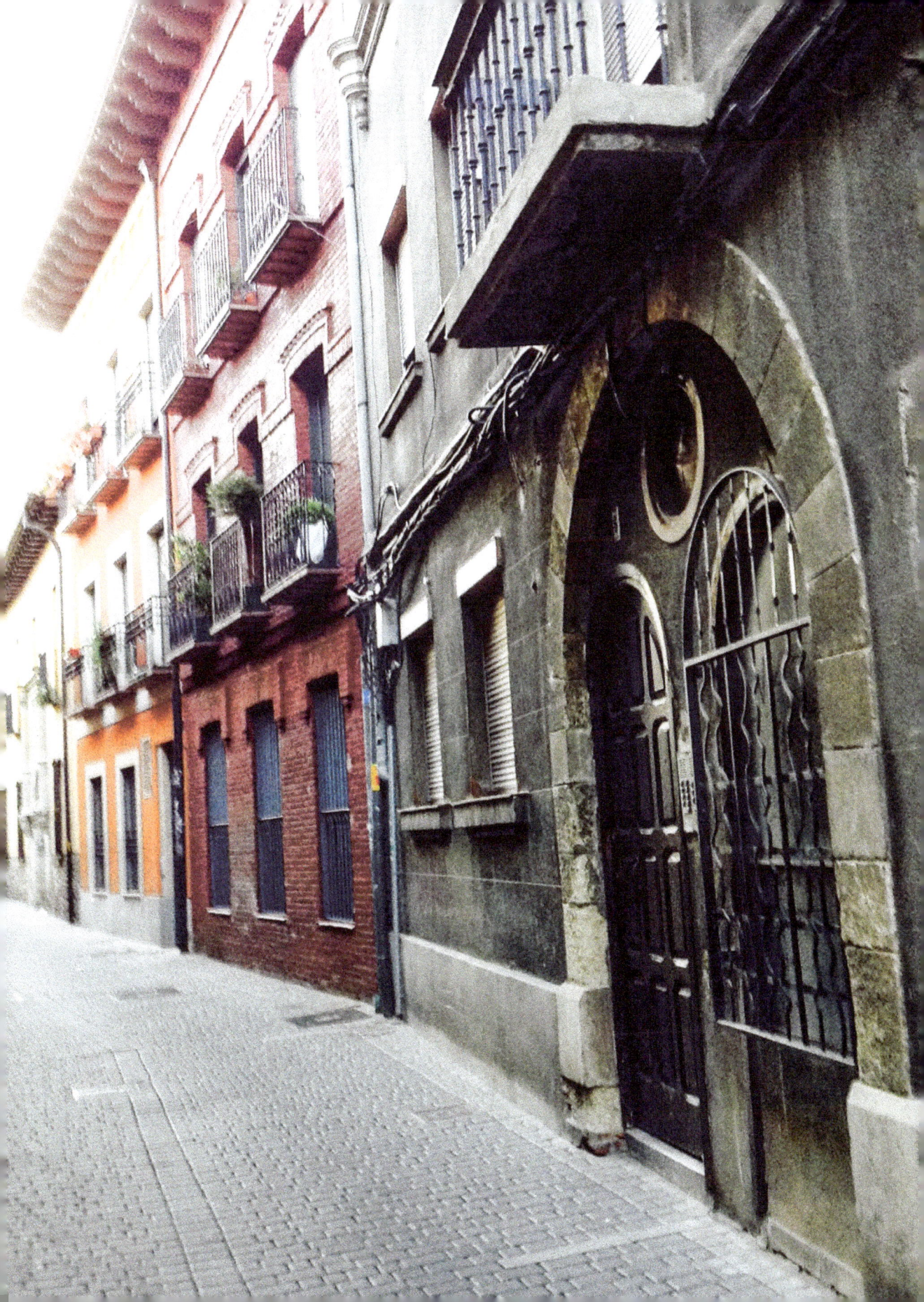

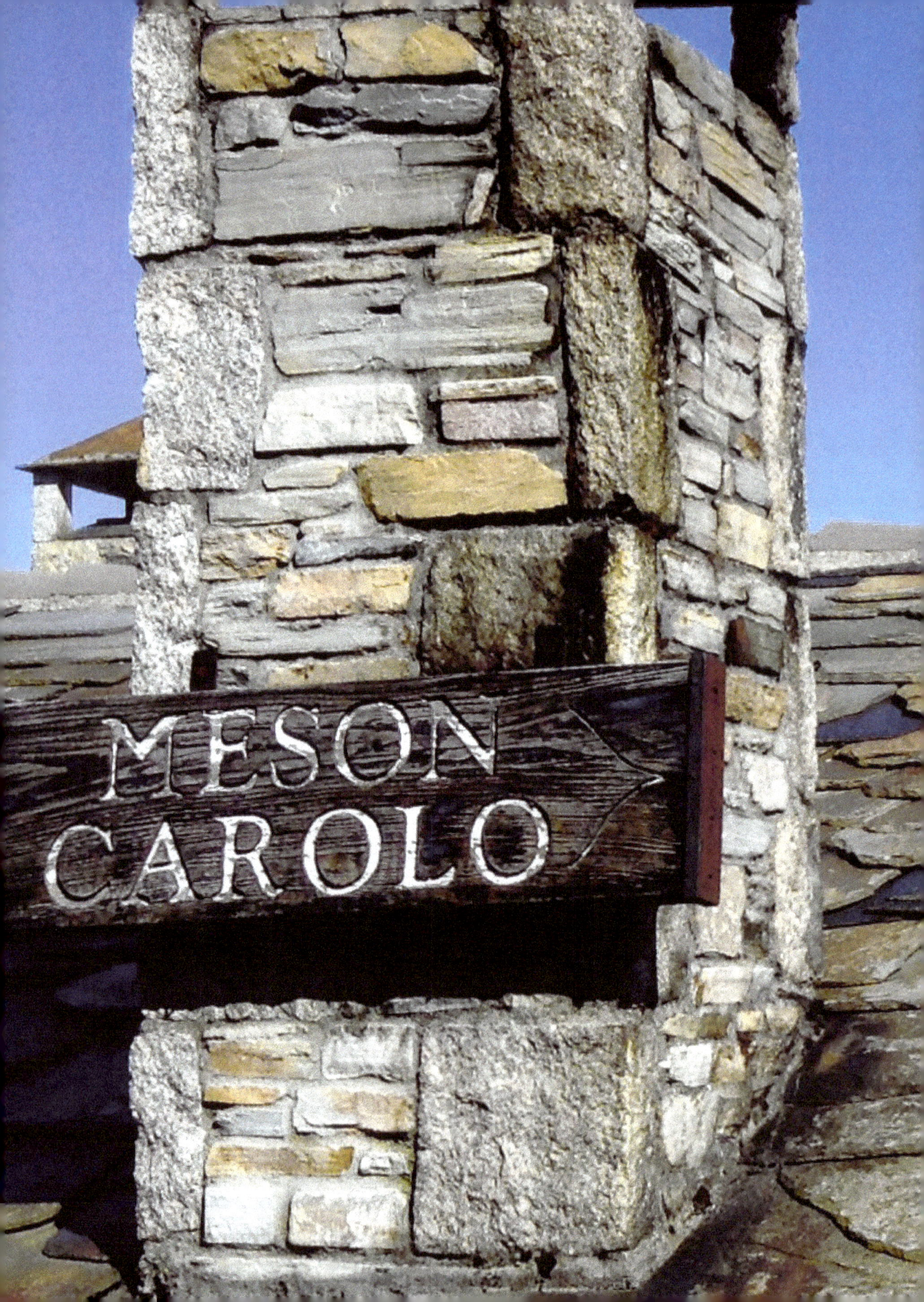
MESON
CAROLO

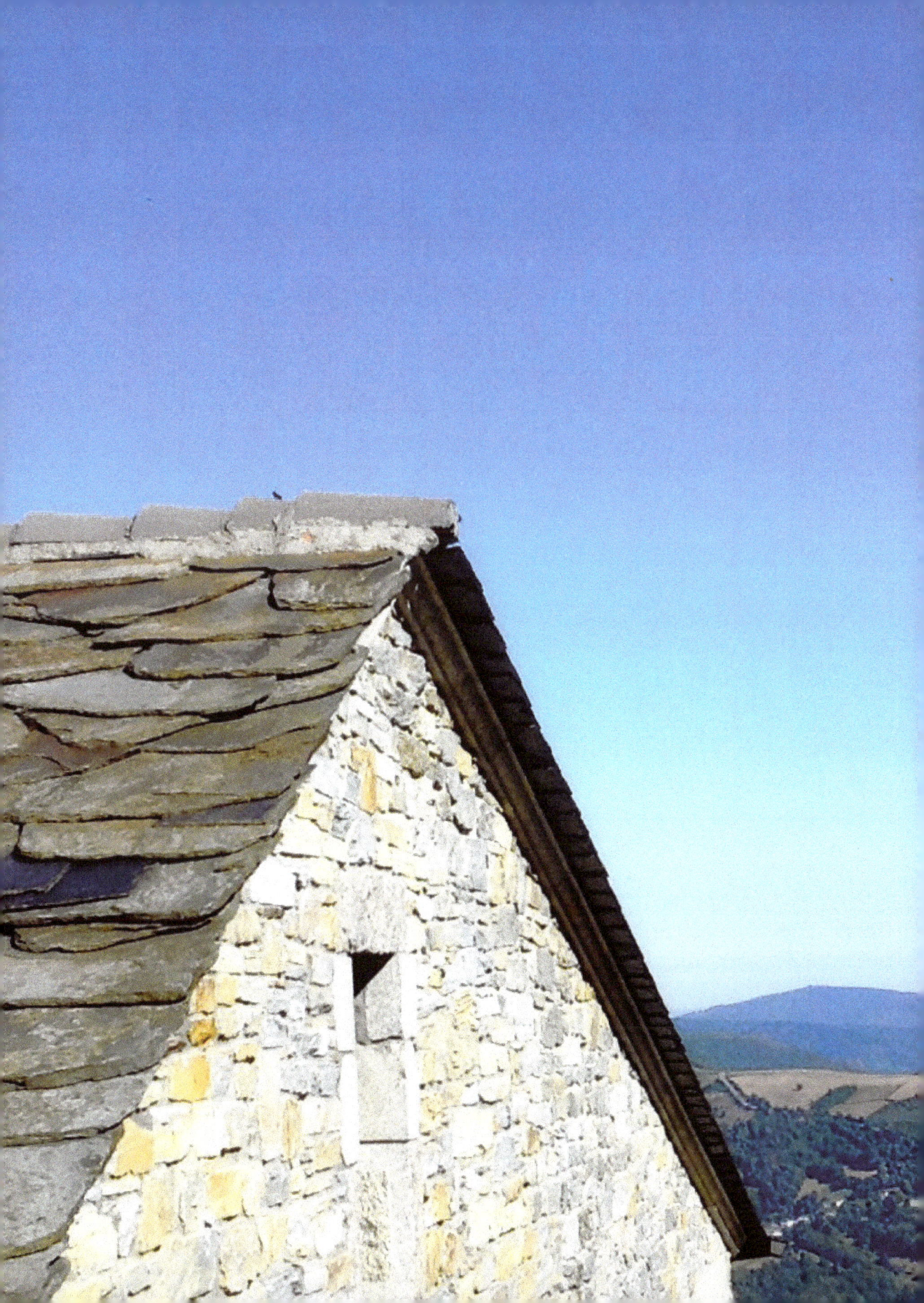

"Nature - like an artist - ever working
toward beauty higher and higher."
-John Muir

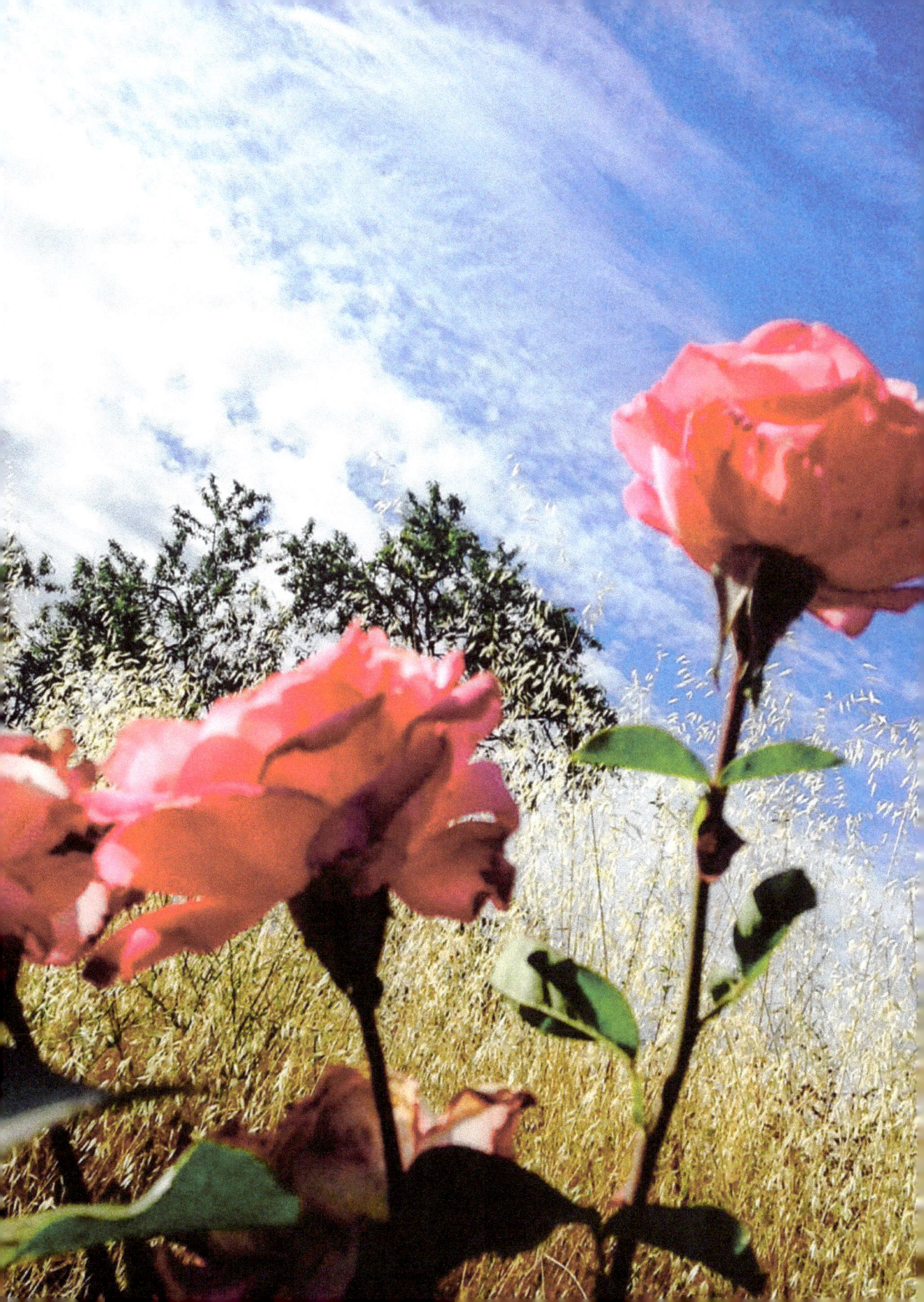

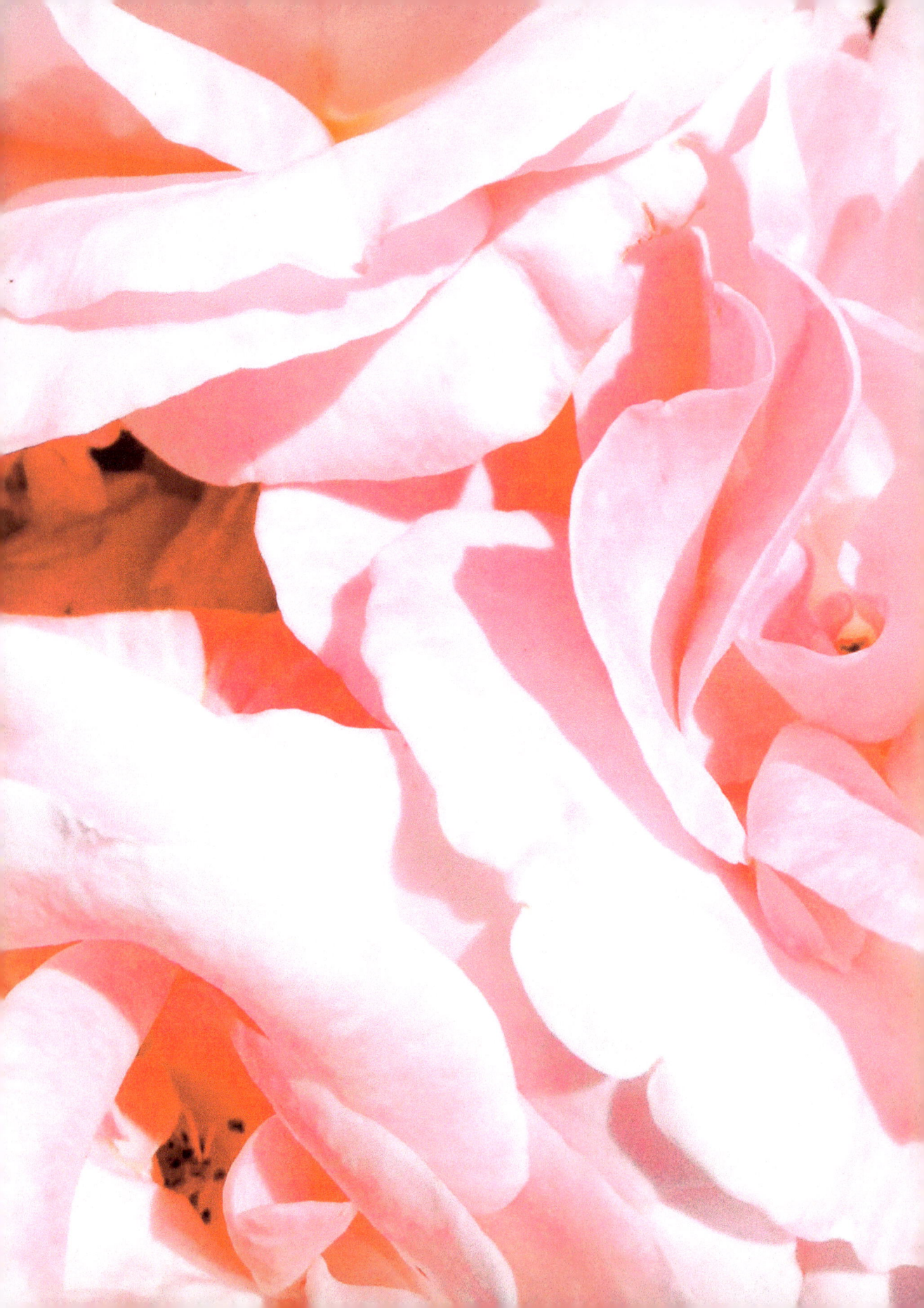

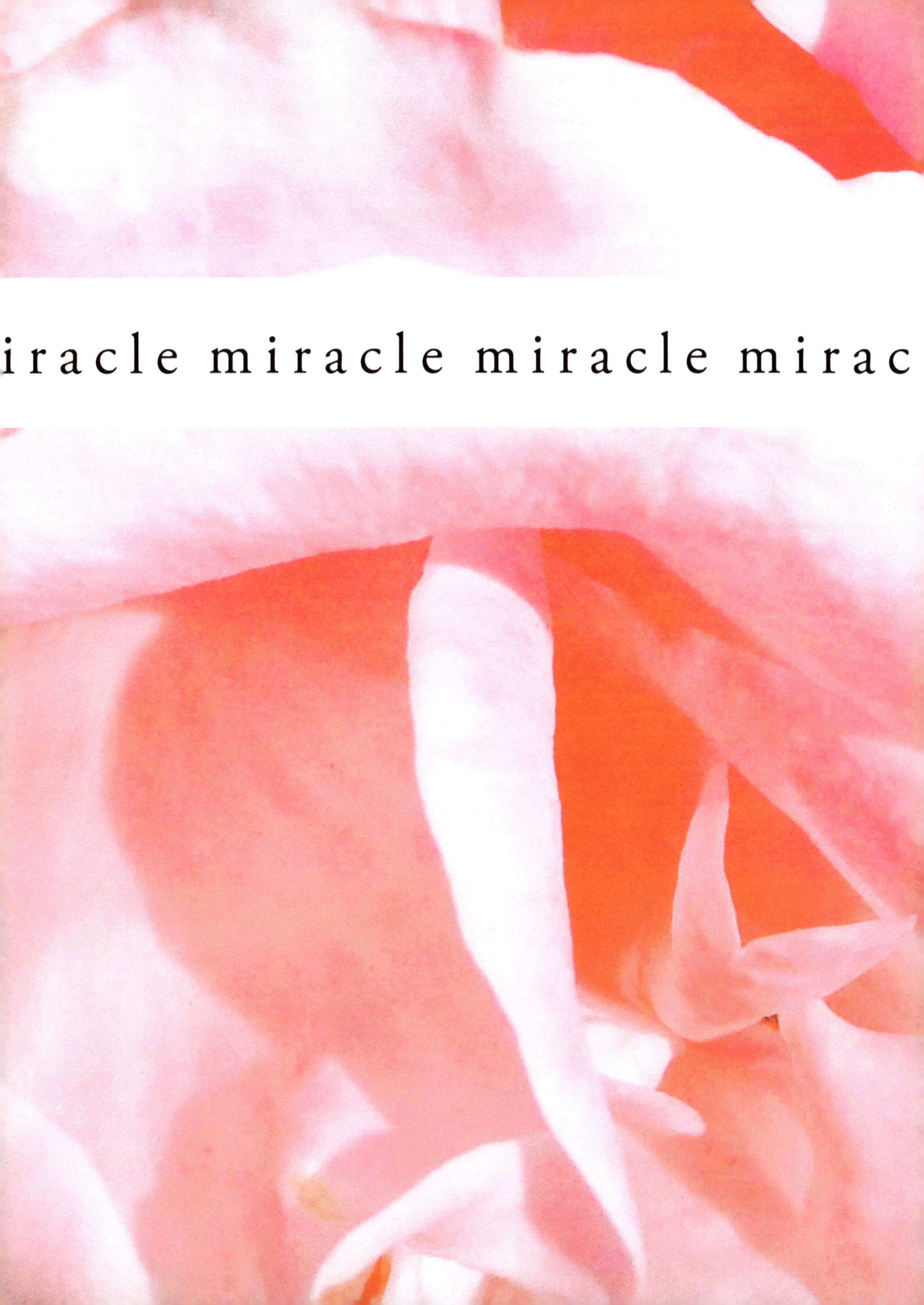

iracle miracle miracle mirac

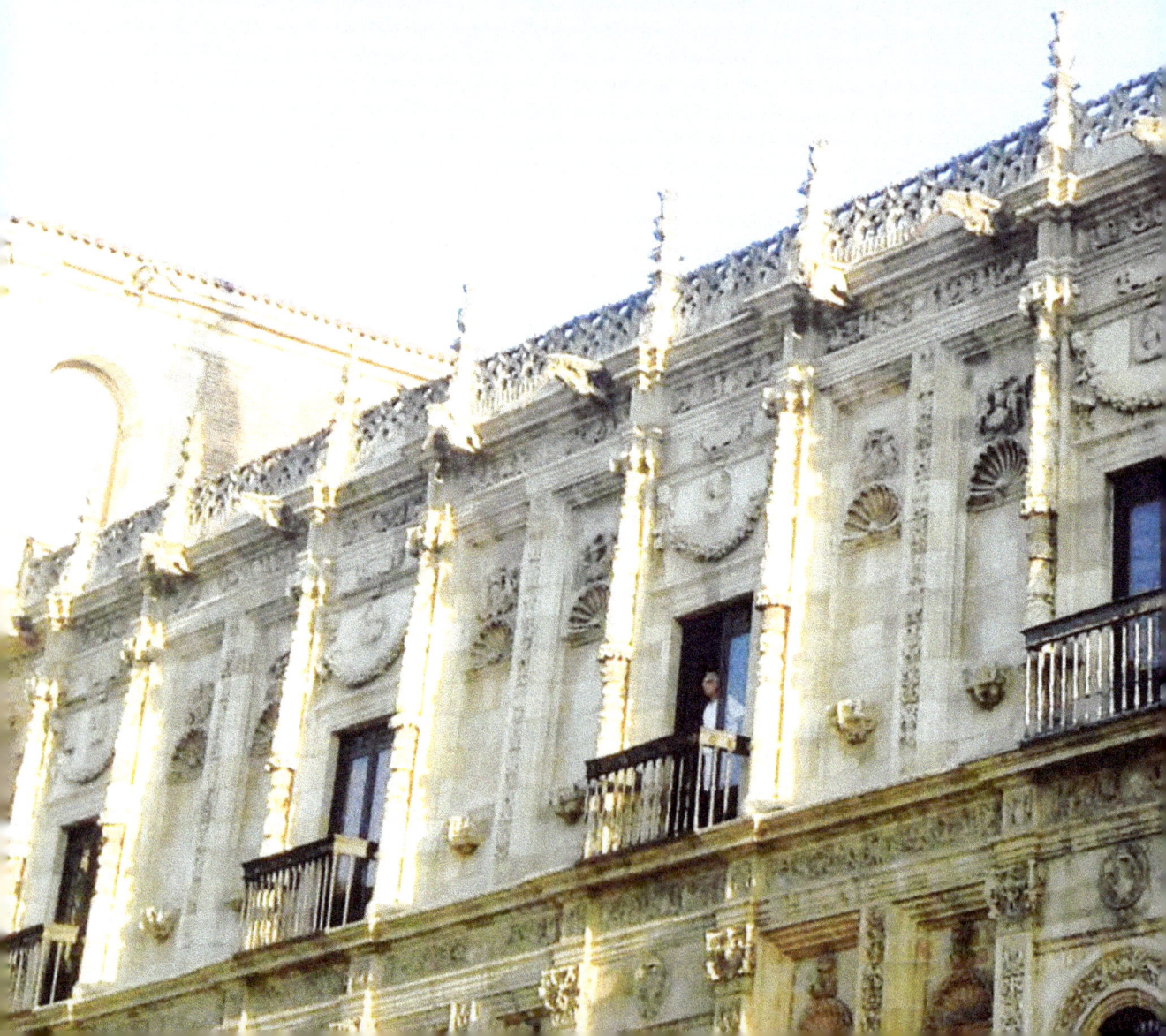

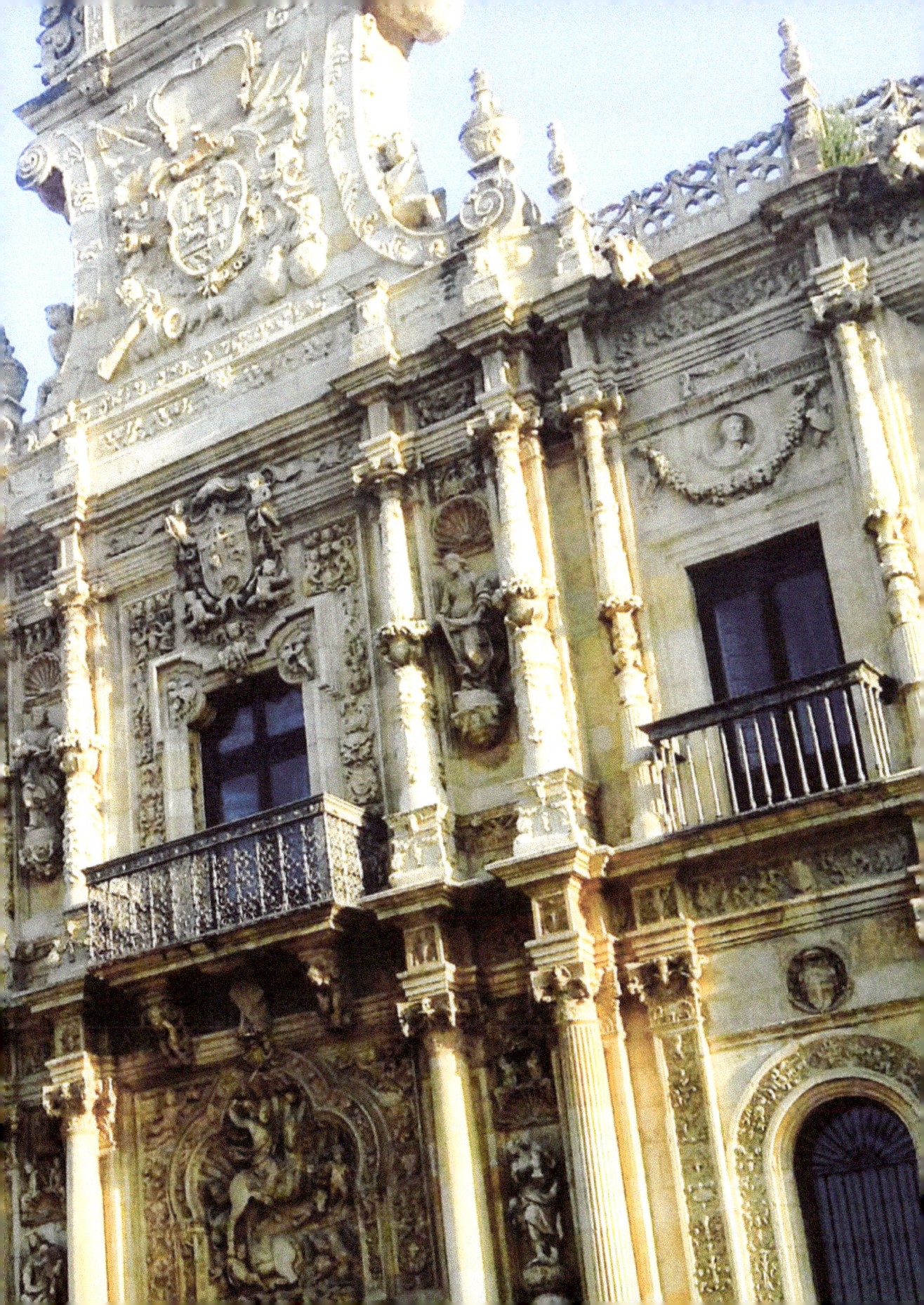

ALBERGUE
SAN LAZARO

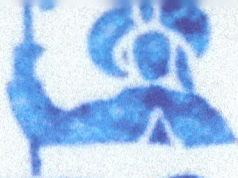

K 82

... Ga .... 27600 SARRIA (Lugo)

cha: __7-7-15__

Fecha: __0__

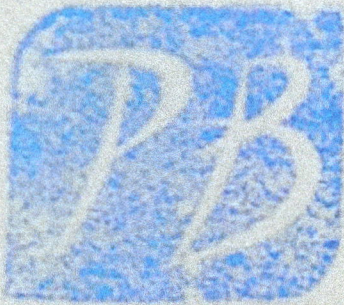

ENSIÓN
ERENGUELA
MELIDE

TERES
Y OTR
C.I.F.: G-
Tfno./Fax:
C/. Ba
15800 MELI...

07/07/2015

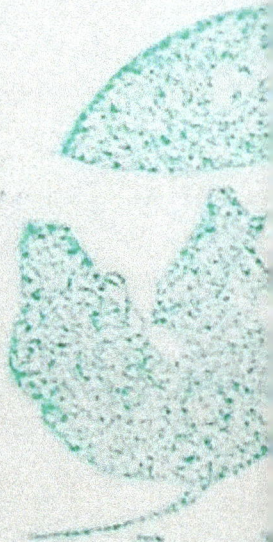

En e...
A Rúa, kn...

cha: __9-7-15__

Fecha: __V...__

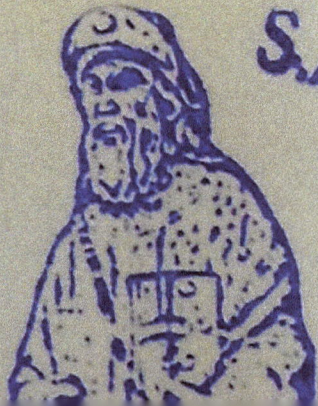

EREGRINO   S.A.M.I. CATED...

One significant miracle for me was finding my way. Although I spent many months planning my route and daily miles, I was completely uninterested in reading the specific directions ("turn right at the large Oak tree"). I became completely overwhelmed with the minute details, so I decided to skip them and then wondered just how I was going to find my way across Spain. I kept reading other accounts of pilgrims and trusted that I would somehow find my way. It was unnerving to have this looming unknown for a place I had not seen and a place I did not know the language. To be going alone without specific directions, navigational skills and tools was a concern. I kept reading. Not knowing exactly what to expect (the terrain, the weather, the directions, the language, the accomodations, the food, the water, et cetera) was an opportunity to become paralyzed by fear. I kept reading. Learning and reading about all of the endless experiences of people before me who somehow made it (one from England who left home with only a hunk of cheese) gave me the courage to go. To them, I am eternally grateful.

"There are always flowers
for those who want to see them."
-Henri Matisse

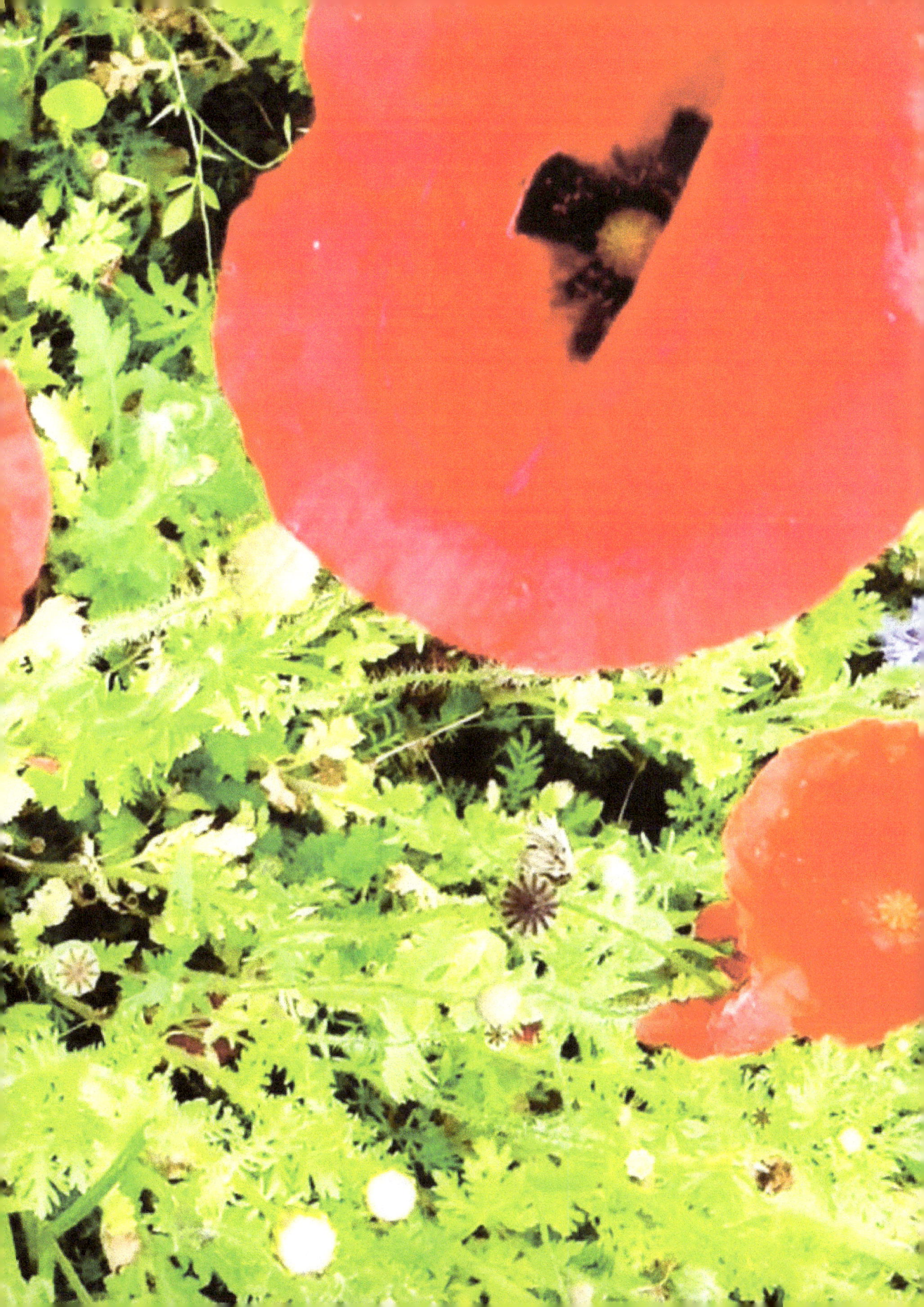

I am also eternally grateful for all of the people of Spain who look out for the wandering pilgrims and who maintain the trails and arrows showing us the way. Their kind, watchful and encouraging greetings, their smiles, nods and "buen caminos," their patience with and acceptance of so many wandering strangers through their hometowns, this and much more is why I consider finding my way, every step, every mile, alone and not knowing anything, across Spain truly a most unforgettable M I R A C L E !

The trail from Santiago to Finisterre is much less traveled these days. I was aware that there would be less guidance and help, but also less crowds making it a different but glorious experience. After successfully hiking 500 miles and learning how to locate the arrows even if they were not immediately visible, I did not know what to expect with less arrows. Also, at this point, all of the pilgrims that I had met were stopping after Santiago or taking a bus to the coast. I was uncertain about how I would do it, but I was determined to continue. I remember feeling excited when I saw the first familiar Camino arrow. It was just like the first 500 miles! I did notice a difference in the amount of arrows and found myself consulting an iPod application that I had downloaded, but I was still advancing! ¡Ultreia! Just like the readings described, I exulted in the beautiful and isolated trail. Then, I literally came to a "T" in the road in a tiny village. I looked up, down, to the left and to the right but could not find direction. For the first time, I was perplexed and had no idea which direction to walk. I was curious about what to do when suddenly I saw a small hand in the window pointing left. A woman in her house was the arrow! M I R A C L E !

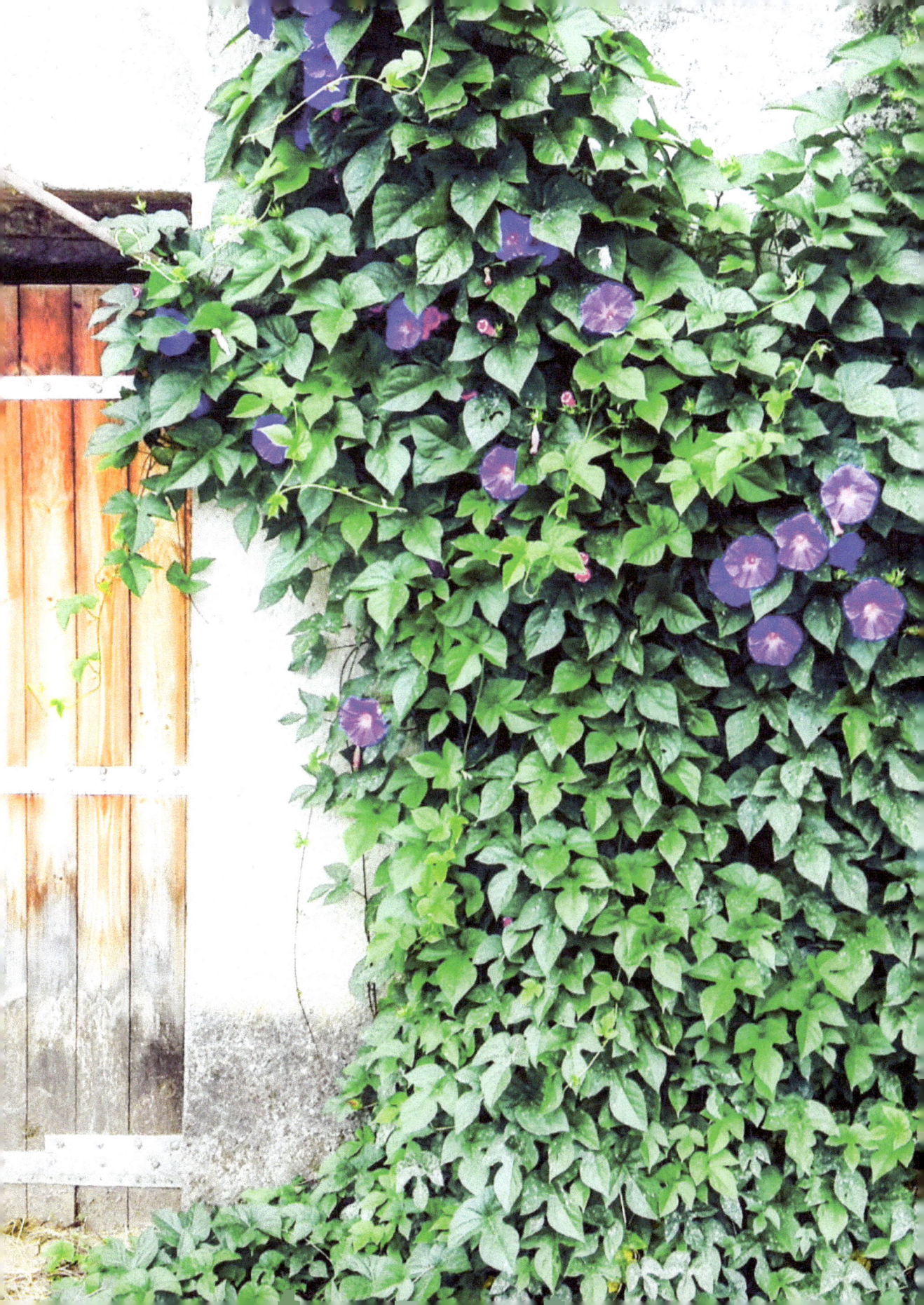

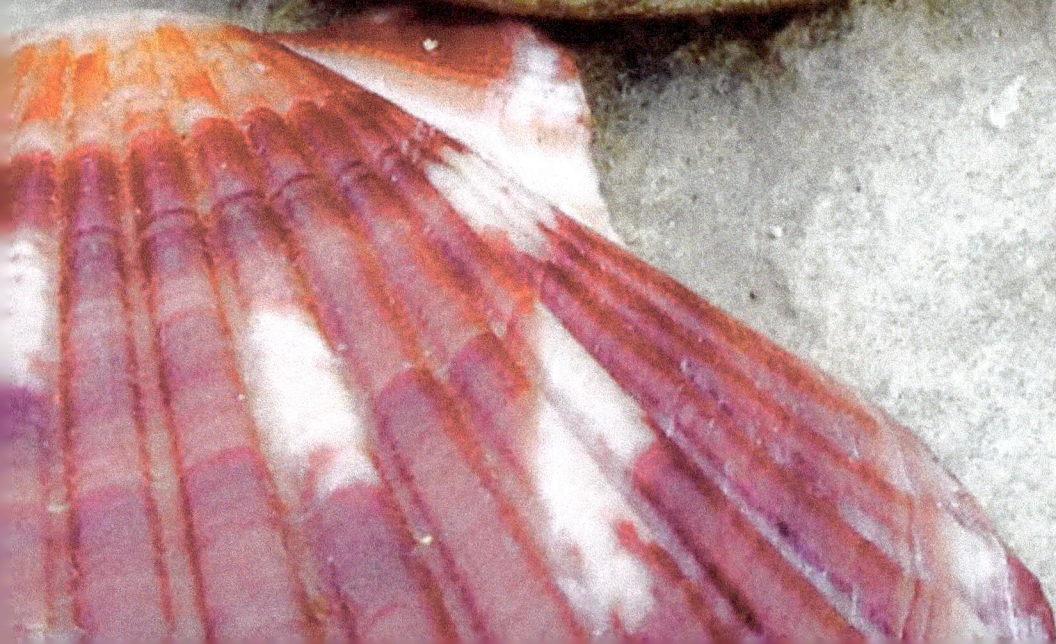

Carry a small pebble from home (rub all your cares and worries into the pebble) and leave it at the base of the Cruz de Ferro near Foncebadon

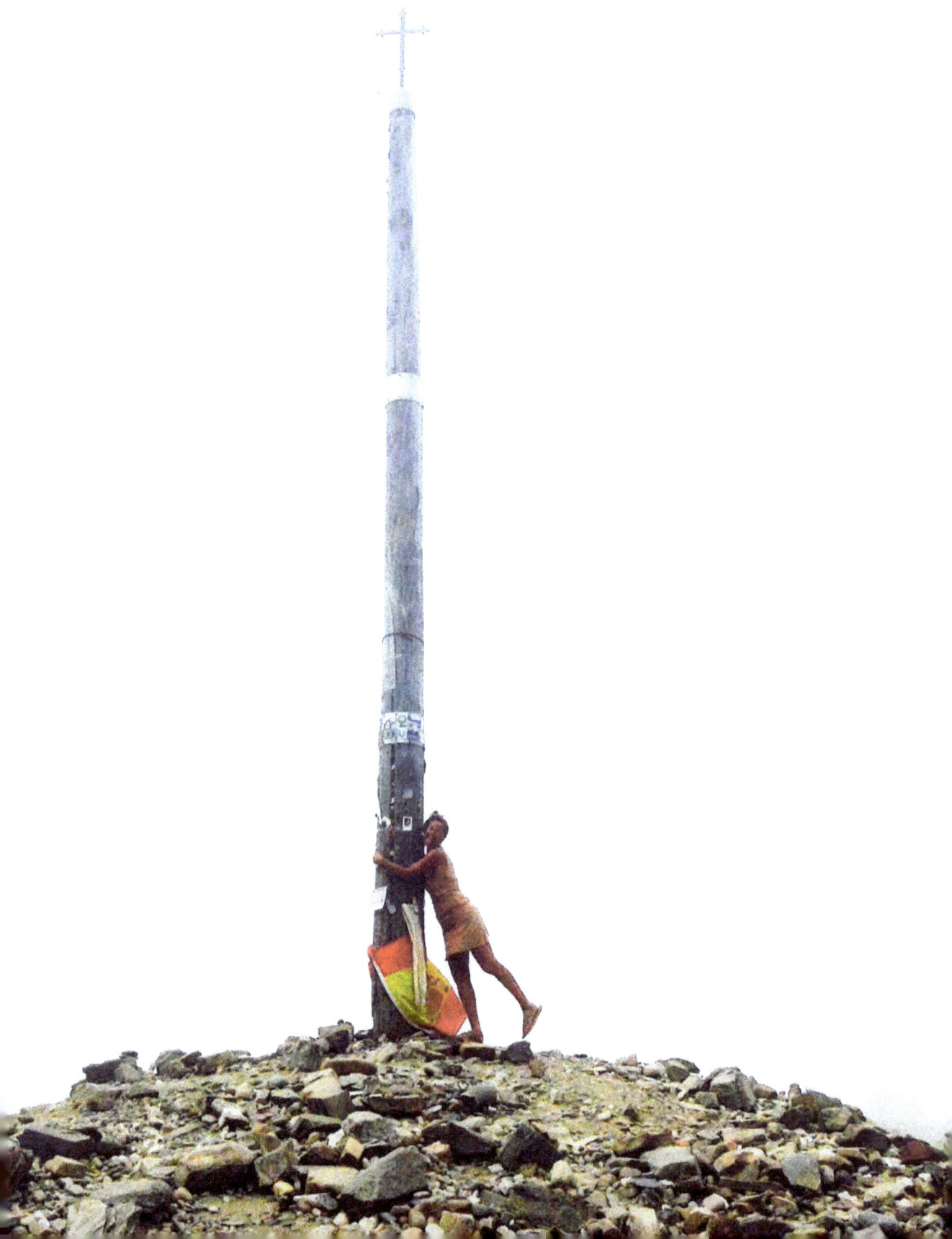

I WILL ALWAYS REMEMBER

-helping a pilgrim push his baby in a stroller up a steep mountain

-the shop owner who gave me a pair of her flip-flops to wear when mine were beyond repair

-the cab driver who drove me to León and helped me find new flip-flops in a department store

-Pamplona

-Villafranca

-washing my hair in a mountain stream

-always arriving just in time and on the right day to the post offices

-when a friend told me sternly to go to the Pilgrim Mass (I would have missed it!)

-the fashion, the outdoor cafes, Burgos University, the historic centres

-the pilgrims who left their homes in Germany and had been walking for three months

-the pilgrims traveling with a donkey

-the awe-inspiring vistas

-the nature

-the endless beauty of Spain and its people...M I R A C L E S

dinero (money)

comida (food)

agua (water)

baño (bathroom)

cama (bed)

dormir (sleep)

ducha (shower)

huevos (eggs)

aceite de oliva (olive oil)

orgánico (organic)

de la forma artesanal (made the traditional way)

queso (cheese)

leche cruda (raw milk)

alimentados con pasto (grass-fed)

sin pasteurizar (unpasteurized)

por favor (please)

gracias (thank you)

buenos días (good morning)

muy agradecido (so grateful)

te agradeceria mucho (I appreciate it so much)

computadora (computer)

¿cuánto cuesta? (how much?)

¡buen camino! (good way!)

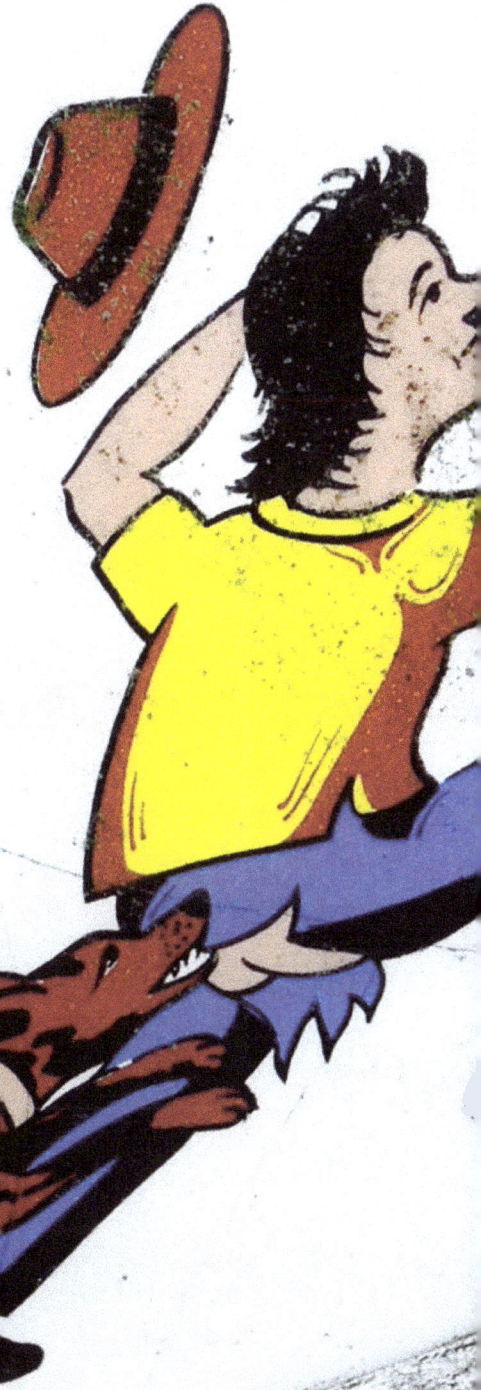

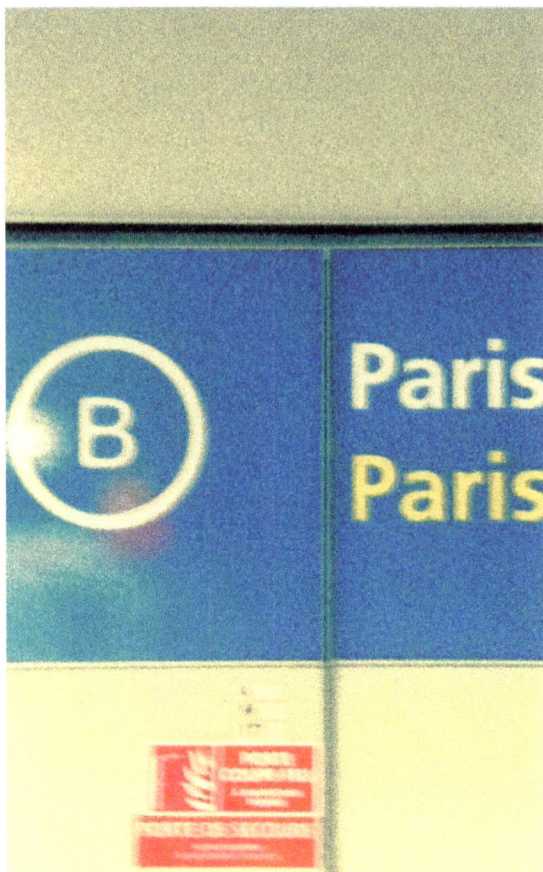

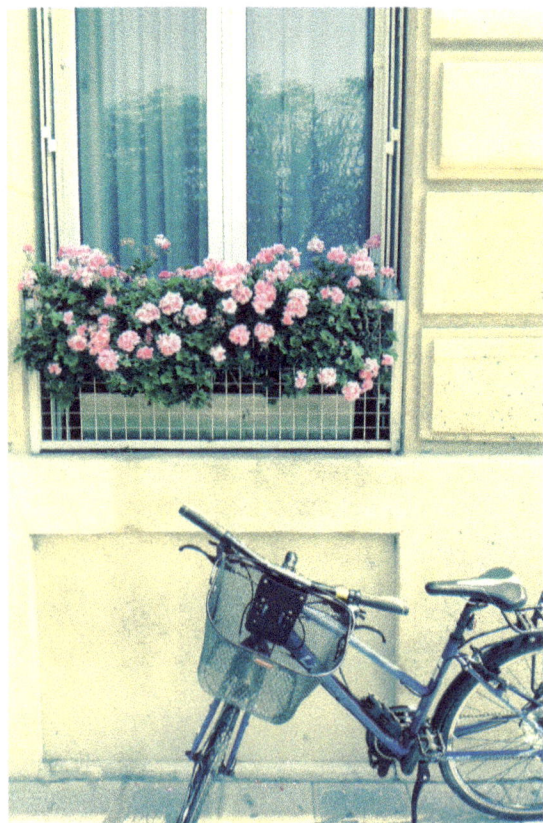

Wednesday 10 June 2015
Mpls to Paris
depart: 1:15pm
arrive: 7:50am (11 June)
DELTA $1508.97

....

Thursday 11 June 2015
Airport to Notre-Dame
HOTEL-DIEU €139
www.hotel-hospitel.fr

....

Friday 12 June 2015
Paris
www.louvre.com

....

Saturday 13 June 2015
TGV train to Bayonne €60
(5 hours)
mountain train to
St-Jean-Pied-de-Port €10
(1 1/2 hours)
www.voyages-sncf.com
Gîte Ultreia €18 (prepaid online)
www.ultreia64.fr/en

....

Sunday 14 June 2015
walk to Roncesvalles (Navarra)
Albergue de Roncesvalles
€15 (prepaid online)
www.alberguederoncesvalles.com

....

Monday 15 June 2015
walk to Larrasoaña
Hostel Bide Ederra €16
667 406 554 (Cristina)
www.hostelbideederra.com
call to confirm reservation

....

Tuesday 16 June 2015
walk to Pamplona
www.casaibarrola.com €18
call to confirm: 692 208 463
"spend time in Pamplona"

....

Wednesday 17 June 2015
walk to Puente La Reina
www.albergueamalur.com €10

....

Thursday 18 June 2015
walk to Villamayor de Monjardin
www.oasistrails.org €7
(no reservations taken)

....

Friday 19 June 2015
walk to Viana
Albergue Parroquial Santa María €donation
phone: 948 645 037
library research to find traditional chorizo
purchase chorizo & cheese
"delightful walled town with a bustling down-
town and many attractive cafes"

....

Saturday 20 June 2015
walk to Sotes via Logroño
Logroño: DeTorre Gourmet
Ibérico de bellota, raw-milk cheese, 100%
cacoa, bottled asparagus
mail ahead at post office before noon
walk to Sotes
www.alberguesotes.com €10
650 962 625 (Ana Alonso)

....

Sunday 21 June 2015
walk to Azofra
Albergue de Peregrinos €7
phone: 941 379 220
2-person room albergue

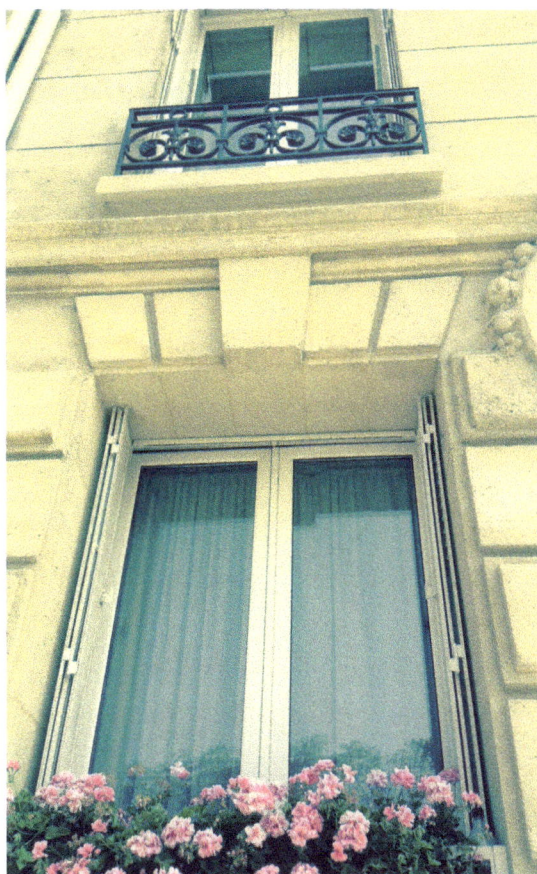

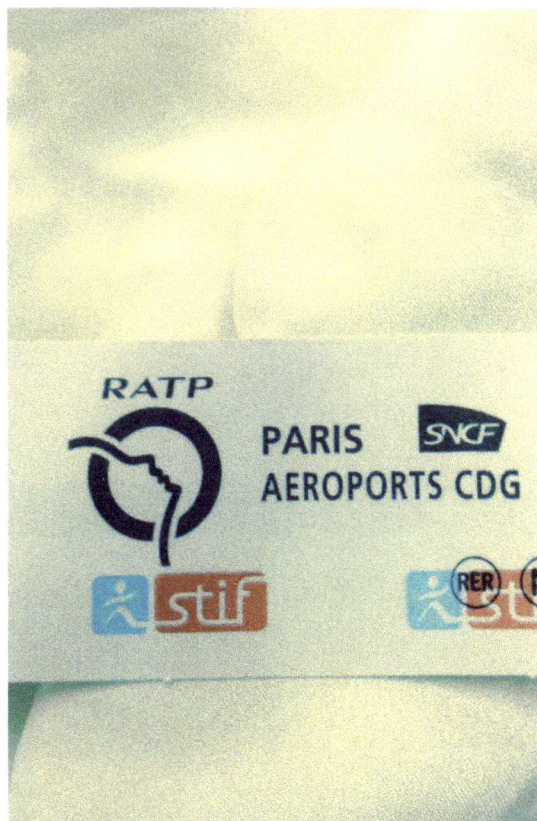

....

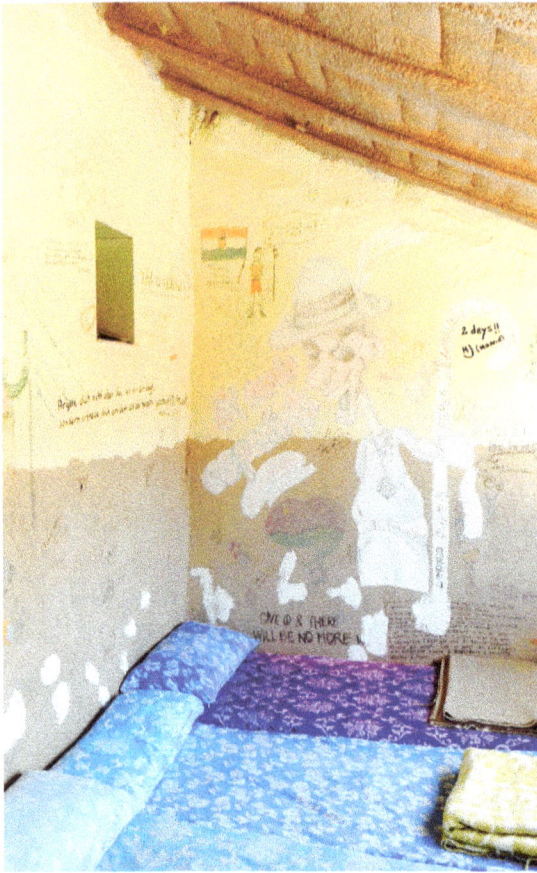

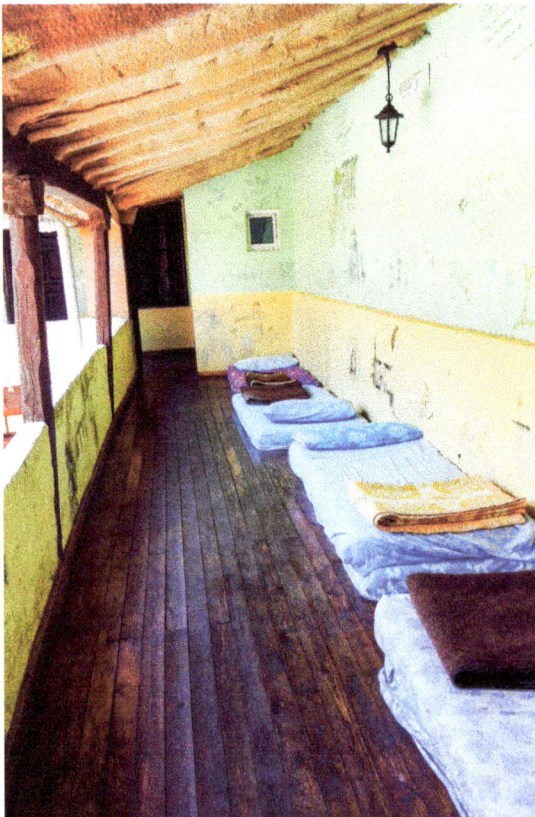

Monday 22 June 2015
walk to Belorado
Cuatro Cantones €11
www.alberguecuatrocantones.com
phone: 947 580 591

....

Tuesday 23 June 2015
walk to Agés
El Pajar de Agés €9
phone: 947 400 629

....

Wednesday 24 June 2015
walk to Burgos
Divina Pastora €donation
Calle de Laín Calvo, 10
phone: 947 207 952
Delicatessen Ojeda
bought Ibérico de bellota, raw-milk cheese,
bottled vegetables & mailed ahead

....

Thursday 25 June 2015
walk to San Anton
Hospital de Peregrinos de San Antón
€donation
"special experience in ruins of convent"
no electricity & no hot water

....

Friday 26 June 2015
walk to Población de Campos €4

....

Saturday 27 June 2015
walk to Ledigos
El Palomar €8
phone: 979 883 614

....

Sunday 28 June 2015
walk to Cazadilla
Vía Trajana €15
www.albergueviatrajana.com

....

Monday 29 June 2015
walk to Arcahueja
La Torre €8
www.alberguetorre.es
phone: 987 205 896

....

Tuesday 30 June 2015
walk to Villar de Mazarife
El Refugio de Jesús €5
phone: 987 390 697
took a taxi to León to buy flip-flops

....

Wednesday 1 July 2015
walk to Astorga
San Javier €7
phone: 987 618 532
bought more food &
mailed ahead with new flip-flops
visited chocolate museum & sent ahead more
100% cacao

....

Thursday 2 July 2015
walk to Rabanal del Camino
Gaucelmo €donation
phone: 987 691 901

....

Friday 3 July 2015
walk to Molinaseca
Casa Pichin €10
(they drove me to a different one because I did
not call ahead to confirm, so I walked back to
walk the steps I missed)
phone: 987 453 162

....

Saturday 4 July 2015
walk to Villafranca
Albergue de la Piedra €8
www.alberguedelapiedra.com
phone: 987 540 260

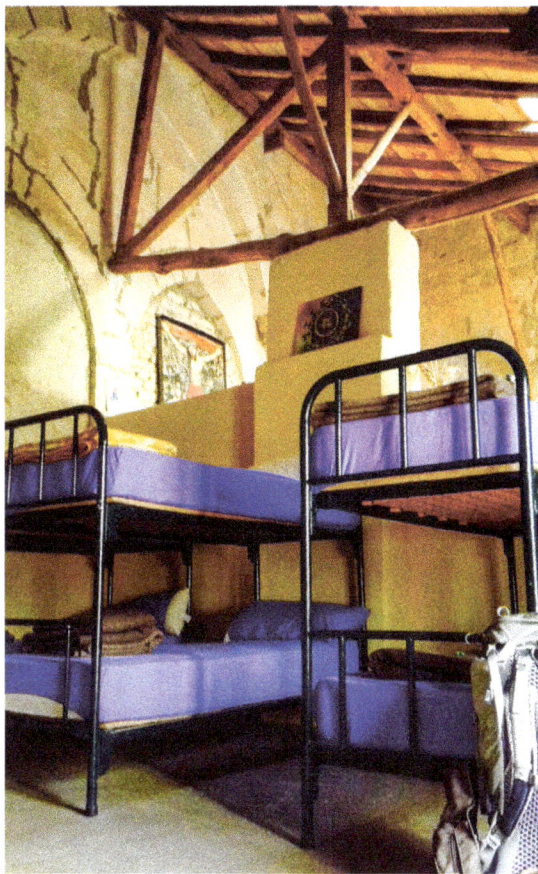

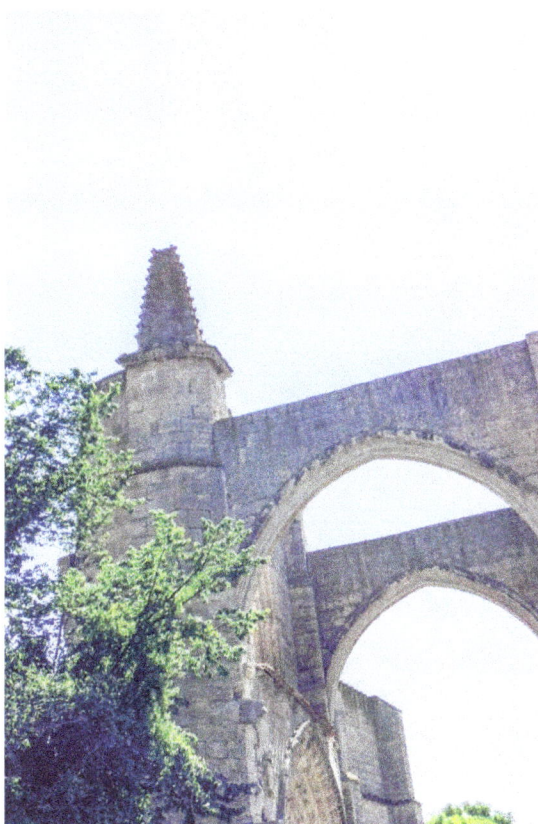

....

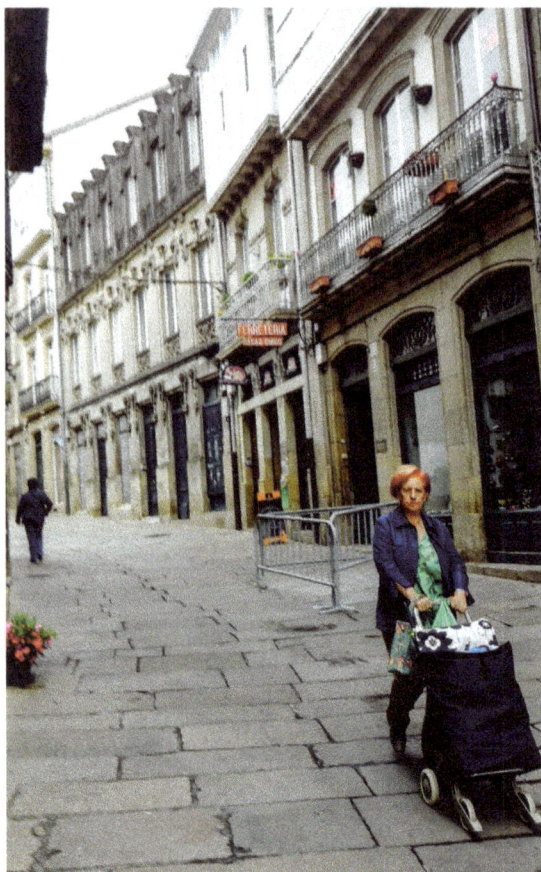

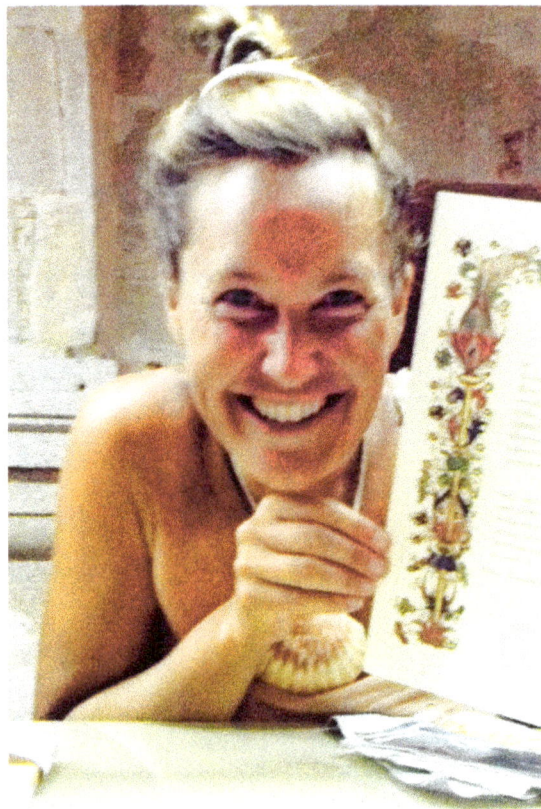

Sunday 5 July 2015
walk to Ruitelán
Pequeño Potala €5
phone: 987 561 322

....

Monday 6 July 2015
walk to Fonfría
A Reboleira €13
phone: 982 181 271

....

Tuesday 7 July 2015
walk to Sarria
San Lázaro €10
www.alberguesanlazaro.com

....

Wednesday 8 July 2015
walk to Gonzar
Casa García €10
phone: 982 157 842 call to confirm

....

Thursday 9 July 2015
walk to Melide
Pension Berenguela €30
Pulpo restaurant: Pulpería Ezequiel €14

....

Friday 10 July 2015
walk to Arca do Pino
Hotel Restaurante O Pino €75
including dinner of squid in its own ink

....

Saturday 11 July 2015
walk to Santiago!!!
Azabache €20
Calle Azabachería, 15
phone: 981 071 254
pilgrim's office to receive compostela

....

Sunday 12 July 2015
walk to Vilaserío
O Rueiro €15
www.restaurantealbergueorueiro.com

....

Monday 13 July 2015
walk to Logoso
Albergue O'Logoso €12
phone: 981 727 602
worth finding the natural spring waterfall/
swimming hole

....

Tuesday 14 July 2015
walk to Finisterre
Albergue Do Mar €17
Rúa de San Rogue
phone: 981 74 02 04
www.alberguedomar.com
fresh barnacles, crab, octopus, razor clams at
Pedra Do Rei €43
walk to Cabo Fisterra
walk to Monte Facho/San Guillerme (Celtic
sun & fertility altar)

....

Wednesday 15 July 2015
earliest bus to Santiago 8:00am-11:00am
(purchase ticket from driver) €15
www.monbus.es/en
explore Santiago
Albergue Azabache €20

....

Thursday 16 July 2015
enjoy last day in Spain!
explore Santiago & send gifts home
Hospedería San Martín €45
So helpful with packages, getting to airport,
and finding gifts

....

Friday 17 July 2015
taxi to Santiago airport 5:00am
fly to Madrid
Iberia Airlines €30
Madrid to Mpls
Delta Airlines
11:35am-6:23pm

....

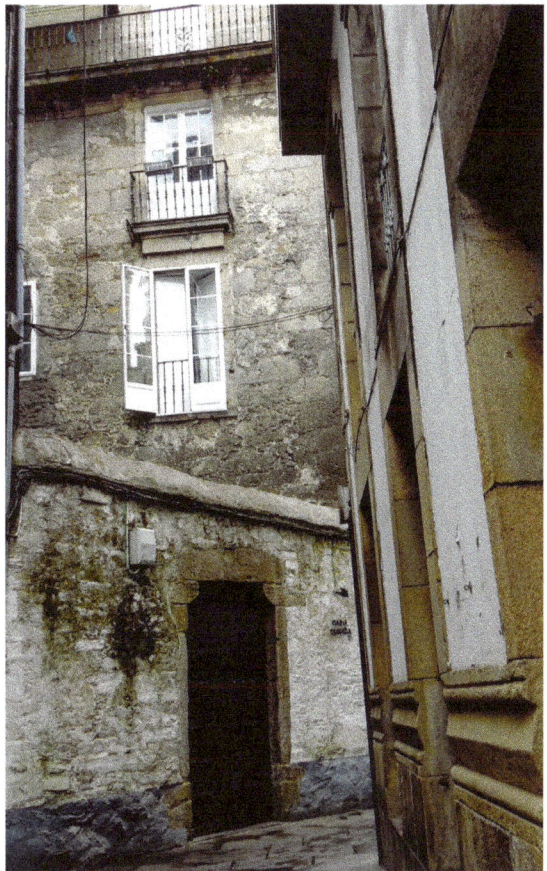

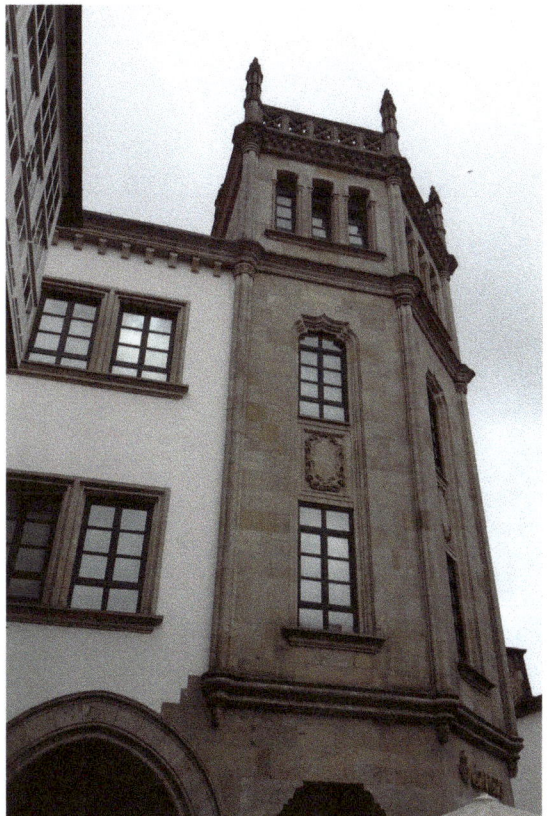

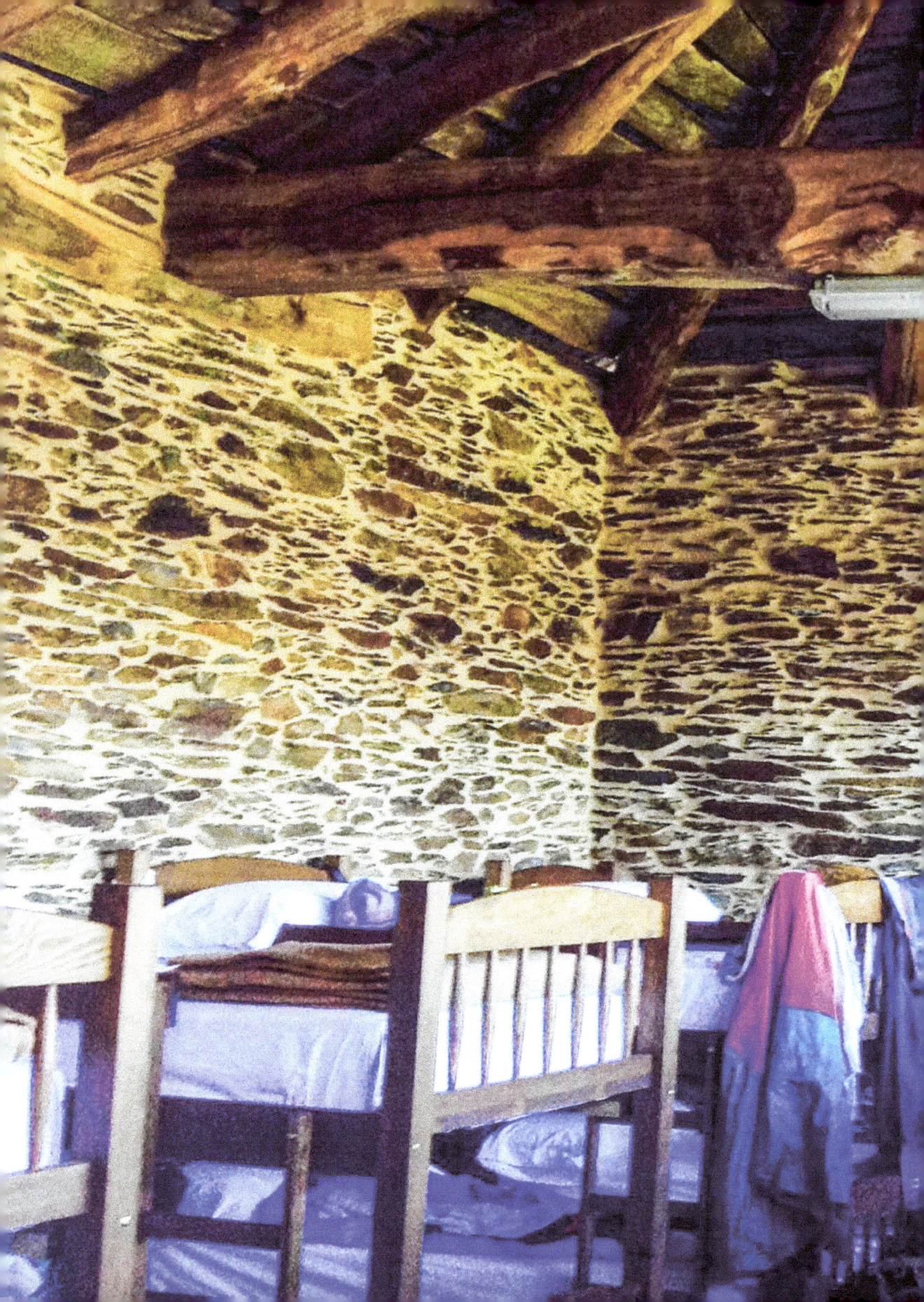

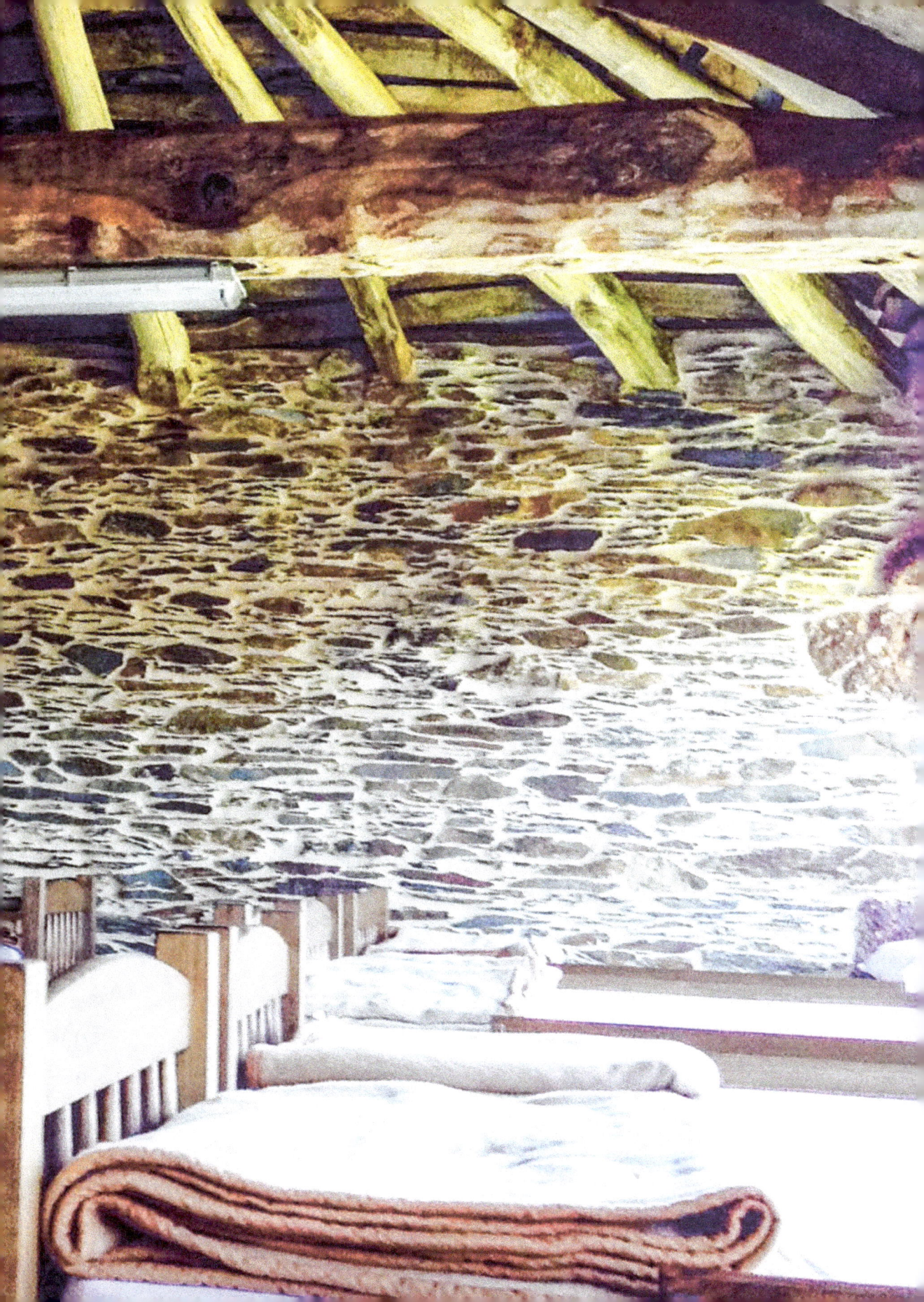

¡ultreïa!

keep going! onward! persevere!

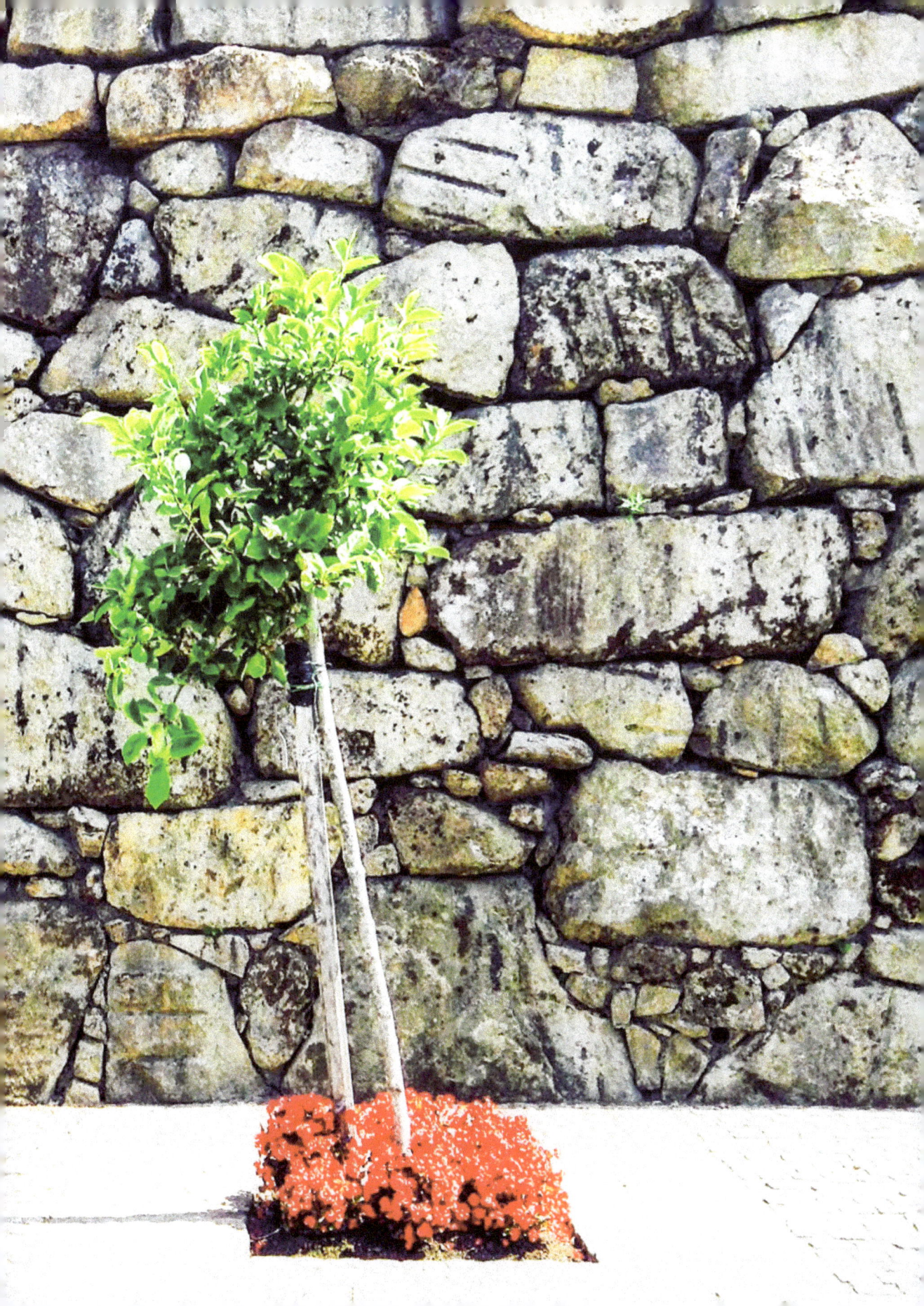

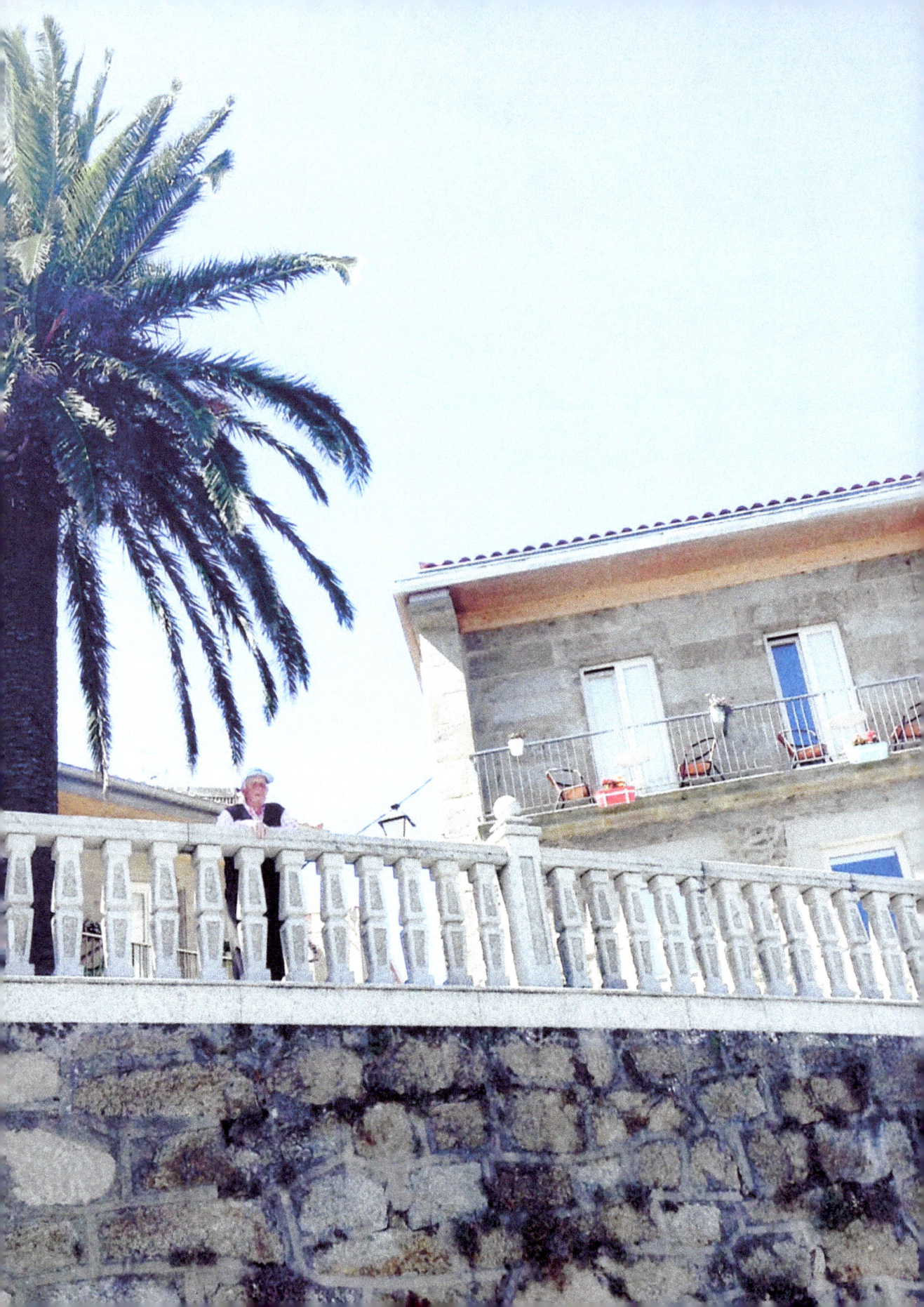

TRAVEL TIPS I USED

-registering my trip with https://step.state.gov
-syncing my breathing with the sound of snoring to help myself fall asleep
-earplugs
-staying hydrated before/during/after flights using a filtered water bottle
-immediately adapting to current time zone
-carrying an extra passport photo for easy emergency replacement
-photographing and then emailing myself photos of all documents (credit cards, ID, passport)
-photographing and then emailing myself photos of everything in backpack
-bedbug spray (lavender/tea tree oils and water)
-mailing purchases and provisions
-public transportation
-using Facebook Messenger and iPod messaging instead of a phone
-making advanced reservations whenever possible and calling to confirm
-learning basic words to communicate in Spanish, French, German
-purchasing train tickets online
-opening an account with Andrews Federal Credit Union
-using several different payment options (cash, credit cards, debit cards)
-using debit and credit cards with no foreign transaction fees
-adapter for iPod charger (a few savvy pilgrims brought multi-outlet adapters)
-ITIC (International Teacher Identity Card) discounts
-reading/learning as much as possible about Spain, the Camino and travel
-downloading map, currency, time zone and translation apps
-registering travel information/dates/times with credit card companies and banks before departing

Finisterre (called "finis terrae") used to be considered the farthest edge of the north westerly land mass and was described as "the end of the earth" (in Latin, "finis terrae" means "end of the world").

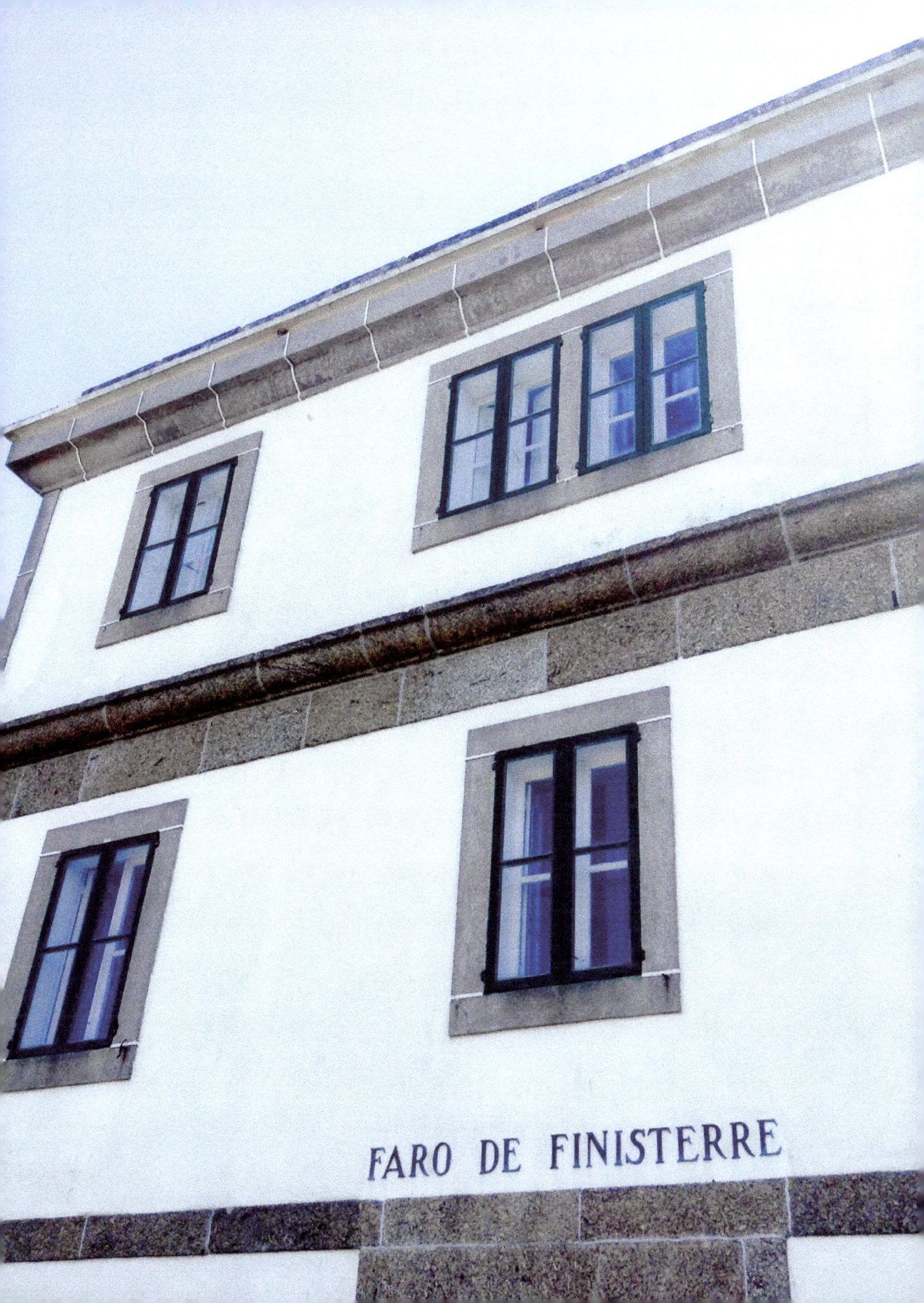

FARO DE FINISTERRE

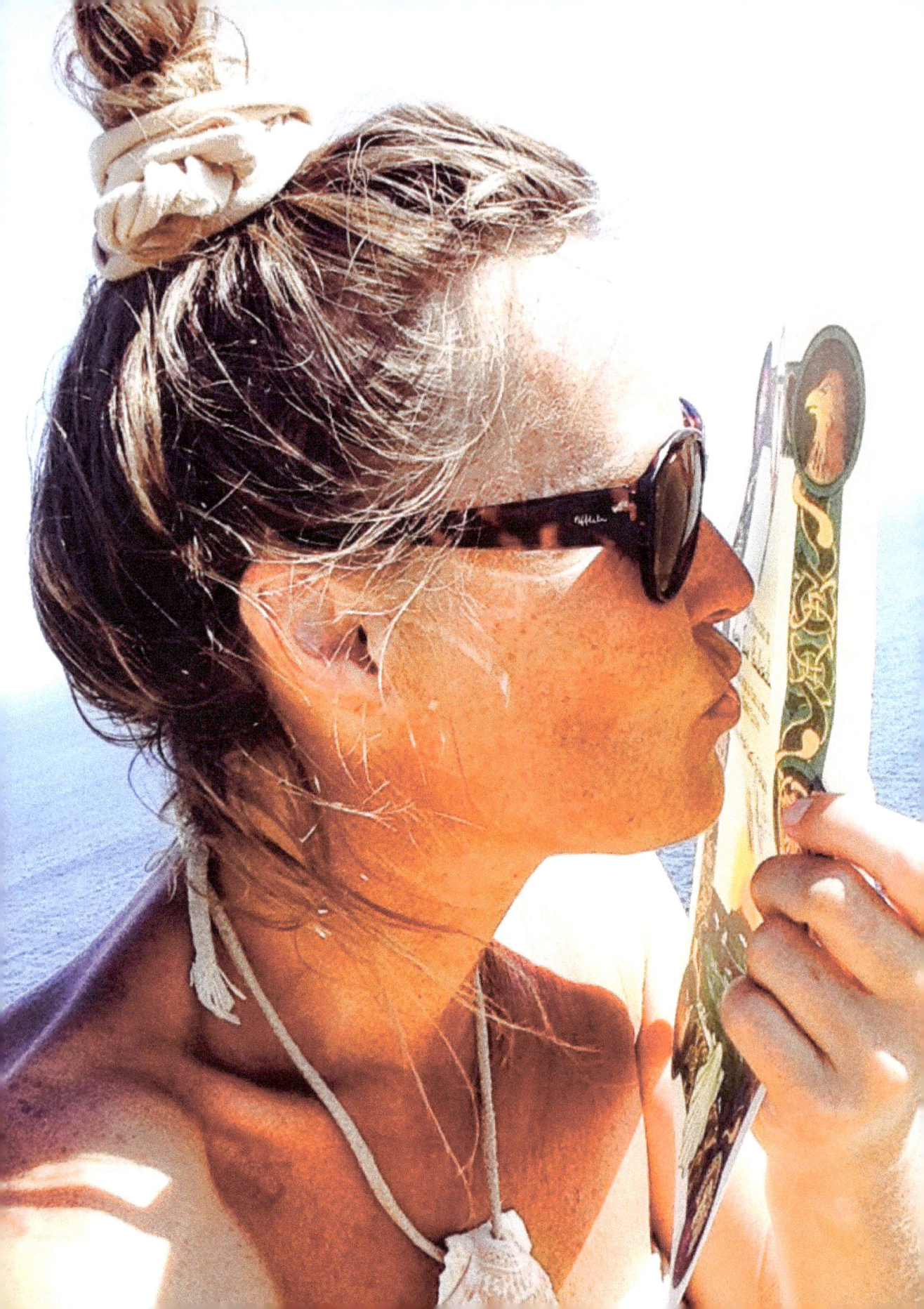

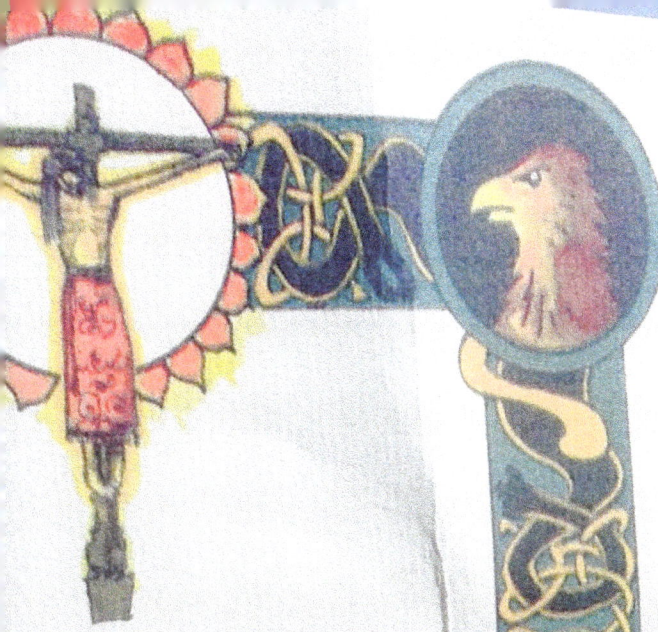

de Fisterra acredita que

Jane Paulisich

s terras da Costa da Morte
do Camiño Xacobeo

14/07/2015 O Alcalde

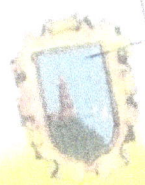

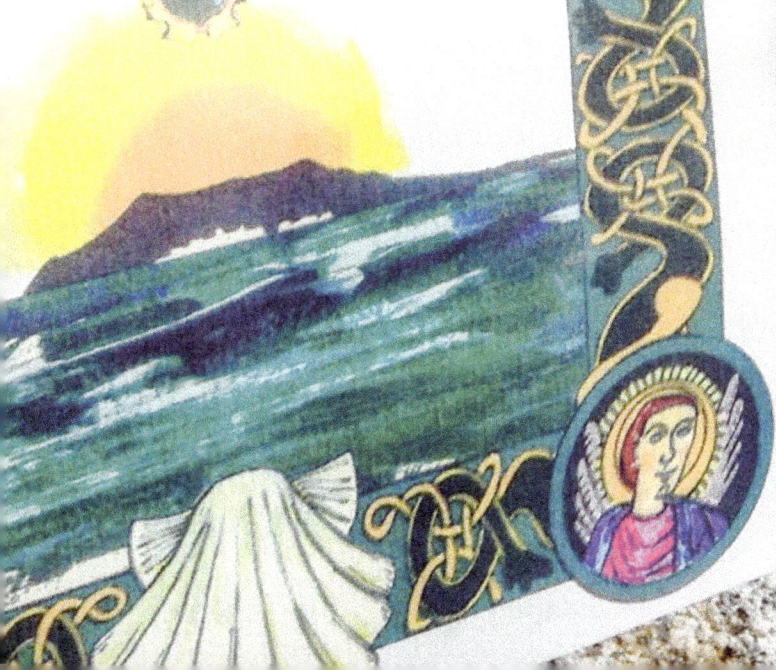

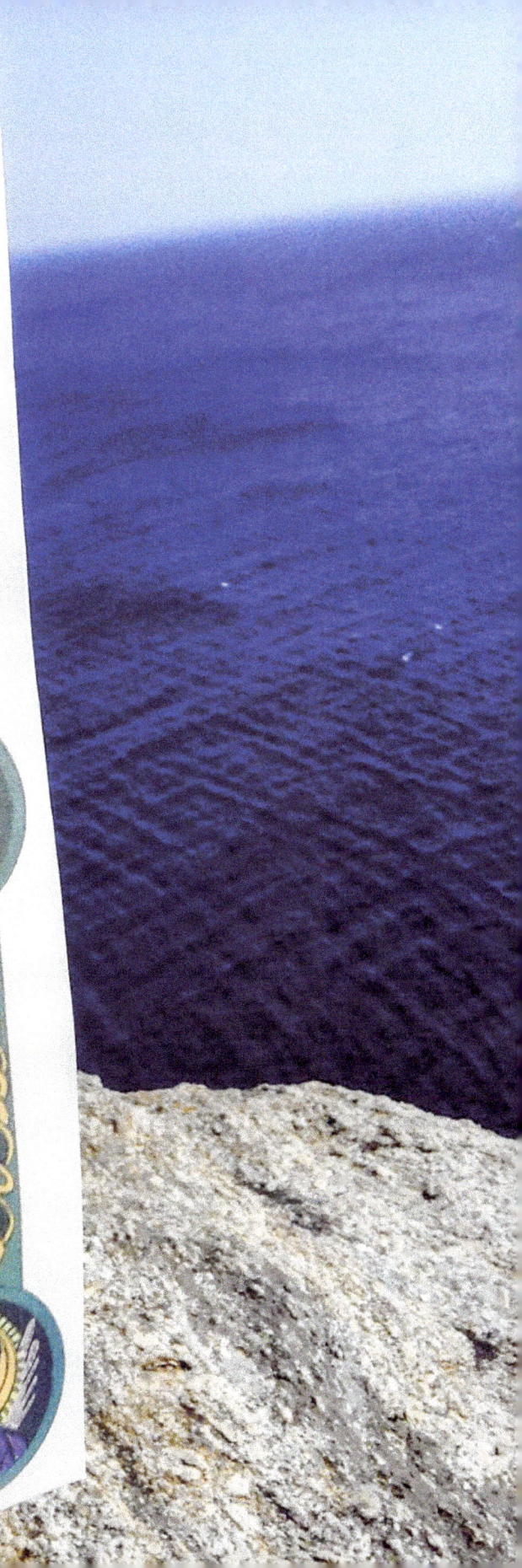

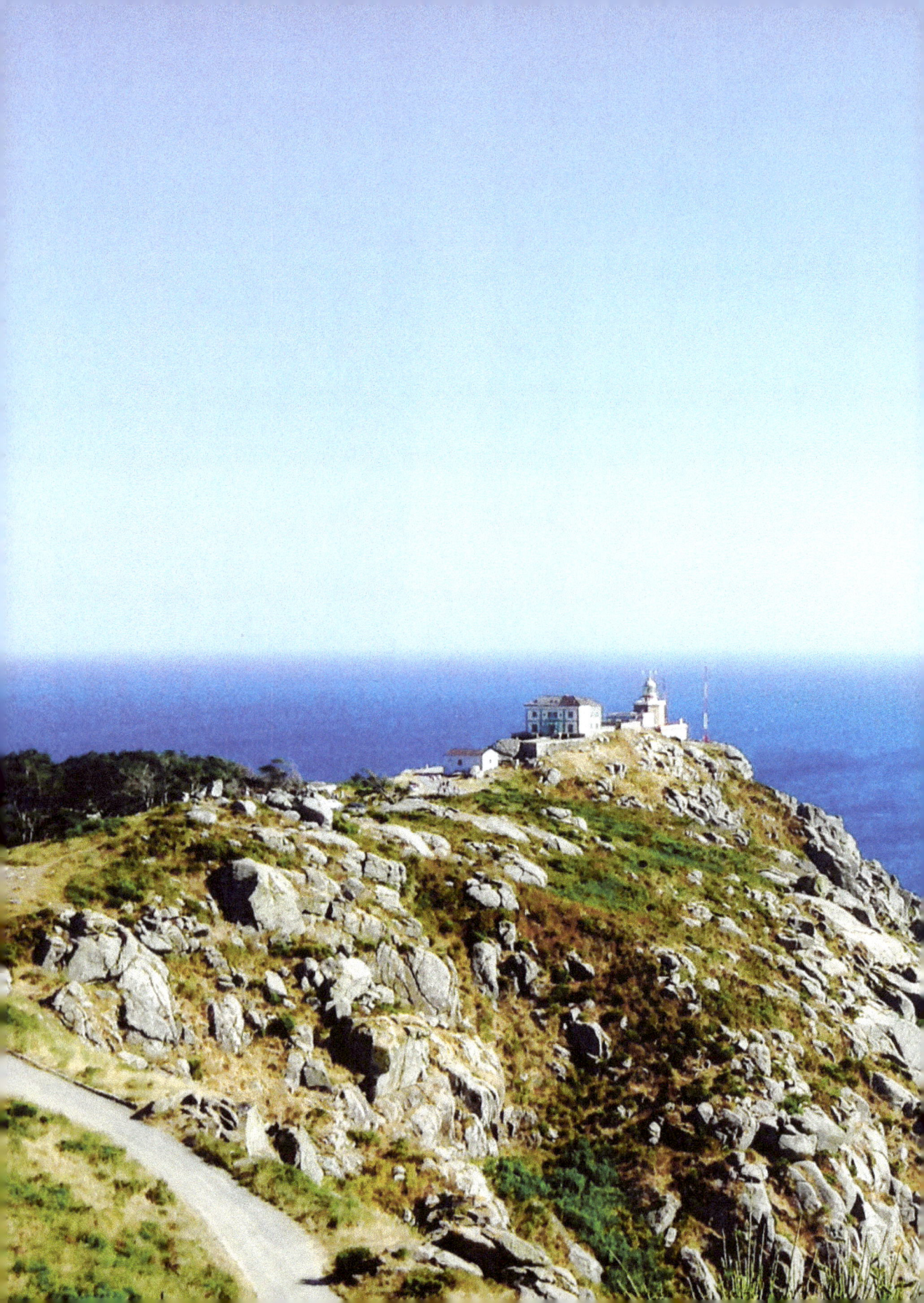

I still struggle to always have faith, hope, positive thoughts and to live each moment as it happens. Walking the Camino was a PhD-level crash course with built-in immediate feedback to grow more habituated in living life with these graces. If I let my mind wander or worry, I easily and quickly lost my way, my direction, my guidance. I learned to keep going, to keep trusting, to watch the signs, to listen to my body and to rely on the goodness of others. I learned to make sure to keep trying, to always move in a forward and positive direction, and to rely on something greater than myself to always be there for repair and provisions. I realized that every moment is a miracle, every person is a miracle, and I am a miracle always and forever.

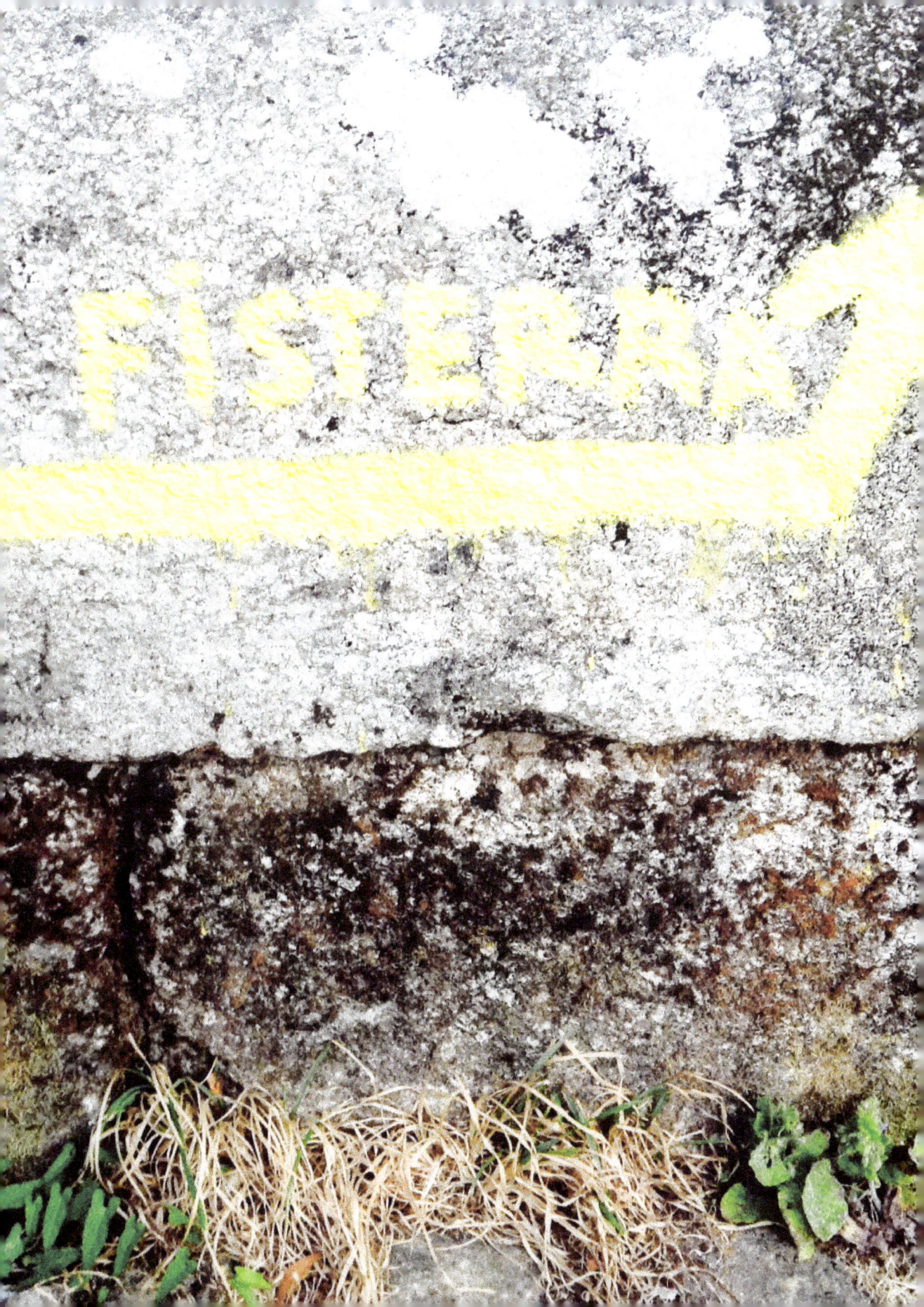

FISTERRA

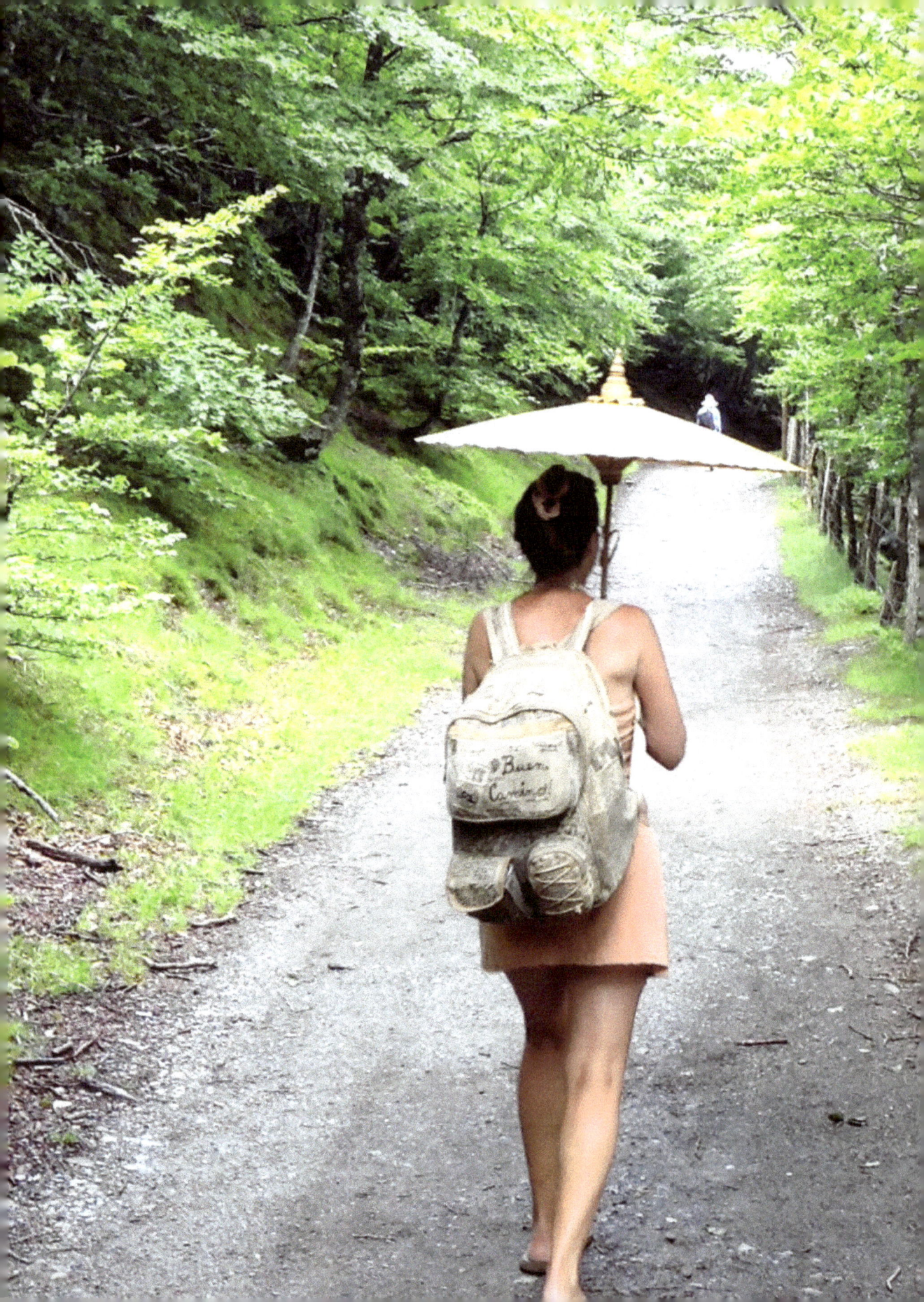

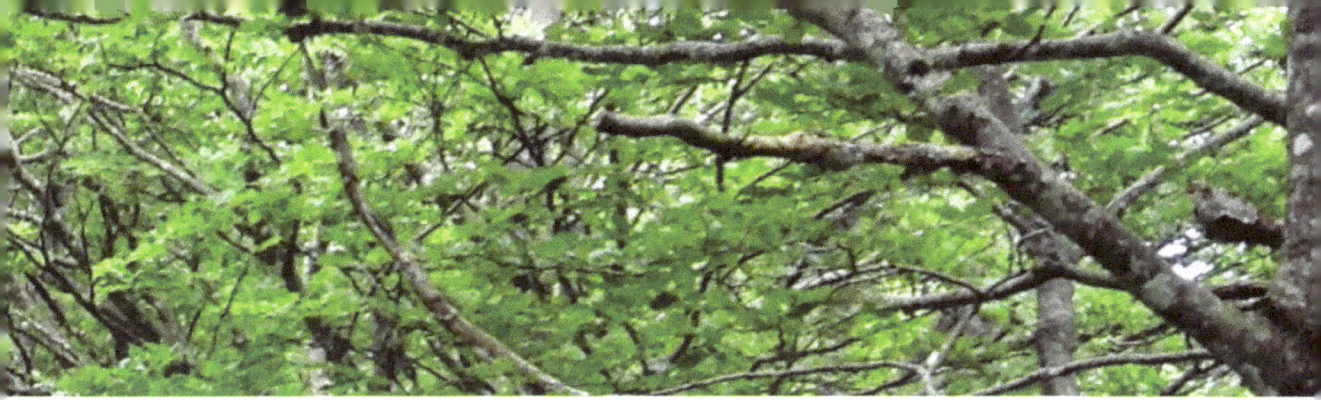

"Throw your dreams into space like a kite, and you do not know what it will bring back, a new life, a new friend, a new love, a new country." -Anaïs Nin

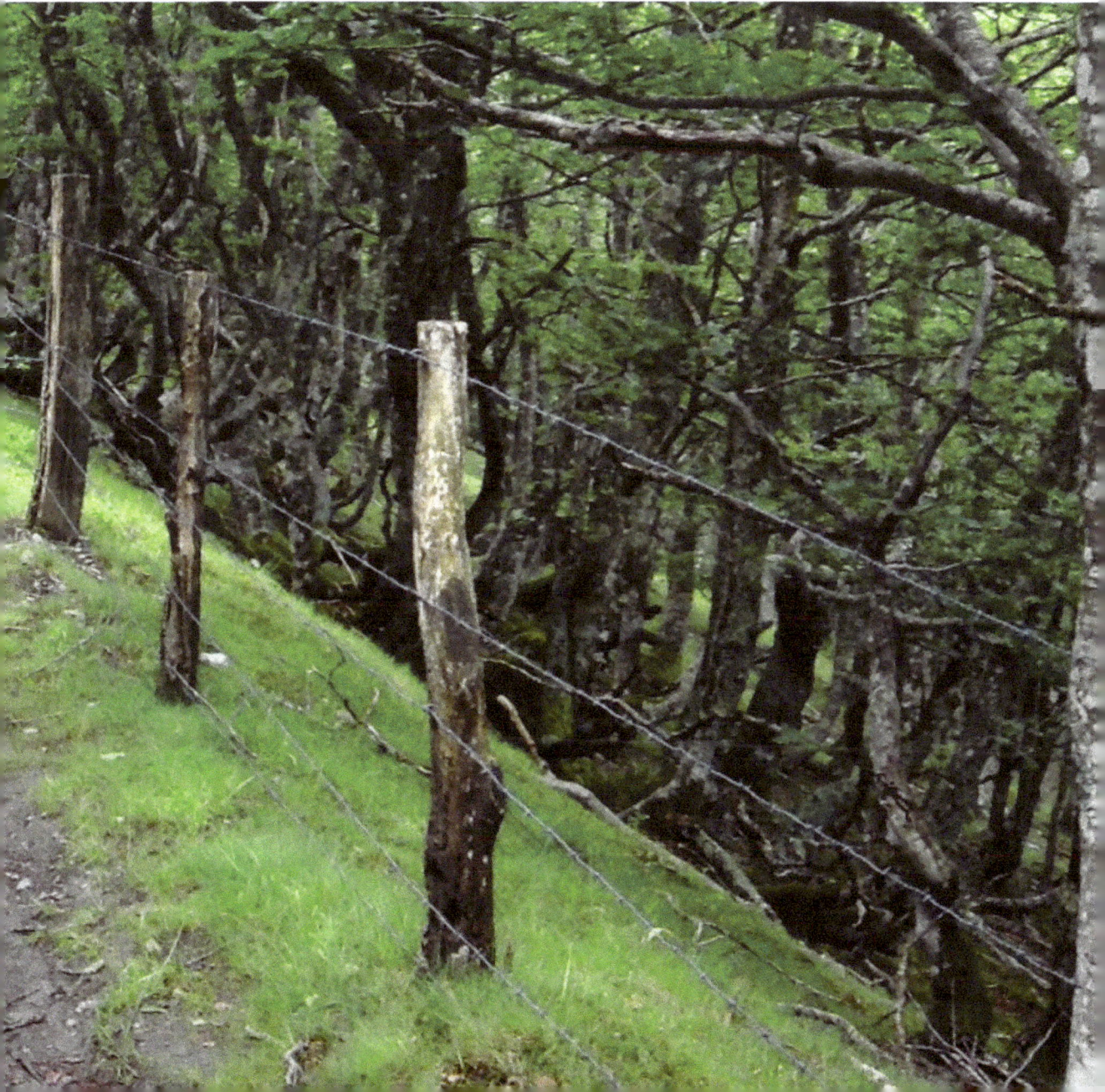

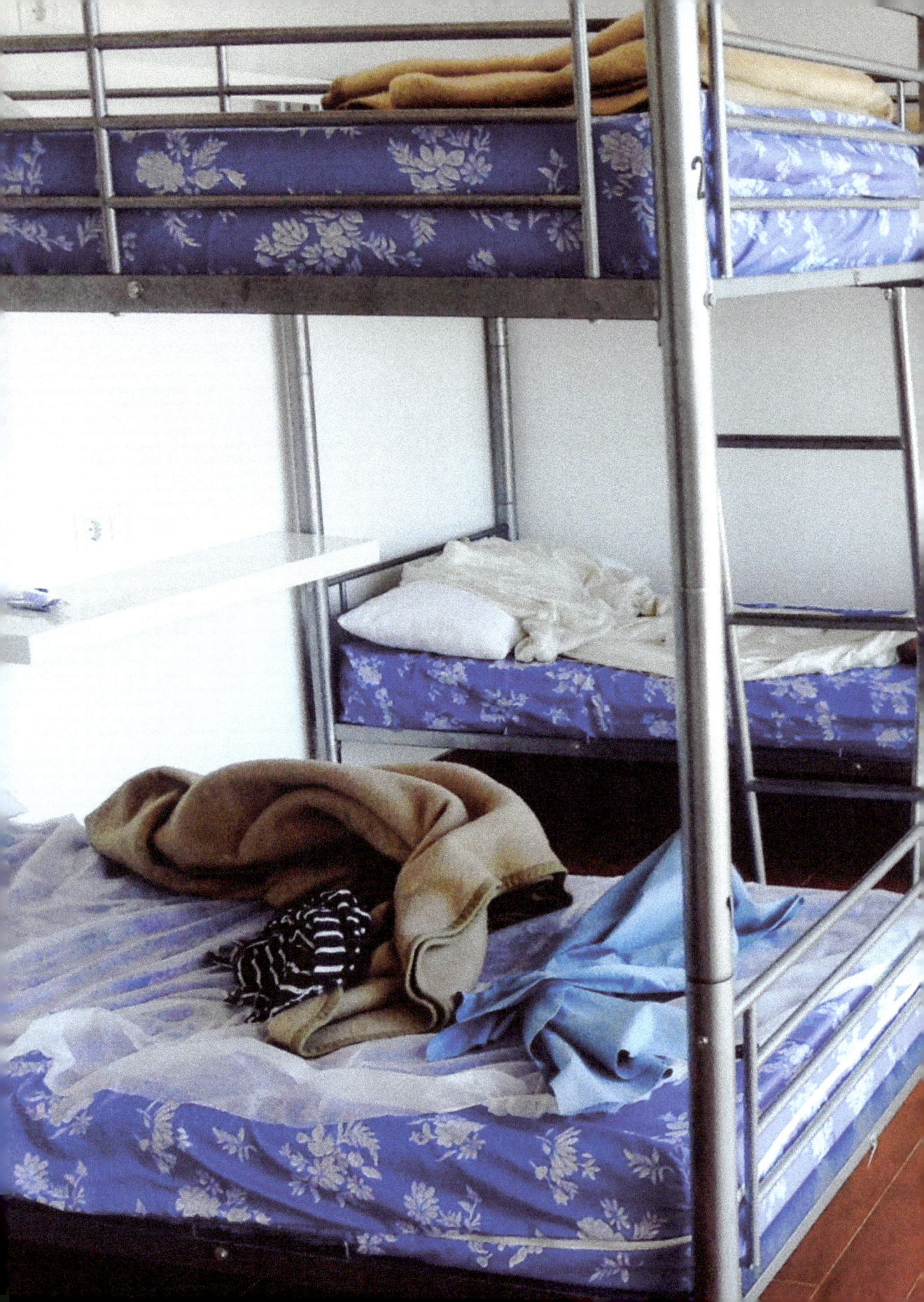

Thank you

Eternal and enormous gratitude for **Jane F Ebeling, Henry J Paulisich,** Gene Murphy, Maria Emmerich, friends & family. I am wordless for how honored I am to receive your encouragement, enthusiasm and LOVE!!! To Lynn & Corinna for your emergency rescues! To "Elliot the smallest angel" for his gigantic generosity, knowledge, humor, heart, enthusiasm, creativity and good will! An unforgettable and extreme privilege to share the Camino path with June 14-July14 2015 pilgrims and all past, current and future pilgrims! ¡Buen Camino! To all of the people who serve the Camino and its pilgrims. Thank you so much for the wide and impeccably groomed paths, the endless encouragement along the way, the welcoming and unexpected hospitality always offered and the generous sharing of your beautiful country! Your munificent example has imprinted me forever! I hope this book honors you and Spain. To the employees of the Pamplona, Burgos, Astorga, Sarria, and Santiago Correos. I am overwhelmed with gratitude for your kindness and patience! To the employees and owners of Casa Torrens and Delicatessen Ojeda who so meticulously helped me pack and mail the most nutritious and delicious food while hiking the Camino. And to all the gracious store/albergue owners along the way. ¡Muy agredecido! To Hudson Public Library and all libraries: I LOVE YOU and would be lost without you! YOU MAKE EVERYTHING POSSIBLE!

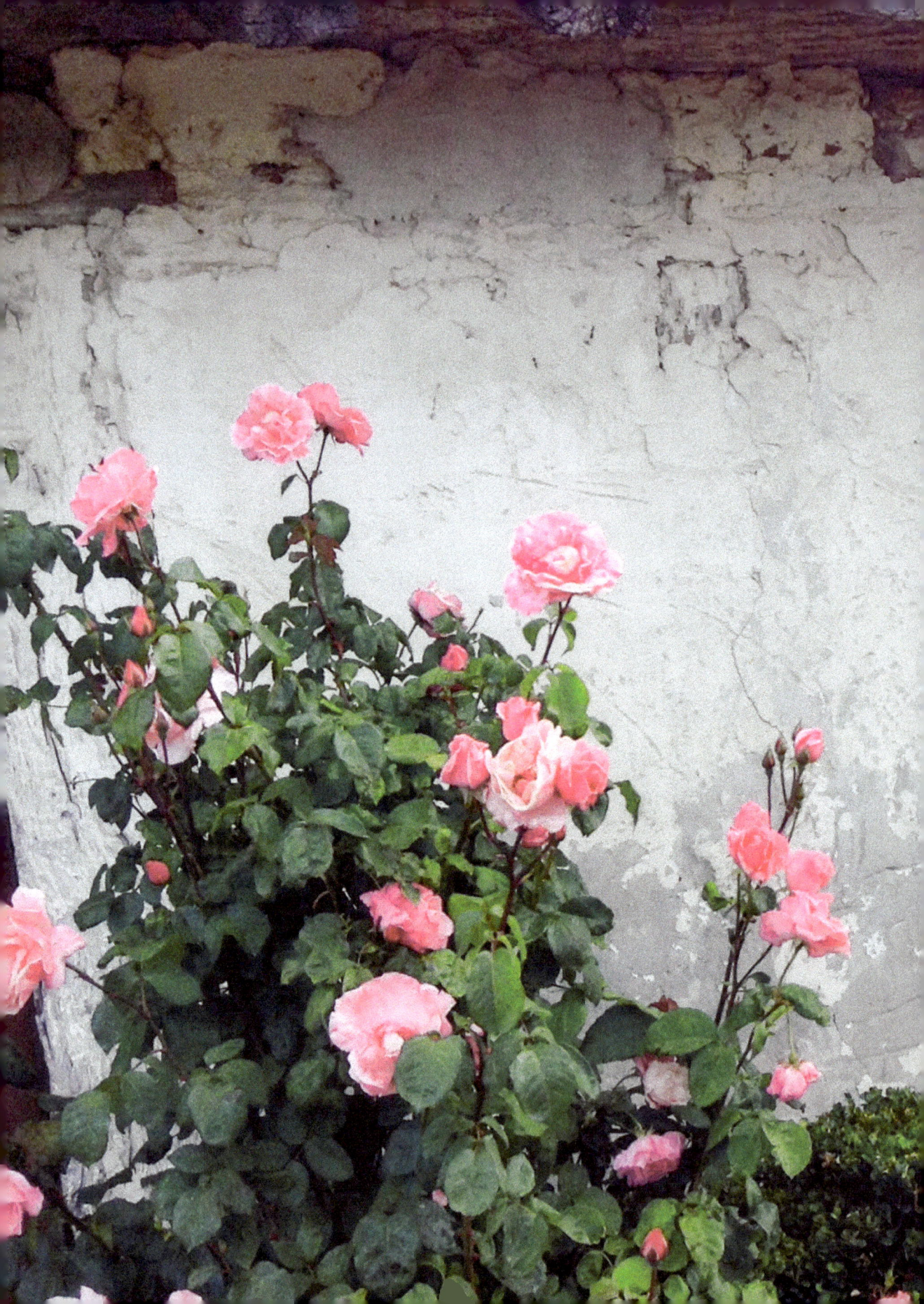

¡buen camino!

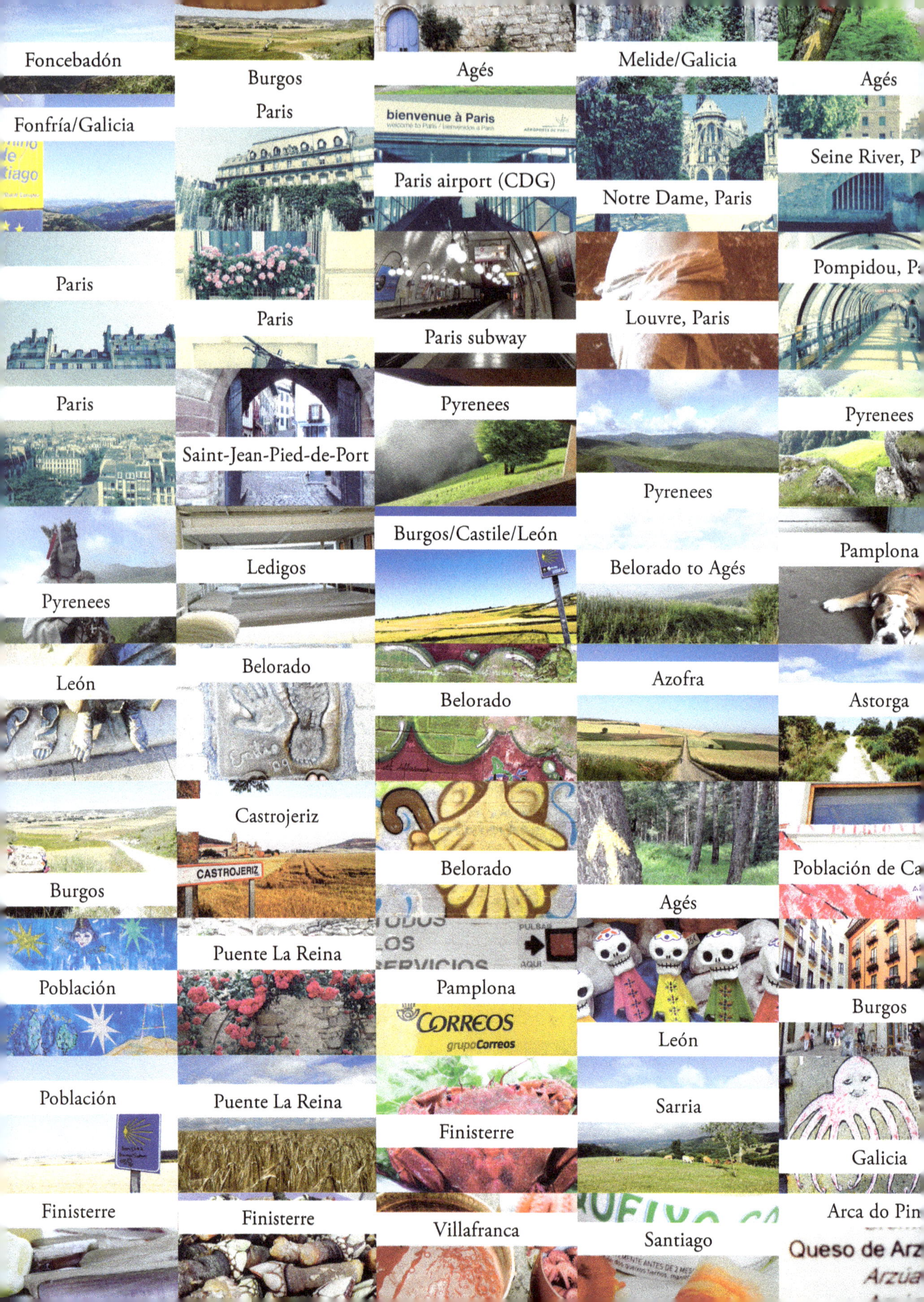

Foncebadón

Burgos

Agés

Melide/Galicia

Agés

Fonfría/Galicia

Paris

Paris airport (CDG)

Notre Dame, Paris

Seine River, P

Paris

Paris

Paris subway

Louvre, Paris

Pompidou, P

Paris

Paris

Pyrenees

Pyrenees

Saint-Jean-Pied-de-Port

Pyrenees

Belorado to Agés

Pamplona

Pyrenees

Ledigos

Burgos/Castile/León

León

Belorado

Belorado

Azofra

Astorga

Castrojeriz

Burgos

Belorado

Agés

Población de Ca

Puente La Reina

Población

Pamplona

León

Burgos

Población

Puente La Reina

Sarria

Finisterre

Finisterre

Finisterre

Villafranca

Santiago

Arca do Pin

Queso de Arz

Arzúa

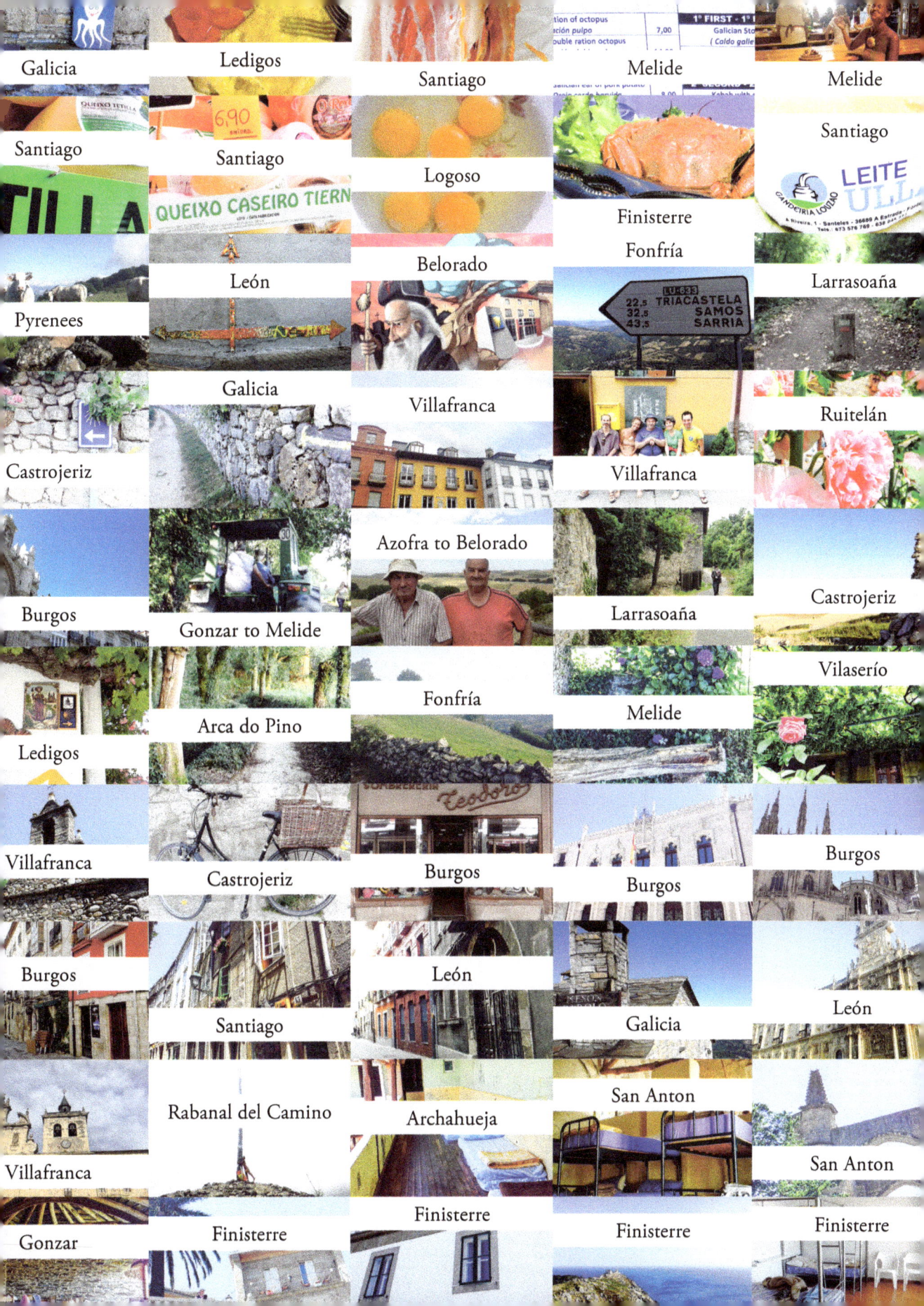

Galicia

Ledigos

Santiago

Melide

Melide

Santiago

Santiago

Logoso

Finisterre

Santiago

León

Belorado

Fonfría

Larrasoaña

Pyrenees

Galicia

Villafranca

Ruitelán

Castrojeriz

Villafranca

Burgos

Gonzar to Melide

Azofra to Belorado

Larrasoaña

Castrojeriz

Arca do Pino

Fonfría

Melide

Vilaserío

Ledigos

Villafranca

Castrojeriz

Burgos

Burgos

Burgos

Burgos

Burgos

León

León

Santiago

Galicia

San Anton

Villafranca

Rabanal del Camino

Archahueja

Finisterre

San Anton

Gonzar

Finisterre

Finisterre

Finisterre

Finisterre

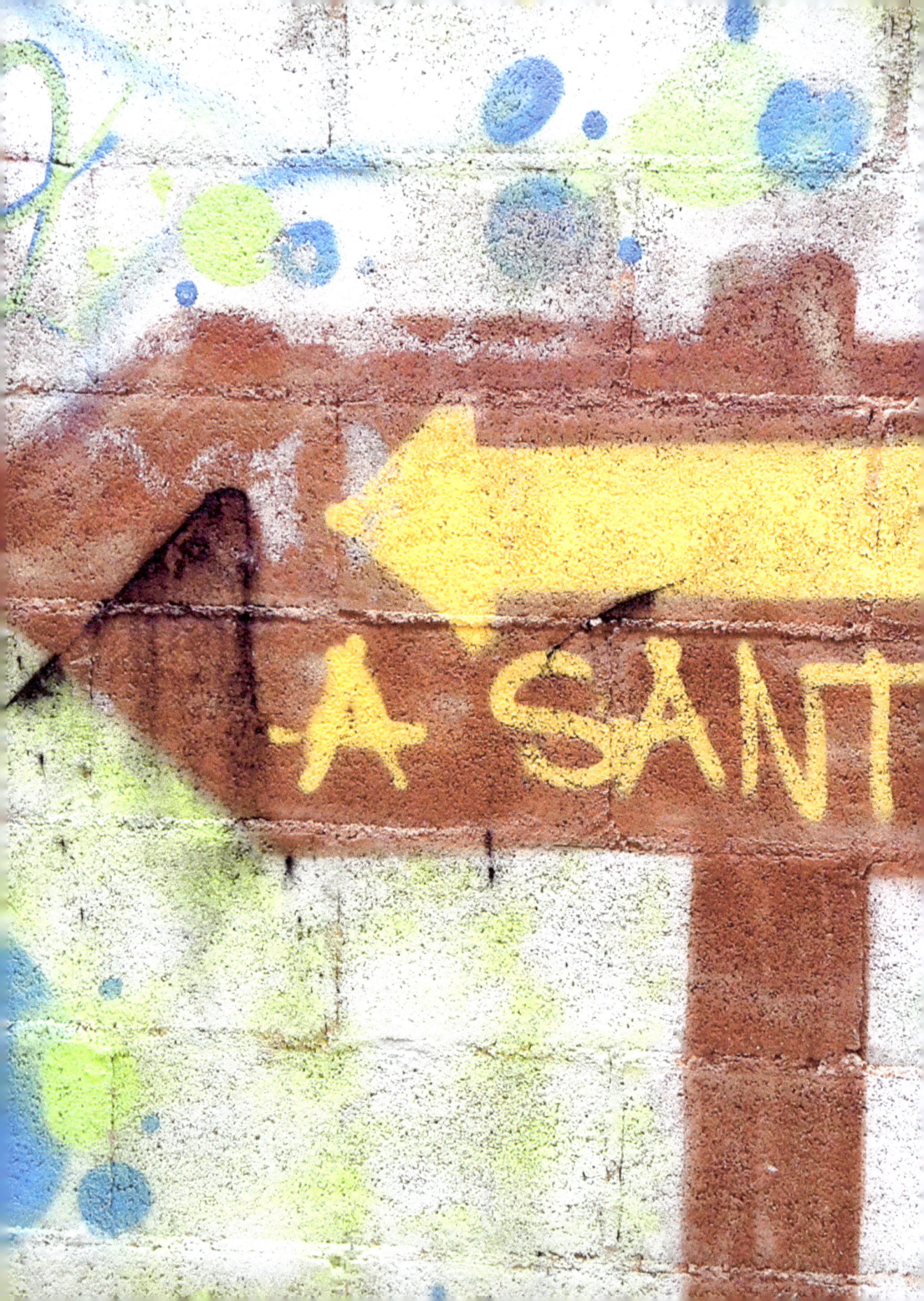